Peter K. Sand and Donald R. Ostergard

# Urodynamics and the Evaluation of Female Incontinence:

## A Practical Guide

With 106 Figures

Springer
London Berlin Heidelberg New York
Paris Tokyo Hong Kong
Barcelona Budapest

Peter K. Sand MD
Associate Professor of Obstetrics and Gynecology,
Director, Division of Urogynecology, Evanston Continence Center, Evanston Hospital,
Northwestern University Medical School, 2650 Ridge Ave, Evanston, Illinois, USA

Donald R. Ostergard MD
Professor of Obstetrics and Gynecology,
Director, Division of Urogynecology, Long Beach Memorial Hospital,
University of California at Irvine,
701 E.28th St, 212 Long Beach, California, USA

British Library Cataloguing in Publication Data
Sand, Peter K.
Urodynamics and the Evaluation of Female Incontinence: Practical Guide
I. Title II. Ostergard, Donald R.
616.620082

Library of Congress Cataloging-in-Publication Data
Sand, Peter K., 1956–
Urodynamics and the evaluation of female incontinence : a practical guide / Peter K. Sand and Donald R. Ostergard.
p. cm.
Includes bibliographical references and index.
ISBN-13: 978-3-540-19904-5 e-ISBN-13: 978-1-4471-2109-1
DOI: 10.1007/978-1-4471-2109-1

1. Urinary stress incontinence—Diagnosis. 2. Urodynamics. 3. Urinary incontinence—Diagnosis. I. Ostergard, Donald R., 1938–. II. Title.
[DNLM: 1. Urodynamics. 2. Urinary Incontinence. 3. Genital Diseases, Female. 4. Urinary Tract—physiopathology. 5. Urethral Diseases—diagnosis. WJ 190 S213u 1995]
RG485.S7S26 1995
616.6'2—dc20
DNLM/DLC
for Library of Congress 94–24640



28/3830-543210 Printed on acid-free paper

# Preface

Urodynamic evaluation of the incontinent female has come of age. It is no longer acceptable to subject women to surgical procedures for urinary incontinence based solely on the physician's clinical impression of the cause of the urine loss. Multiple studies in the urogynecological literature have told us that the error rate for stress incontinence is about 25% and the error rate for the unstable bladder is 50% when these diagnoses are based solely on historical data obtained from the patient. Unfortunately the patient is a poor witness to her bladder's activities and diagnoses arrived at without further evaluation are subject to error. Urodynamic testing allows the establishment of precise diagnoses using procedures that have been proven to be accurate.

For the physician who has not had the opportunity to have fellowship training, the urodynamic tracing is sometimes more of a mystery than a diagnostic aid. Physician training in the reading of urodynamic tracings is limited to piecing together information from the literature, textbooks and postgraduate courses. Unfortunately none of these sources can provide the experience necessary to become an expert in the interpretation of the physiological and pathophysiological events depicted on the tracing. Artifacts occur commonly and may lead to misinterpretation of these events and even misdiagnosis if the reader of the tracing is not careful and fully informed on the nuances of the testing procedures. This is why this text was conceived as an atlas of urodynamic testing procedures. It embodies a comprehensive reference source, not only for normal events but also for those abnormalities which form the backbone of urodynamic diagnoses. Artifacts are depicted extensively in relation to concurrent urodynamic events in order to show how they may confuse the physician and his/her interpretation of the pathophysiological events depicted thereon.

This atlas should be of great aid to those laboratories where urodynamic technicians are employed to actually perform the studies. Unless the technician is equally as well informed as the physician, artifacts will not be recognized and the physician who reads the tracing may not even recognize the potential existence of an artifact. It is incumbent upon the physician to maintain constant communication with the technician in order to make the best possible use of the testing process and to allow accurate interpretation. This text will allow the physician more fully to train the technician to minimize this type of interpretive error.

The authors of this atlas hope that the reading of urodynamic tracings will be simplified through this study and that common errors in the interpretive process may be avoided through a more thorough understanding of the process of urodynamic testing.

# Contents

## Section III: MULTICHANNEL URODYNAMICS: NORMAL STUDIES



## Section IV: MULTICHANNEL URODYNAMICS: PATHOLOGIC STUDIES

APPENDICES

# Section I
# Routine Office Evaluation

Chapter 1

# The Female Urologic History

In most medical conditions, a detailed history will help to establish the underlying diagnosis in the vast majority of patients. In addition, a careful history will often suggest how to treat the patient. Unfortunately, a urologic history is not as helpful in determining the underlying diagnosis. Work in our laboratory and others has demonstrated that the urologic history is less than 60% accurate in establishing the underlying cause of urinary incontinence. Many urinary tract symptoms are non-specific and overlapping. There are no truly pathognomonic symptoms. For example, urgency, frequency and dysuria are the hallmarks of lower urinary tract infections. However, many women with these same symptoms may have the urethral syndrome and no detectable urinary infection. In addition, frequency and urgency may signify uninhibited detrusor contractions rather than inflammation or infection. Although a detailed history is necessary, it should never be considered diagnostic. Operating or initiating therapy on the basis of the urologic history alone will lead to a high incidence of failure.

However, a detailed urologic history will guide the clinician in the performance of appropriate testing to determine the underlying diagnosis. Some have suggested that premenopausal women with complaints of only stress incontinence in the absence of urgency, frequency and nocturia, almost always have genuine stress incontinence. Such a history, with evidence of urethral hypermobility on physical examination, documented urinary leakage and a negative simple cystometry study may be all that is necessary before treatment is initiated. However, patients who complain of urgency, frequency, nocturia and stress incontinence need a more detailed workup including endoscopy and possibly multichannel urodynamic investigation.

It is also important to recognize that many urinary symptoms may arise from non-urologic and non-neurologic disease processes. Diabetes, thyroid disease, psychiatric disorders and congestive heart disease may all cause urinary symptomatology in the absence of lower urinary tract disease. For this reason, review of the patient's past medical history and symptoms is crucial. In addition, it is important to obtain a thorough drug usage and allergy history from the patient. Parasympatholytic drugs and alpha-adrenergic drugs will tend to promote urinary retention, whereas parasympathomimetic and alpha-adrenolytic drugs may cause urgency and urine loss. Numerous other types of medications may also have profound effects on the lower urinary tract.

We routinely obtain a detailed history from the patient by asking her to fill out a programmed history questionnaire before coming to her first visit. These forms are found in Appendix C. A programmed history avoids the majority of errors inherent in the history-taking process. Because the questions are detailed, little information is missed. It also allows the patient to take the time to review information from medical records at home and also to obtain a detailed family medical history. The history questionnaire reviews topics such as prior urologic treatment, prior urologic disease, family medical history, prior surgery and the details of the patient's current urologic problem. This programmed history form is then rapidly reviewed by the physician before the patient is seen. Confirmation of pertinent positives is then used to initiate a detailed description of the patient's current symptomatology. At each visit, a review of the patient's symptoms is made. This allows the physician to assess not only how the patient is feeling, but how she is progressing with her current treatment course.

## Bibliography

Cardozo LD, Stanton SL: Genuine stress incontinence and detrusor instability – a review of 200 patients. Br J Obstet Gynecol 87:184, 1980.

Farrar DJ, Whiteside CG, Osborne JL et al: A urodynamic analysis of micturition symptoms in the female. Surg Gynecol Obstet 141:875, 1975.

Ostergard DR: The effect of drugs on the lower urinary tract. Obstet Gynecol Surv 34:424, 1979.

Sand PK, Hill RC, Ostergard DR: The incontinence history as a predictor of detrusor stability. Obstet Gynecol 71:257, 1988.

Wein, AJ: Non-surgical treatment of lower urinary tract dysfunction. In Raz S (ed) Female urology. Philadelphia, W.B. Saunders, 1983, pp. 161–188.

# Chapter 2
# Voiding Diaries

Voiding diaries are a simple way to ascertain the true frequency of a patient's voiding. We routinely ask new patients to record the volumes they drink and void, with the times of these events for a 24–48 h period. In addition, we also ask them to chart if any urine was lost during this period of evaluation and if it was associated with urgency.

Comparing these objective results with a patient's symptoms of frequency often reveals that the patient has over estimated her urinary frequency. It may also reveal the patient who voids with abnormal frequency during the day but who sleeps all night. This may indicate a psychogenic origin of her urinary tract symptoms (i.e. sensory urgency). In addition, a voiding history may help reveal a problem with psychogenic water intoxication or diabetes insipidus. It may also demonstrate patterns of urine loss associated with different periods during the day. Such a pattern is frequently seen in patients with unstable bladders who are taking diuretics in the morning. Their urine loss is commonly found during the hours before noon and will resolve in the afternoon. Such a record may help us adjust a patient's anticholinergic therapy to match her urinary incontinence history. Knowledge of the patient's normal voiding intervals may be used to alter these intervals if behavior modification is selected for therapy. Timed voiding, used in the treatment of detrusor instability (Appendix A), should initially be done more frequently than the patient's routine interval.

Others have suggested that knowledge of the patient's voided volume and frequency may help to establish the presence or absence of unstable bladder contractions. We have been unable to confirm the accuracy of this in our laboratory, but find voiding diaries helpful in objectively corroborating the patient's history and establishing the patient's normal voiding interval. The form used for patient recording of her voiding diary may be found in Appendix C.

## Bibliography

Larsson G, Abrams P, Victor A: The frequency/volume chart in detrusor instability. Neurourol Urodynam 10:533, 1991.

Larsson G, Victor A: Micturition patterns in a healthy female population, studied with frequency/volume charts. Scand J Urol Nephrol Suppl 4:53, 1988.

# Chapter 3
# Uroflowmetry in the Female

## 3.1 Normal Uroflowmetry (Genuine Stress Incontinence)

Uroflowmetry is the study of voiding velocity. This can be measured eloquently with electronic uroflowmetry as demonstrated in Fig. 3.1, or can be measured simply by using a stopwatch to time the patient's voiding effort and calculating a mean flow rate when the volume is measured. However, since uroflowmetry is usually used to determine obstructive voiding, mean flow rates do not have as much significance as maximal flow rates.

Fig. 3.1, demonstrates a uroflowmetry study from a 21-year-old primipara with genuine stress incontinence. This uroflow is a normal study. The curve is bell shaped with a peak flow rate >25 ml/s and a total flow time <20 s. The peak flow rate is reached in <10 s and there is no residual urine. These factors define a normal uroflowmetry study. Normal parameters for uroflowmetry have been described elsewhere in the literature and are volume dependent.

An important calculation in uroflowmetry which is not demonstrated here, is the residual urine. Many define normal residuals as <30 ml, whereas others choose a cut off of 50 ml. Residuals must be evaluated in relationship to the volume voided. A residual of 30 ml after a void of 45 ml is not normal. However, the same residual might be reasonable after a patient voided 500 ml of urine.

Uroflowmetry in the female has not been shown to be diagnostic for specific disorders. Uroflowmetry in the male patient may demonstrate an obstructive outflow problem, but in the female, physical obstruction to flow is unlikely. More often, an abnormal uroflow will indicate a functional obstruction. For this reason, uroflowmetry in the female should be looked upon as an adjunctive or screening test which when viewed with other data may suggest the need for further evaluation. Uroflowmetry cannot be used independently in the female to make a diagnosis of the underlying etiology of urinary retention nor of incontinence. Uroflowmetry is also suspect, because of problems with reproduceability of the test for an individual patient. Uroflowmetry is highly volume dependent and peak flow rates will increase as the volume voided rises in normal women. For this reason, uroflowmetry studies with volumes less than 150 ml are often misleading and should be repeated.

## 3.2 Normal Uroflowmetry (Detrusor Instability)

Fig. 3.2 demonstrates a normal uroflow curve, which is not qualitatively different from the curve seen in Fig. 3.1. This patient is a 32-year-old $G_2$ $P_2$ female who has detrusor instability. Again, in this figure, there is a bell-shaped curve with a maximal flow rate >25ml/s and a time to peak flow <10 s. In comparison to Fig. 3.1, there is both a higher peak and average flow rate. This is most likely due to the higher total volume voided. Again, there is minimal residual urine. Although the underlying diagnosis is different in these two

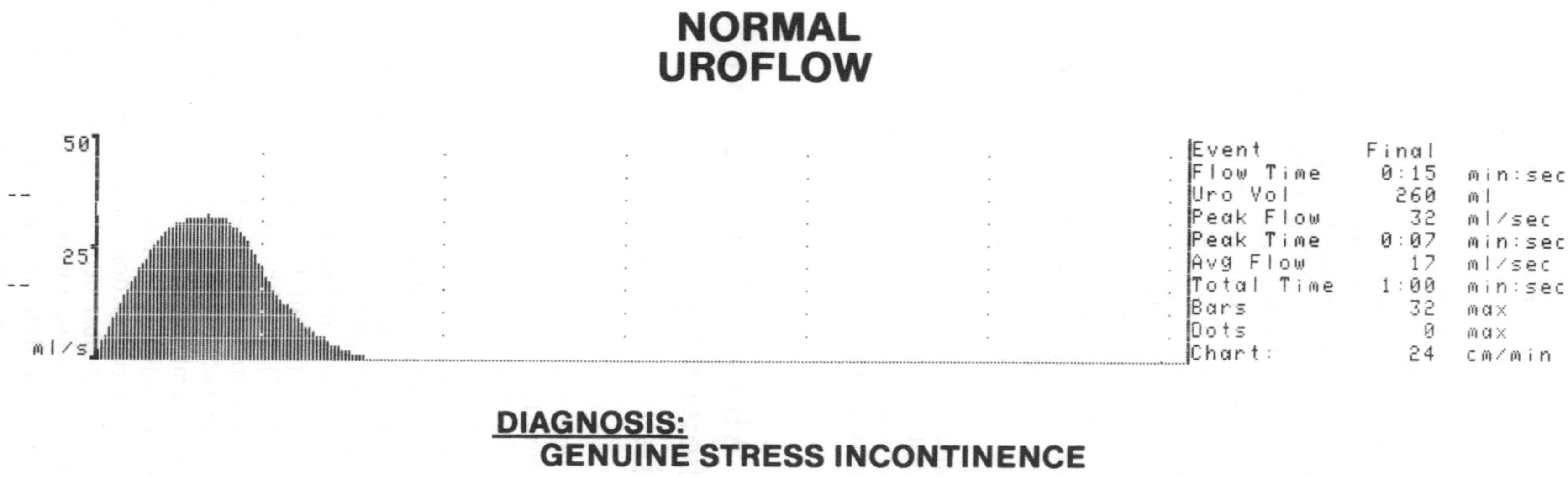


**Fig. 3.1.** Normal uroflowmetry in a woman with genuine stress incontinence.

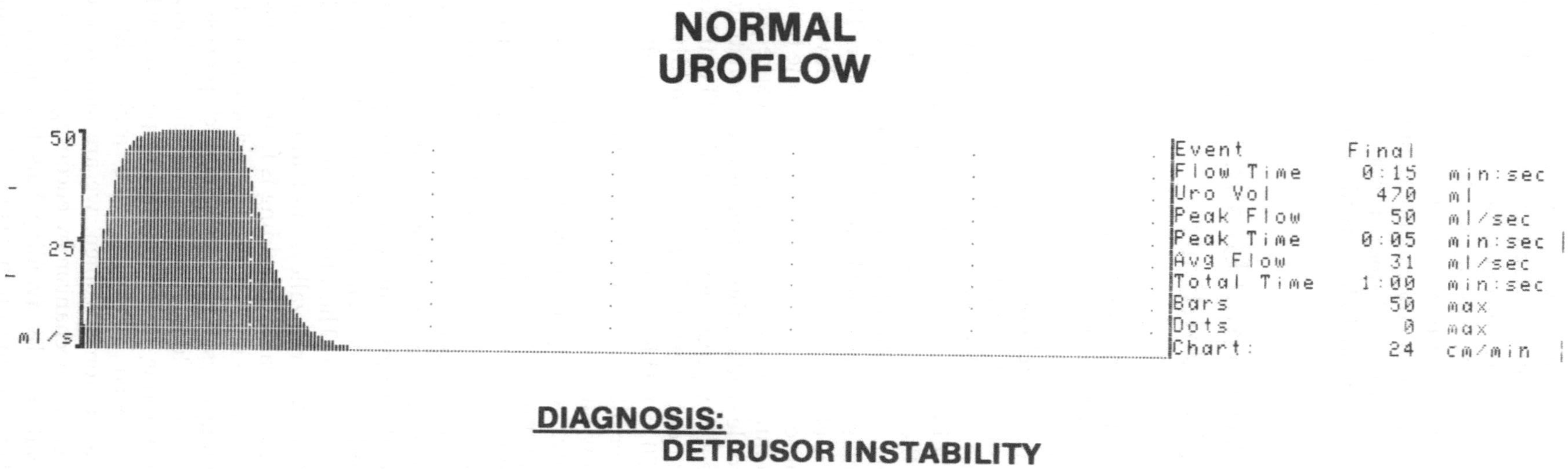


**Fig. 3.2.** Normal uroflowmetry in a woman with detrusor instability.

patients (Figs. 3.1 and 3.2), the uroflow patterns take on the same appearance. This underscores the inability of uroflowmetry to diagnose the etiology of urinary incontinence. However, this patient's problem was not voiding dysfunction, but rather a dysfunction of the storage phase. Whereas uroflowmetry was not diagnostic in this patient with a normal study, it may be helpful in those patients who do have voiding dysfunction.

## 3.3 Abnormal Uroflowmetry (Valsalva Voiding)

In contrast to the previous normal studies, the patient shown in Fig. 3.3 does not have a bell-shaped uroflow curve. Instead, she has an intermittent flow or roller coaster-type pattern. She is a 54-year-old $G_5$ $P_5$ female who has genuine stress incontinence and a low pressure urethra (Chapter 29). In addition to the abnormal shape of this curve, the flow time is also prolonged (33 s). However, the patient has a normal peak flow rate of 34 ml/s and a normal time to peak flow. This patient is able to generate a normal peak flow rate in the absence of a detrusor contraction due to her low urethral resistance. On urethral closure pressure profile studies, the patient was demonstrated to have a low pressure urethra ($CP \leq 20$ $cmH_2O$). This patient's residual urine is also mildly elevated (50 ml). This uroflow would be described as both intermittent and retentive despite the normal peak flow rate.

Valsalva voiding in the female is capable of generating normal maximal flow rates. These can be achieved in the female because of the relatively short urethra. A short urethra with reduced outlet resistance can be overcome by large intravesical pressures that occur during Valsalva. This overwhelms the reflex contraction of the pelvic floor and periurethral striated muscles that occurs during Valsalva. The uroflow curve is typically one of peaks and valleys, not unlike that of a roller coaster. Valsalva voiding is frequently associated with an elevated residual urine due to the underlying physiologic "dyssynergic" process of reflex pelvic floor contraction with Valsalva. Double voiding may be useful in patients who have elevated residual urine and void by Valsalva. In some women, we are able to alter their voiding mechanism by encouraging them to avoid Valsalva. By avoiding Valsalva, many can alter their voiding mechanisms and void by urethral relaxation alone or in association with a detrusor contraction. This is especially important in women who are to undergo surgery for genuine stress incontinence. Retropubic urethropexies are known to increase urethral resistance by mechanical means. The goal of this surgery is to avoid urine loss during increases in intra-abdominal pressure (i.e. Valsalva). Obviously, attempts to void with Valsalva will be relatively unsuccessful after such surgery. In patients who have retropubic suburethral sling procedures, Valsalva voiding almost always leads to elevated residuals during the postoperative period. Therefore, it is important to consider the patient's voiding pattern before surgery. Uroflowmetry or uroflowmetry combined with voiding pressure studies are helpful in counseling patients before incontinence surgery.

Many females who void by Valsalva, can switch to other voiding mechanisms when counseled properly. Sometimes, education is all that is necessary. Other patients require biofeedback during voiding efforts to avoid this. A simple method, suggested to us by a patient, is to have the patient void while blowing bubbles with a straw into a glass of water. By doing this, patients do not increase their abdominal pressure during voiding.

## 3.4 Abnormal Obstructive Uroflowmetry (Detrusor Sphincter Dyssynergia)

The patient in Fig. 3.4 is a 35-year-old primipara with multiple sclerosis who has detrusor hyperreflexia and detrusor sphincter dyssynergia. The patient is incontinent and also has problems with urinary retention and recurrent urinary tract infections. In contrast to the previously noted uroflowmetry studies, this uroflow demonstrates a low peak flow rate (12 ml/s), a prolonged flow time (61 s) and a reduced average flow rate. In addition, the patient has an elevated residual urine (150 ml). Voiding pressure studies with EMG demonstrated that this patient voids with a dyssynergic pattern. Instead of undergoing coordinated urethral relaxation followed by a detrusor contraction, this patient has concurrent detrusor and urethral contractions. Dyssynergic voiders typically have obstructive uroflows with prolonged flow times, intermittent flow patterns, decreased peak flow rates and increased urinary residuals. A markedly abnormal uroflow like this may suggest some underlying pathology.

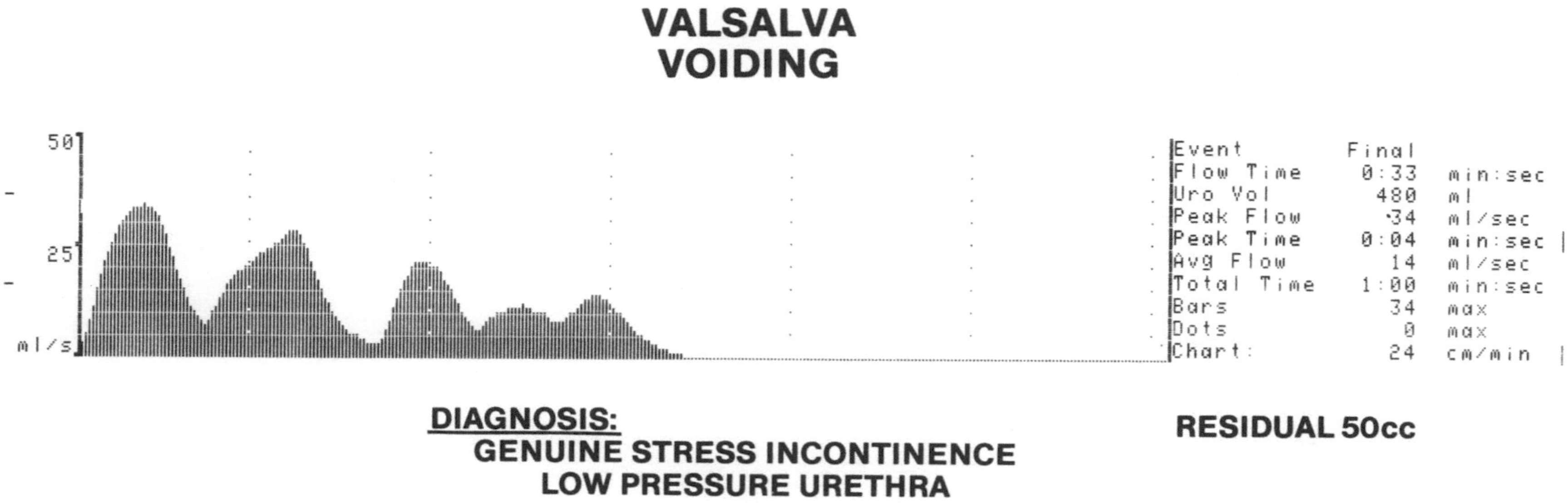


**Fig. 3.3.** Valsalva voiding during uroflowmetry in a woman with genuine stress incontinence and reduced urethral resistance.

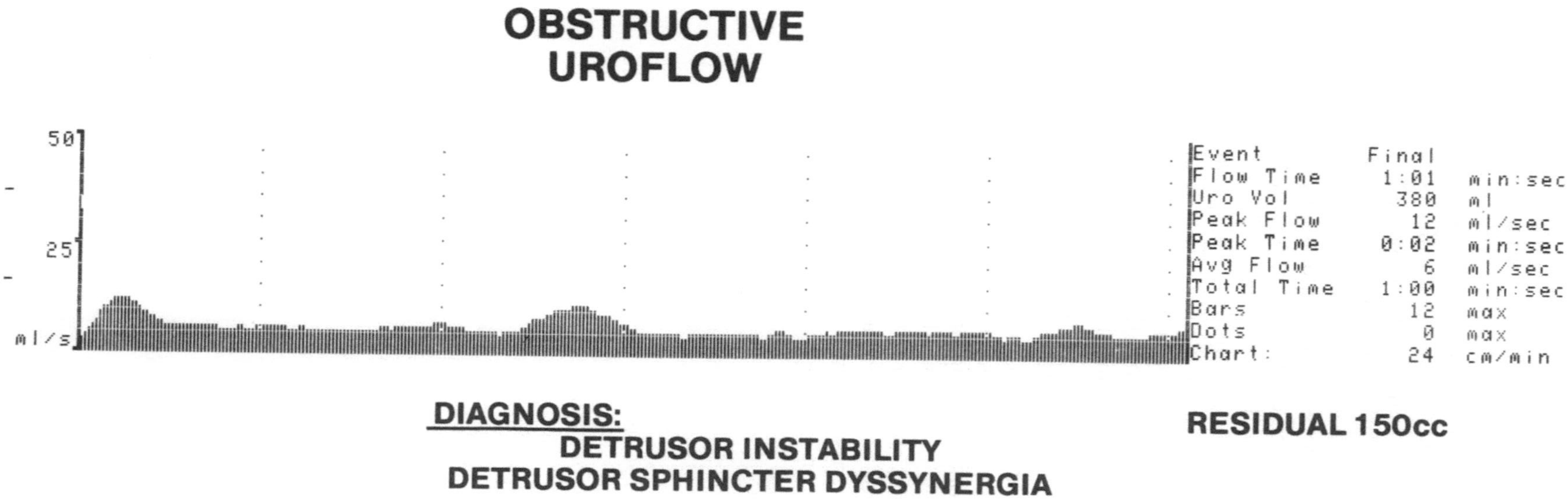


**Fig. 3.4.** Obstructive uroflowmetry in a woman with detrusor sphincter dyssynergia.

Although this study is not diagnostic of detrusor sphincter dyssynergia, it clearly indicates the need for more sophisticated studies.

Detrusor sphincter dyssynergia is usually a problem of neurologically abnormal patients with "upper motor neuron" lesions. However, in some patients who are neurologically normal, we theorize that dysfunctional voiding (concurrent detrusor and urethral contractions in neurologically normal patients) represents habituation of a continuous process of trying to avoid urinary incontinence associated with detrusor instability. During involuntary detrusor contractions urine is forced into the proximal urethra. The patient then voluntarily attempts to squeeze her pelvic floor musculature in an effort to milk this urine back into the bladder. Frequently these efforts are successful in preventing urinary incontinence. Repetitive contraction of the pelvic floor musculature in response to urine in the proximal urethra might theoretically lead to habituation of this response. Such an abnormal response may lead to a dysfunctional voiding pattern by interrupting normal voiding reflexes. It is theorized that during voiding, urine in the proximal urethra leads to urethral relaxation and further augmentation of the detrusor contraction. Although these arguments are theoretical, they may help to explain why some neurologically normal women with detrusor instability end up being dyssynergic voiders. If this theory is true, one would expect that treatment of the underlying detrusor instability would eventually correct the detrusor sphincter dyssynergia. This can be accomplished in some individuals.

## Bibliography

Abrams P, Blaivas JG, Stanton SL, Andersen JT: The standardization of terminology of lower urinary tract function. Int Urogynecol J 1:45, 1990.

Bhatia NN, Bergman A: Use of preoperative uroflowmetry and simultaneous urethrocystometry for predicting risk of prolonged postoperative bladder drainage. Urology 28:440, 1986.

Drach GW, Ignatoff J, Layton T: Peak urinary flow rate observations in female subjects and comparison to male subjects. J Urol 122:215, 1979.

Fantl JA, Smith PJ, Schneider V et al: Fluid weight uroflowmetry in women. Am J Obstet Gynecol 145:1017, 1983.

Lose G, Jorgensen L, Mortensen SO et al: Voiding difficulties after colposuspension. Obstet Gynecol 69:33, 1987.

Sand PK, Bowen LW, Panganiban R, Ostergard DR: The low pressure urethra as a factor in failed retropubic urethropexy. Obstet Gynecol 69:399, 1987.

Chapter 4

# The Lumbosacral Neurologic Examination

It is important to establish whether the patient's urinary symptomatology is due to underlying neurologic disease. Patients with underlying neurologic disease may not be amenable to certain therapies. In order to rule out a neurologic etiology in the otherwise apparently normal patient, one needs to do a careful screening neurologic exam. This neurologic exam involves testing the lumbosacral nerve roots, with regards to sensation, motor function and reflexes. Sacral cord segments $S_2$ to $S_4$ contain the most important neurons involved with micturition, however, the sympathetic nervous system (originating from $T_{10}$ to $L_2$) also significantly influences both the storage and voiding phases. A clinical screening examination aimed at discovering abnormalities is outlined below. Neurologic consultation may be necessary when the exam is abnormal.

Initially, the sensory dermatomes from $L_2$ to $S_2$ are evaluated by pinprick testing around the knee. As can be seen in Fig. 4.1, this allows for complete sensory evaluation of these dermatomes. Next, motor function is tested. Fig. 4.2 demonstrates testing $L_3$–$S_1$ with knee extension and flexion. $L_{2-5}$ can be tested by hip extension and flexion. Ankle abduction and adduction are used to test $L_4$–$S_1$. Flexion and extension of the ankle will also test these same nerve roots. Deep tendon reflexes are also tested in the lower extremities, as is the Babinski reflex. The bulbocavernosus and clitoral reflexes, as shown in Fig. 4.3, are used to evaluate $S_{2-5}$. Anal tone may be directly tested at the time of pelvic examination. The bulbocavernosus reflex involves stroking the labia majum which causes contraction of the pelvic floor and anal sphincter. The clitoral reflex is elicited by gently tapping on the clitoris which leads to a pelvic floor contraction. A similar reflex may be evoked by coughing or touching the transitional epithelium of the lower urinary tract. If these reflexes are intact, they confirm the integrity of $L_5$–$S_5$.

When clinical assessment with this simple neurologic examination reveals abnormalities, the patient should be referred for more complete neurologic testing. In the majority of patients where this examination is normal, the assumption may be made that the patient's problem is non-neurologic. However, experimental work with evoked potentials and nerve conduction velocities suggests that this may be an oversimplification.

## Bibliography

Bradley WE: The urologically oriented neurological examination. In Ostergard DR, Bent AE (eds) Gynecologic urology and urodynamics, 3rd edn. Baltimore, Williams & Wilkins, 1991, pp. 102–107.

Snooks SJ, Badenoch DF, Tiptaft RC et al: Perineal nerve damage in genuine stress urinary incontinence. Br J Urol 57:422, 1985.

Snooks SJ, Swash M: Abnormalities of the innervation of the urethral striated sphincter musculature in incontinence. Br J Urol 56:401, 1984.

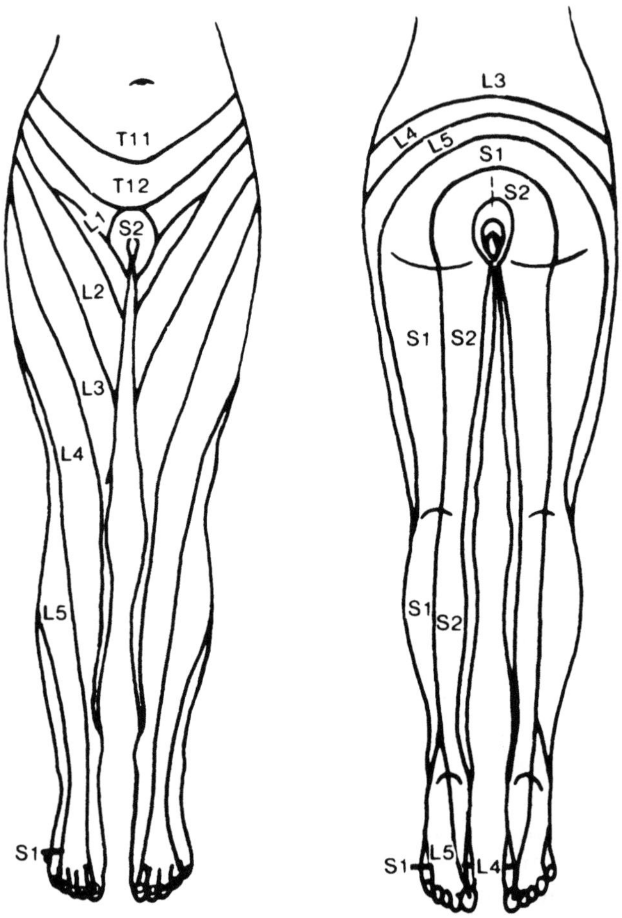


**Fig. 4.1.** Lumbosacral sensory dermatomes. Reprinted by permission of the author and Williams & Wlkins, Baltimore. From Ostergard, D.R., Bent, A.E. (Eds.) Urogynecology and Urodynamics: Theory and Practice, Third Edition, 1991

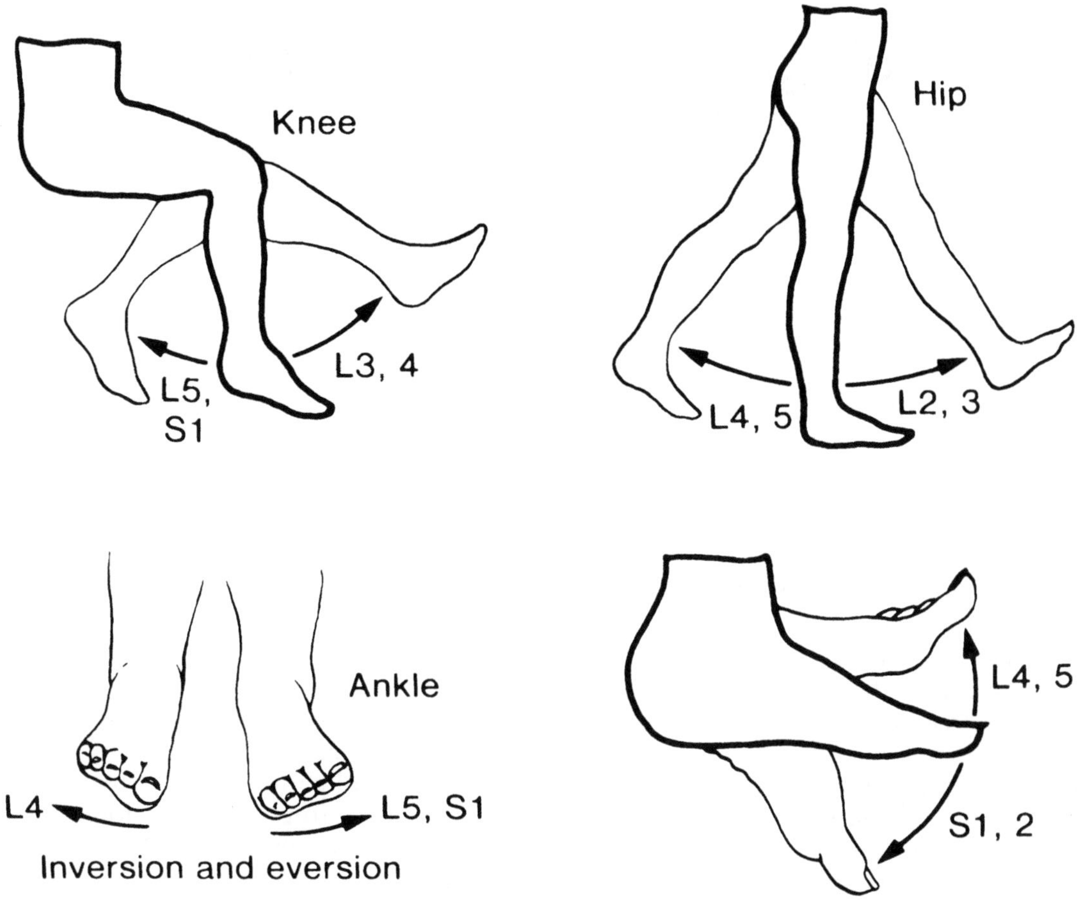


**Fig. 4.2.** Lumbosacral motor testing. Reprinted by permission of the author and Williams & Wilkins, Baltimore. From Ostergard, D.R., Bent, A.E. (Eds.) Urogynecology and Urodynamics: Theory and Practice, Third Edition, 1991

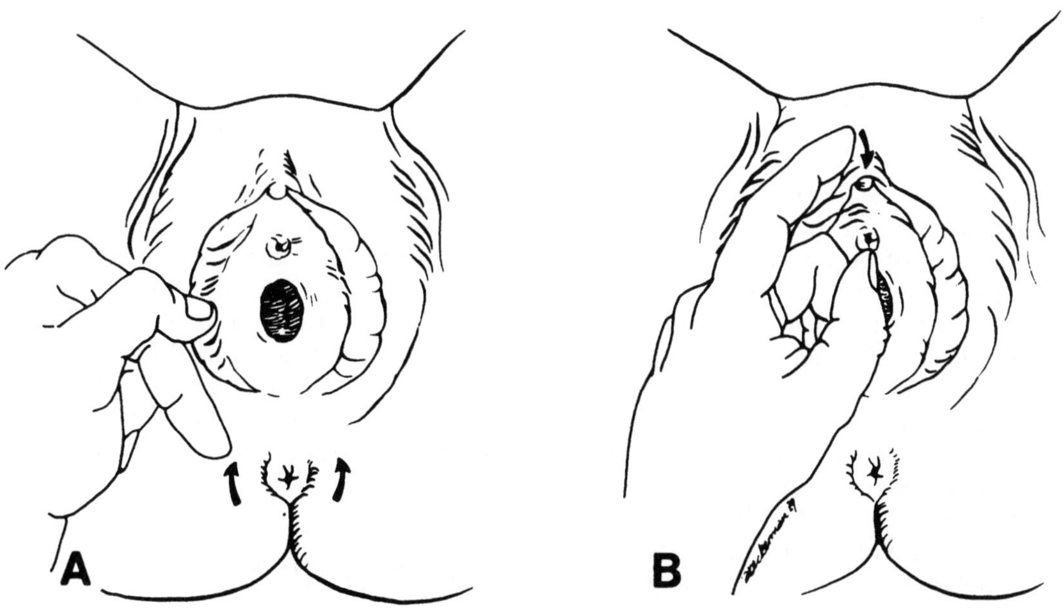


**Fig. 4.3.** Bulbocavernosus (A) and clitoral (B) sacral reflexes. Reprinted by permission of the author and Williams & Wilkins, Baltimore. From Ostergard, D.R., Bent, A.E. (Eds.) Urogynecology and Urodynamics: Theory and Practice, Third Edition, 1991

# Chapter 5
# The Gynecologic Pelvic Examination

All incontinent patients should undergo a complete gynecologic pelvic examination. Care is taken to examine the estrogenic condition of the vulva and vagina and the structural integrity of these organs. Decreased estrogen effect found on examination of the lower genital tract directly parallels the changes seen in the urethra on cytologic examination. Such estrogen deficit may have a profound effect on lower urinary tract function. In addition, observations are made of any pelvic relaxation that may be present. The anterior, posterior and apical vaginal walls are all examined for prolapse. These can be examined independently by the use of a Sims speculum or the posterior blade of a bivalve speculum to isolate first the anterior and then the posterior wall of the vagina. Central and paravaginal defects may be analyzed. The degree of prolapse and its effect on the voiding and storage phases may be evaluated with "pessary testing" as discussed in Chapter 34. Bimanual examination allows for further confirmation of vaginal wall prolapse and the rectovaginal examination is used to help identify the presence or absence of an enterocele. Speculum examination also allows the observer to look for fistulae. If there is a suspicion of vesicovaginal fistula, dye or sterile milk may be placed in the bladder and observations made for extrusion of this media into the vaginal cavity. The patient can also be evaluated after walking around with a tampon or cotton pack placed in the vagina to see if there is any leakage of dye into the upper vaginal vault at the top of the pack. This will help differentiate between urethral leakage and leakage from a vesicovaginal fistula. Cervical or vaginal cytology may also be evaluated at this time. All women undergoing this evaluation should also have a rectovaginal examination looking for rectal pathology and the presence of any blood on hemoccult or guaiac screening. Anal incontinence and dysfunction should be sought out and evaluated where indicated. Fecal incontinence may be found in as many as one-third to one-half of all patients with urinary incontinence.

It is also important to look for anatomic abnormalities which could lead to abnormal voiding or recurrent infection. Women with relative hypospadias may notice post-void dribbling because of pooling of urine within the vaginal vault. Other women are noted to have urethral hymenal fusion and on testing may be shown to have relative hypospadias during simulation of intromission. Patients with relative hypospadias and urethral hymenal fusion may have coitally related bacteriuria leading to recurrent urinary tract infection or dyspareunia. Some patients may need to undergo a urethroplasty (modified O'Donnell procedure) with or without a perineoplasty if antibiotic suppression does not relieve their recurrent urinary tract problems or conservative therapy does not relieve dyspareunia. Vaginal examination may also help in the identification of a urethral diverticulum. Compression of a protruding vaginal bulge may lead to a urethral discharge from the meatus suggesting the presence of a urethral diverticulum or a Skene's duct cyst.

## Bibliography

Bhatia NN, Bergman A, Karram MM: Effect of estrogen on urethral function in women with urinary incontinence.

Am J Obstet Gynecol 160:176, 1989.
Haaden K, Dahlstrom JA, Bengtsson M et al: Sphincter function in the urethra and anal canal: a comparison in women with manifest urinary incontinence. Int Urogynecol J 2:85, 1991.
Lee RA, Symmonds RE, Williams TJ: Current status of genitourinary fistula. Obstet Gynecol 72:313, 1988.
Munsick RA: Introital operations for dyspareunia. Clin Obstet Gynecol 23:243, 1980.
Shull BL, Baden WF: A six year experience with paravaginal defect repair for stress incontinence. Am J Obstet Gynecol 160:1432, 1989.

Chapter 6

# The Q-tip Test

The Q-tip test is a simple clinical test used to evaluate urethral mobility. Fig. 6.1 shows an intraoperative example of the test as it is being used to estimate the relative position of the urethrovesical junction during a modified Pereyra procedure.

The Q-tip test is performed by placing a sterile Q-tip applicator, which has been moistened with 2% xylocaine jelly, into the urethra. It is inserted gently until there is no further resistance, suggesting that the Q-tip has entered the bladder. The applicator is slowly withdrawn until it is felt to pull snugly up against the urethrovesical junction. This is followed by measurements of the resting angle of the Q-tip in relation to the horizontal with a compass or goniometer with an attached carpenter's level. The patient is then asked to repetitively Valsalva and cough until the maximal deflection is measured during an increase in intra-abdominal pressure. Although not well established in the literature, we assume that a normal Q-tip angle should be –10° to –30° at rest and should rise to no more than +30° during straining. Straining angles greater than +30° suggest that there is urethral hypermobility. Straining Q-tip angles greater than +30° suggest a descent of the urethrovesical junction of 1–1.5 cm which could potentially be corrected by surgery. Because the urethral meatus is fixed to the skin and will not move, movement of the Q-tip upward during Valsalva or coughing implies descent of the urethrovesical junction. Although the Q-tip test does not allow for a direct measurement of prolapse posteriorly away from the pubic symphysis, it does allow for indirect measurement of descent below the symphysis.

The Q-tip test, initially described by Crystle et al. (1971) was shown to reproduce accurately the results obtained by a bead chain cystourethrogram. Contrary to some reports in the literature, the Q-tip test is not meant to be diagnostic of stress incontinence. Indeed, it is well established that the Q-tip test is a non-specific, but fairly sensitive test used in the diagnosis of genuine stress incontinence. We use it as a negative test to indicate the need for further testing in those patients felt to have genuine stress incontinence who do

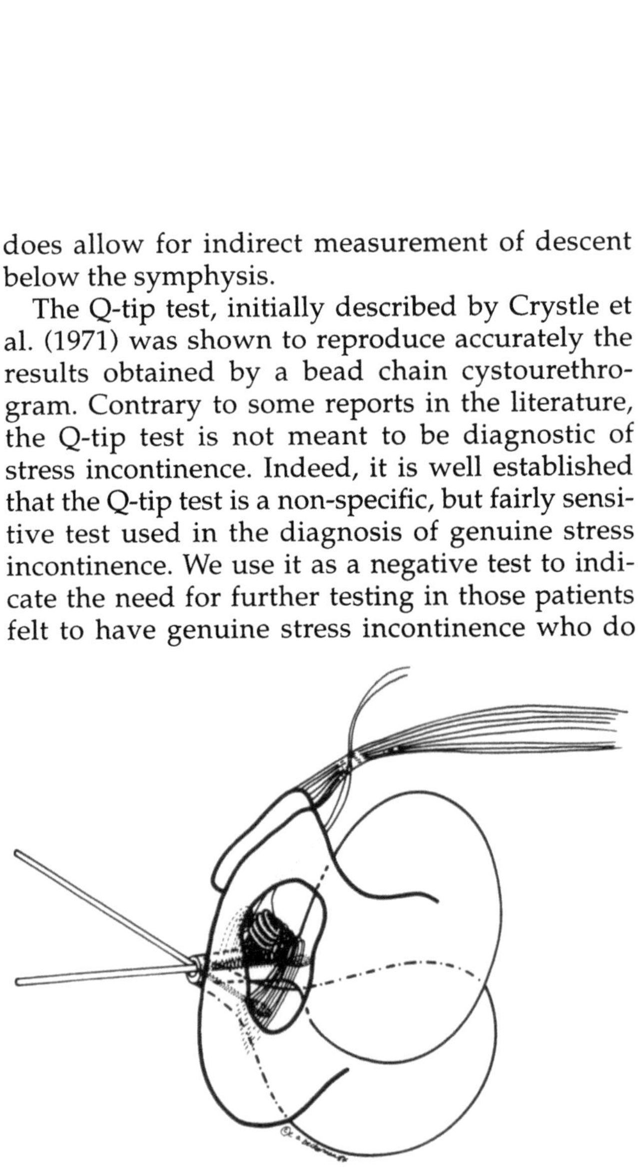

**Fig. 6.1.** Intraoperative Q-tip testing. Reprinted by permission of the author and Williams & Wilkins, Baltimore. From Ostergard, D.R., Bent, A.E. (Eds.) Urogynecology and Urodynamics: Theory and Practice, Third Edition, 1991

not have a positive Q-tip test (straining deflection <+30° from the horizontal). In these patients we are suspicious that retropubic urethropexy, which attempts to elevate the urethrovesical junction, may not be successful. If the urethrovesical junction is already elevated as demonstrated by a negative Q-tip test, then consideration must be given to some other pathophysiology which has not yet been identified to explain the patient's incontinence. Patients with rigid, fixed urethras or Type III incontinence (Chapter 53) may have negative Q-tip tests, yet lose large amounts of urine in the absence of detrusor contractions. Patients who have negative Q-tip tests, therefore, may warrant further radiographic analysis of their lower urinary tract.

We have also used the Q-tip test intraoperatively to demonstrate adequate elevation of the urethrovesical junction at the time of retropubic urethropexy, suburethral sling or needle suspension procedures. This is demonstrated in Fig. 6.1, where elevation of the modified Pereyra sutures leads to a decrease in the straining deflection of the Q-tip.

It is important to remember that the Q-tip test should not be used to establish the presence or absence of genuine stress incontinence. Instead it is used as a simple, safe and inexpensive substitute for the bead chain cystourethrogram and other radiographic measures of urethral mobility.

## Bibliography

Bergman A, Koonings PP, Ballard CA: Negative Q-tip test as a risk factor for failed incontinence surgery in women. J Reprod Med 34:193, 1989.

Crystle CD, Charme LS, Copeland WE: Q-tip test in stress urinary incontinence. Obstet Gynecol 38:313, 1971.

Karram MM, Bhatia NN: The Q-tip test: standardization of the technique and its interpretation in women with urinary incontinence. Obstet Gynecol 72:807, 1988.

McGuire EJ: Urodynamic findings in patients after failure of stress incontinence operations. Progr Clin Biol Res 78:351, 1981.

Montz FJ, Stanton SL: Q-tip test in female urinary incontinence. Obstet Gynecol 67:258, 1986.

# Chapter 7
# Urethral Calibration

Urethral calibration or measurement of the urethral diameter may be useful in women with irritative voiding symptoms (urgency, frequency, dysuria and post-void fullness) who are being evaluated for urinary incontinence. Some of these women may be found to have voiding dysfunction, the urethral syndrome or sensory urge incontinence. These disorders in women are usually associated with functional rather than physical obstruction. Hole (1972) showed that the urethral caliber in women with the urethral syndrome was no different from that of controls. However, it is important to rule out true urethral stenosis as a cause of obstructive voiding or detrusor overactivity. Relative urethral stenosis associated with atrophic urethritis or the urethral syndrome is not uncommon. Women who have urethral stenosis and suffer from voiding dysfunction, urge incontinence or the urethral syndrome may benefit from dilatation.

Urethral calibration is accomplished using Walthard female dilators. Calibration is done with topical anesthesia using 2% xylocaine jelly or a bladder pillar block if topical anesthesia is inadequate. Progressively larger dilators are used until blanching is seen around the urethral meatus or resistance to passage of the dilator is encountered in the proximal urethra. Urethral caliber is established as the largest dilator that could be passed without blanching or obvious proximal resistance. Urethral calibration may be done as a clean procedure and patients are given prophylactic antibiotics after evaluation. Calibration may be associated with a small amount of pain and bleeding as the largest calibrating dilator is passed. This will usually resolve spontaneously, but where persistent bleeding is noted a smaller dilator may be placed intraurethrally with or without transvaginal compression to gain hemostasis.

## Bibliography


Farrar DJ, Whiteside CG, Osborne JD et al: A urodynamic analysis of micturition symptoms in the female. Surg Gynecol Obstet 141:875, 1975.

Gustenberg TC, Lykkegaard Nielsen M, Lindberg J: Spastic striated external sphincter syndrome imitating recurrent urinary tract infection in females. Eur Urol 9:87, 1983.

Hole R: The caliber of the adult female urethra. Br J Urol 44:68, 1972.

## Chapter 8
# Stress Testing

Stress testing is essential to the diagnosis of genuine stress incontinence. Urinary incontinence is defined by the International Continence Society (ICS) as a condition where there is involuntary leakage of urine that is objectively demonstrable and represents a social and hygienic problem. Before any patient can be said to be incontinent there needs to be some objective demonstration of this urinary loss.

One of the simplest means of demonstrating urinary leakage in the patient complaining of stress incontinence is to fill their bladder to their maximum cystometric capacity (the point at which they can no longer tolerate any more bladder filling) and then, after the removal of the filling catheter, have them cough and Valsalva repetitively. If this does not cause urinary leakage the patient is asked to either jump up and down, do deep knee bends or lift objects off the floor. If these exercises do not result in urinary leakage we ask the patient to suggest what might reproduce her urinary leakage. Any urinary leakage during this testing is documented as a positive stress test. Stress testing may be positive in the patient with genuine stress incontinence, but also may be positive in patients who have stress-induced detrusor overactivity. Therefore, it cannot be used accurately as a discriminative tool but merely as an indicator of whether patients have urinary incontinence. Typically, urinary leakage that is coincident with increased intra-abdominal pressure and stops as soon as the increased intra-abdominal pressure stops is usually due to genuine stress incontinence. Negative stress testing does not necessarily rule out the presence of urinary incontinence and may need to be augmented by pad tests as described in Chapter 9.

Stress testing may be done in a number of different positions. The more upright the position, the more stressful it will be on the patient and the more sensitive the test. For this reason we routinely use standing stress testing in all patients. Comparisons between supine and standing results may help to assess the relative severity of the urinary leakage.

## Bibliography


Sand PK: Evaluation of the incontinent female. Curr Probl Obstet Gynecol Fertil 15:107, 1992.

Scotti RJ, Myers DL: A comparison of the cough stress test and single-channel cystometry with multichannel urodynamic evaluation in genuine stress incontinence. Obstet Gynecol 81:430, 1993.

# Chapter 9
# Pad Testing

Pad testing is a method which allows for the quantification of urinary leakage and is useful for monitoring a therapeutic effect during a clinical trial. Pad testing may also be useful to document urinary incontinence when it is not discovered on clinical or urodynamic evaluation. Up to 10% of all patients undergoing a urodynamic evaluation may fail to leak urine during testing in the office despite complaints of urinary incontinence in their normal environment. Pad testing may help to document this urinary leakage either in the office or in the patient's home setting. There are several pad tests that have been described in the medical literature ranging from short 20 min tests to 24 or 48 h home pad tests which attempt to reproduce the amount of urinary leakage occurring during the patient's normal activities. Fig. 9.1 shows a time line representation of the ICS approved one hour pad test which is described in greater detail in Appendix B. Pad tests all basically operate by measuring the differential change in weight of some pad or collecting device which is worn over a given period of time during which the patient is performing either their normal routine activities or a set series of activities, such as that listed in Fig. 9.1 The pad or collecting device is weighed before being applied to the patient's perineum and then is weighed at the end of the study. If the difference in weight is greater than 1 g after a one hour pad test, most authors would agree that this is probably a representation of the volume of urine lost. False positive pad tests may occur from excessive perspiration or vaginal discharge. However, most studies have shown that the volume of these secretions is usually less than 1 ml per hour and would not increase the weight of the pad by more than 1 g. Use of urinary dyes such as pyridium, have not been shown to improve the accuracy of pad testing.

Fig. 9.1 describes a one hour standard pad test where the patient drinks 500 ml of liquid at the beginning of the study. This is done after the patient has emptied her bladder and a diuresis is allowed to occur over the next 30 min. At that time the patient starts the activities listed at the 30 min point. Sometimes these activities may be impossible for patients with arthritis, advanced age or limited mobility. For this reason the pad test may need to be modified and this should be noted in the patient's record.

In our laboratory we use a 20 min modified pad test where sterile water is instilled directly into an empty bladder with a catheter rather than relying on a variable diuresis for a half hour at the beginning of the test. Following this bladder instillation the patient is put through a set series of exercises quite similar to the one hour pad test (Fig. 9.2). They are asked to cough hard in the standing position 10 times in a row, Valsalva 10 times in a row, followed by 10 deep knee bends and then jumping in place 10 times. The patient is then asked to wash her hands in warm water for 1 min followed by walking up and down five flights of stairs. After this, the patient walks in the hall for 10 min and then returns, removes her pad and places it in a sealable bag in which it was originally weighed. It is then re-weighed. This allows for rapid and accurate assessment of urinary loss in patients undergoing therapeutic trials. Patients who fail to demonstrate urinary leakage during a standard urodynamic evaluation may undergo a 20 min pad test at the end of the evaluation or be given a set of 12 pads and asked to do a 12 hour

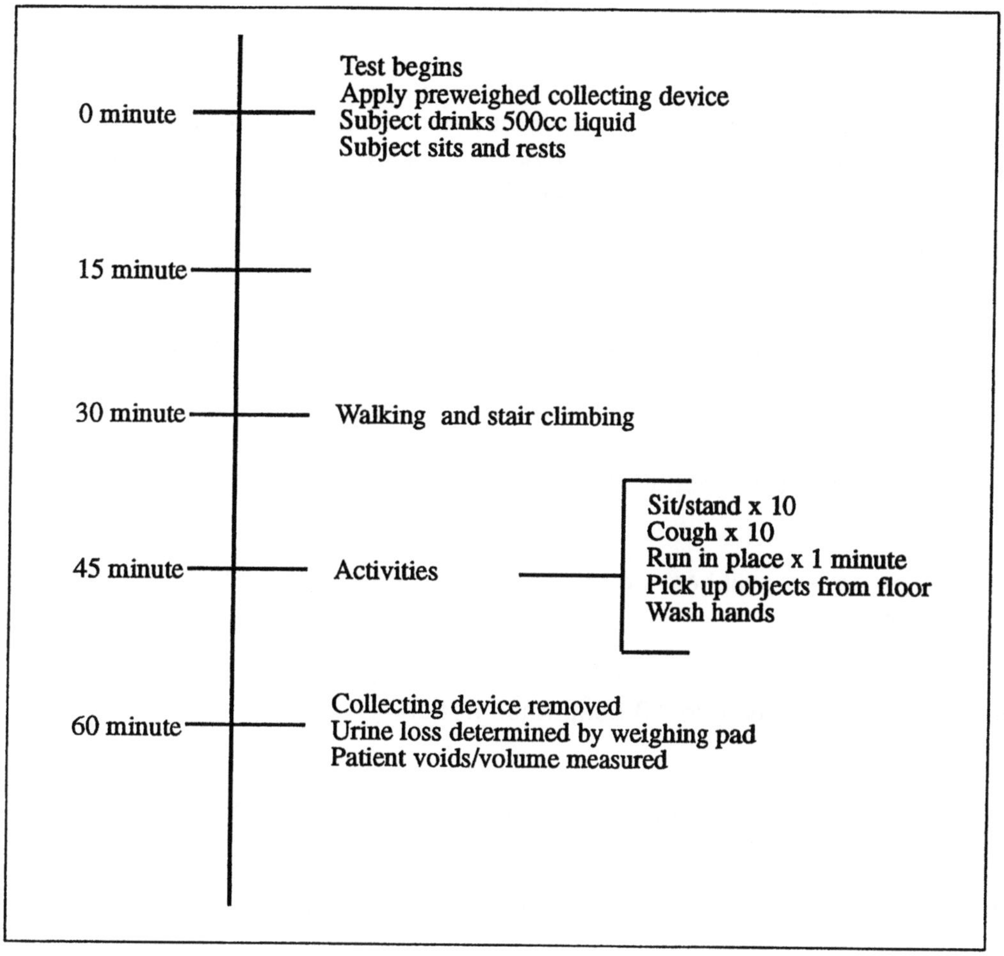


**Fig. 9.1.** ICS one hour pad test. Reprinted by permission of the author and Williams & Wilkins, Baltimore. From Ostergard, D.R., Bent, A.E. (Eds.) Urogynecology and Urodynamics: Theory and Practice, Third Edition, 1991

## MODIFIED 20-MINUTE PAD TEST

This 20-minute pad test is being done to assess the patient's progress with her therapy. It provides Dr. Sand and his coworkers with objective evidence of how much urinary leakage you are currently having. It is important that the test be performed in a standardized fashion at all times. For this reason you will be asked to cooperate with specific instructions listed below during the 20 minutes of the test. The following is an exact list of the procedures which will occur during the 20-minute pad test.

1. The patient's bladder will be emptied with a transurethral catheter and then filled to a bladder volume of 250cc. If this volume cannot be obtained because of uninhibited detrusor contractions the filling volume will be noted and the test will proceed at this lower volume.

2. The catheter will then be removed and the patient will return to the standing position and a preweighed perineal pad will be placed inside the underwear of the patient.

3. The patient will cough (hard) 10 times in a row.

4. The patient will bear down like she is trying to move her bowels 10 times in a row.

5. The patient will do 10 deep knee bends.

6. The patient will jump up and down in place 10 times.

7. The patient will wash her hands under warm water for one minute and then dry her hands.

8. The patient will walk up and down a half flight of stairs (5 stairs) 10 times.

9. At this point the patient will be asked to walk in the halls for 10 minutes and then return and remove the pad.

10. The pad will then be weighed in its Ziploc bag and the wet weight subtracted from the original dry weight to achieve a measure of the total urine loss during the 20-minute exercise. The patient will be informed of this result and the test will end at this point.

**Fig. 9.2.** Twenty minute fixed volume pad test.

home pad test. During this 12 hour pad test they change their pads every hour during their wakeful day while doing their normal activities. The preweighed pads are then replaced into their original resealable bags and placed in a refrigerated area prior to being returned to the laboratory for weighing the following day. A weight increase greater than 1 g per hour may then be interpreted to be representative of urinary leakage. Such pad testing has been demonstrated to correlate well with shorter one hour or two hour pad tests.

## Bibliography


Jorgensen L, Lose F, Andersen JT, One hour pad-weighing test for objective assessment of female urinary incontinence. Obstet Gynecol 69:39,1987.

Kinn AC, Larsson B: Pad test with fixed bladder volume in urinary stress incontinence. Acta Obstet Gynecol Scand 66:369, 1987.

Klarskov P, Hald T: Reproduceability and reliability of urinary incontinence. Assessment with a 60 min test. Scand J Urol Nephrol 18:293, 1984.

Lose G, Rosenkilde P, Gammelgaard J et al: Pad-weighing test performed with standardized bladder volume. Urology 32:78, 1988.

Lose G, Versi E: Pad-weighing tests in the diagnosis and quantification of incontinence. Int Urogynecol J 3:324, 1992.

Mayne CJ, Hilton P: Short pad test: standardization of method and comparison with l-hour test. Neurourol Urodynam 7:443, 1988.

Sutherst JR, Brown MC, Richmond D: Analysis of the patterns of urine loss in women with incontinence as measured by weighing perineal pads. Br J Urol 58:273, 1986.

Sutherst J, Brown M, Shower M: Assessing the severity of urinary incontinence in women by weighing perineal pads. Lancet i:1128, 1981.

Section II

# Cystourethroscopy and Cystometry

## Chapter 10

# Dynamic Urethroscopy

Dynamic urethroscopy, using the Robertson urethroscope, allows the investigator not only to look at the condition of the uroepithelium, but also to observe the dynamic function of the urethral sphincteric unit. The urethroscope, utilizing a 0° lens, allows the investigator to examine the urethra in its natural state as the urethroscope is first inserted. On inspection, the urethral mucosa may be noted to be inflamed and hyperemic in a woman with frequency and dysuria or may be pale and atrophic in the postmenopausal woman. Excessive exudate or glandular secretions may be noted within the lumen of the urethra. Cysts, pseudopolyps, inflammatory fronds and condylomata may also be found in the urethra and on the trigone. With insertion of the scope, the examiner carefully checks the distal urethra for any of these findings. Then the mid urethra and upper urethra are systematically examined and findings noted on a programmed form (Appendix C). Following this, the urethrovesical junction and bladder trigone are examined. Then the operator examines both ureteral orifices as well as the interureteric ridge. Observation of normal ureteral ejaculation of urine and retraction is made and the position and configuration of the ureteral orifices noted.

Following inspection of the urethra and trigone, the operator withdraws the urethroscope into the proximal urethra so that the urethrovesical junction is 50% open. The patient is then asked to squeeze her rectum tight. The examiner should then normally observe closure of the urethrovesical junction in front of the scope. The operator notes whether rectal squeeze leads to total closure, partial closure, no change or opening of the urethrovesical junction. One must be sure the patient understands the request and that the scope does not move relatively forward with downward motion of the patient's perineum. Forward motion of the scope may lead to artifactual funneling of the urethra. This is a common problem when the examiner first begins to do urethroscopy. Following this, the examiner asks the patient to squeeze the urethra closed, as if she were trying to stop urine from leaking out. Once again, closure, partial closure, no change or opening of the urethrovesical junction is noted. The examiner then notes the same changes in response to Valsalva and coughing. The normal response is closure of the urethrovesical junction in response to rectal squeeze, urethral squeeze, Valsalva and coughing. In patients with urethrovesical junction descent, the scope will tend to move forward into the bladder as the urethrovesical junction rotates posteriorly. In an effort to avoid artifactual opening of the urethrovesical junction, the examiner must change the angle of inclination of the scope to meet the downward deflection of the urethrovesical junction. At the same time, the scope may be withdrawn into the mid urethra to be sure there is funneling and opening along the entire proximal urethra in the stress incontinent patient. This mobility of the urethrovesical junction, as well as relative motion of the patient's perineum relative to the examiner and the urethroscope, makes dynamic urethroscopy a challenging procedure. Typically, this examination is accomplished in the supine position. One group found that supine dynamic urethroscopy had a sensitivity of only 60% with a specificity of 79% in diagnosing genuine stress incontinence. However, with the use of a teaching scope or endoscopic camera, one may perform this examination in the sitting upright and standing positions. The most informative and difficult way to perform this examination is to do it in the standing position.

Dynamic urethroscopy theoretically offers the examiner a direct view of the underlying pathology involved in genuine stress incontinence. But, because of the relative difficulty in performing this accurately, this test may have limited application for many examiners.

# Bibliography

Robertson JR: Dynamic urethroscopy. In Ostergard DR, Bent AE (eds) Urogynecology and Urodynamics. Baltimore, Williams & Wilkins, 1991, pp. 115–121.

Scotti, RJ, Ostergard DR, Guillaume AA et al: Predictive value of urethroscopy as compared to urodynamics in the diagnosis of genuine stress incontinence. J Reprod Med 35:772, 1990.

Chapter 11
# Supine Urethroscopic Cystometry

Cystometry is the measurement of the intravesical pressure–volume relationship during filling of the bladder with a distending medium. It allows one to assess the compliance, control, sensation and capacity of the bladder. The distending medium may be sterile water, saline, carbon dioxide or urine. Normal cystometry is defined as the ability to fill the bladder to a normal maximum cystometric capacity in the absence of any involuntary detrusor contractions or voluntary uninhibited contractions. Previously a pressure rise greater than 15 $cmH_2O$ was also considered a measure of detrusor instability (abnormal cystometrogram) but the International Continence Society no longer includes this measure as a necessary part of the definition. However, pressure rises of >15 $cmH_2O$ still indicate an abnormality of storage function. Normal maximum cystometric capacities will differ, depending on the medium used to distend the bladder. In addition, it has been shown that the incidence of detrusor instability will be greater when using carbon dioxide rather than water. This may be related to the formation of carbonic acid in the bladder when carbon dioxide comes into contact with water. This may lead to detrusor contractions from increased afferent sensation. Room temperature solutions will also tend to induce more abnormal detrusor contractions than will saline at 38°C (Chapter 37). Detrusor contractions may also be encountered during supine cystometry in the presence of lower urinary tract infections with Gram negative bacilli. It is theorized that this is related to the production of endotoxins by Gram negative bacilli.

Supine cystometry may be performed through the urethroscope at the time of dynamic urethroscopy or through a Foley catheter attached to a water manometer or a hydrostatic pressure transducer catheter. With simple systems it is a rapid (10 min), simple and inexpensive test. Filling is accomplished at slow, medium and rapid rates, as defined by the International Continence Society(Appendix B).

These studies are usually performed in a retrograde fashion, but may be performed orthograde after water loading and the administration of a diuretic.

In performing cystometry the patient's bladder is initially emptied, then filled at a desired rate. As the patient's bladder is filled, she will state when she first feels like she could urinate (first sensation to void). This is noted and the study continued. The patient then notes when she feels full. We typically ask the patient to wait until she feels full enough that she would get off the freeway and use the restroom at a gas station or restaurant, rather than driving further to her own home. Then the patient is filled until she can stand no more due to pain or extreme discomfort. This is taken as the patient's maximum cystometric capacity. A bladder contraction may be identified during urethroscopy by persistent funnelling of the bladder neck and active opening of the urethra. The urethrovesical junction may be seen in an open position during a bladder contraction even when the urethroscope is withdrawn to the urethral meatus. The bladder contraction may also be visualized directly by noting the interlacing muscle fibers forming a pseudotrabecular pattern within the bladder. During filling, the patient is asked to intermittently cough while in the supine position. If it appears that the patient is having a detrusor contraction, she is asked to inspire to reduce the intra-abdominal pressure. Persistence of an elevated bladder pressure and open bladder neck will help confirm that the pressure rise represents a true detrusor contraction, rather than just a rise in the intra-abdominal pressure which is transmitted to the bladder. Rises in intra-abdominal pressure may lead to false positive perceptions of detrusor contractions during cystometry. Simple supine cystometry using only a single pressure measuring catheter is also susceptible to such artifact. This may be avoided by the addition of a second pressure measuring catheter within the vagina or rectum to estimate the intra-abdominal pressure. Not only is single channel supine cystometry limited by intra-abdominal pressure artifact, but also by the inability to identify as many as 50% of patients who have detrusor instability in the standing position.

## Bibliography

Arnold EP: Cystometry-postural effects in incontinent women. Urol Int 29:185, 1974.

Bhatia NN, Bergman A: Cystometry: unstable bladder and urinary tract infection. Br J Urol 58:134, 1986.

Gleason DM, Bottacini MR, Reilly RJ: Comparison of cystometrograms and urethral pressure profiles with gas and water media. Urology 9:155, 1977.

Jorgensen L, Lose G, Andersen JT: Cystometry: $H_2O$ or $CO_2$ as filling medium? Neurourol Urodynam 7:343, 1988.

Sand PK, Hill RC, Ostergard DR: Supine urethroscopic and standing cystometry as screening methods for the detection of detrusor instability. Obstet Gynecol 70:57, 1987.

## Chapter 12
# Cystoscopy

Cystoscopy is done during the evaluation of the incontinent females with irritative voiding symptoms to rule out any underlying bladder pathology. This may be accomplished with either flexible or rigid cystoscopes. Different lenses may be used to allow for optimal evaluation of all areas of the bladder (0°, 30°, 70°, 110° lenses). Either carbon dioxide or a fluid media, such as water, normal saline or glycine solution may be used to distend the bladder.

The evaluation of the bladder should be done in a systematic fashion to avoid missing any bladder pathology. Evaluation must include a thorough inspection of the dome, lateral walls and posterior wall of the bladder as well as the trigone, bladder neck and ureteral orifices. At the time of cystoscopy, inflammatory changes such as squamous metaplasia, granularity and cystic changes may be noted on the trigone. The rest of the bladder may have chronic inflammatory changes such as diffuse cysts, as in cystitis cystica or cystitis glandularis. Some patients may have evidence of subendothelial hemorrhages (glomerulations), or Hunner's ulcers especially with redistention of the bladder suggestive of interstitial cystitis. This is important to note because many of these patients have sensory urgency and/or urge incontinence. The endoscopist wants to be sure not to miss a transitional cell or adenocarcinoma of the bladder. For this reason, when abnormal lesions are encountered, they should be biopsied. The use of cytologic washings at the time of cystoscopy may also aid in the diagnosis of bladder neoplasia and is more sensitive than the use of urine cytology. Routine diagnostic cystoscopy can usually be accomplished in the office without anesthesia in women. Where biopsies are necessary, anesthesia is often necessary. For small raised lesions anesthesia through bladder instillation with or without bladder pillar block may be all that is necessary. Biopsies must be done carefully by an experienced endoscopist as perforations (although minor) occur as often as 10% of the time.

## Bibliography


Matzkin H, Mimuddin SM, Soloway MS: Value of urine cytology versus bladder washing in bladder cancer. Urology 39:201, 1992.

Uehling DT: Inflammatory diseases of the bladder. In Gillenwater JY, Grayhack JT, Howards SS, Duckett JW (eds) Adult and Pediatric Urology, 2nd edn. St Louis, Mosley Yearbook, 1991, pp. 1101–18.

Walther MM, Campbell WG, O'Brien DP et al: Cystitis cystica: an electron and immunofluorescence microscopic study. J Urol 137:764, 1987.

# Chapter 13
# Standing Single Channel Cystometry

The standing single channel cystometrogram may reveal most of the unstable bladders missed by supine cystometry studies. When compared to multichannel urodynamic studies, some have found the single channel cystometrogram to be remarkably accurate. Our investigations have shown even standing single channel studies to be not only less specific (69%), but also less sensitive (84%) than multichannel urethrocystometry. Despite these limitations, single channel cystometry is an excellent screening method during the evaluation of the incontinent female. Cystometry is an essential part of the workup of all incontinent women who are contemplating anti-incontinence surgery.

Single channel cystometry can be accomplished using carbon dioxide, water and saline through various catheters. Pressure may be measured using simple water manometry, balloon catheters or electronic microtransducers. The study done in Fig. 13.1 was accomplished using a three-way Foley catheter, water manometer and electronic cystometer. Whereas electronic cystometers allow for continuous recording of the bladder pressure, the same qualitative results may be obtained with a far less expensive system consisting of a three-way Foley catheter and a CVP manometer. Besides varying the type of pressure measuring devices and media used to fill the bladder, one can also vary the speed of filling. Slow fill studies involve infusion of media into the bladder at a rate 1–10 ml/min. Medium flow studies infuse fluid at rates of 10–100 ml/min, whereas high flow studies exceed 100 ml/min. In addition, the temperature of the infusing media may vary. Cold and room temperature infusions tend to be more irritating and provocative to the bladder than solutions infused at body temperature.

The study shown in Fig. 13.1 is a single-channel retrograde cystometrogram obtained with a water transducer and electronic cystometer using a medium flow rate with normal saline at 37°C. The study was begun after a three-way Foley catheter was placed in the patient's bladder. The three-way system allows for continuous recording of pressure through one channel while fluid is infused through another. Before the initiation of the study, the water manometer was placed at the level of the patient's pubic symphysis and the electronic cystometer zeroed with no saline in the bladder. Then the infusion was begun at 80 ml/min and markings placed for every 100 ml infused (identified by the Arabic numbers 1 to 5 on this tracing). These each represent 100 ml infused. The patient was asked to note her first sensation to void. This needs to be clearly distinguished from an absolute need to void in the patient's mind. The large narrow peaks seen after each 100 ml infusion represent coughs and heel bounces, which were used to attempt to provoke an unstable bladder contraction. Other provocative maneuvers such as hand washing, seeing and hearing running water and straining may also be used to attempt to trigger involuntary detrusor contractions. During this study, the patient noted first sensation at 225 ml. This is well within the range of normal recognition of first sensation. Next, the patient noted fullness at 450 ml – when she felt she was full enough to get off the freeway and use a bathroom at a gas station rather than continuing on another 15 min to her home. The study was then continued beyond this point until

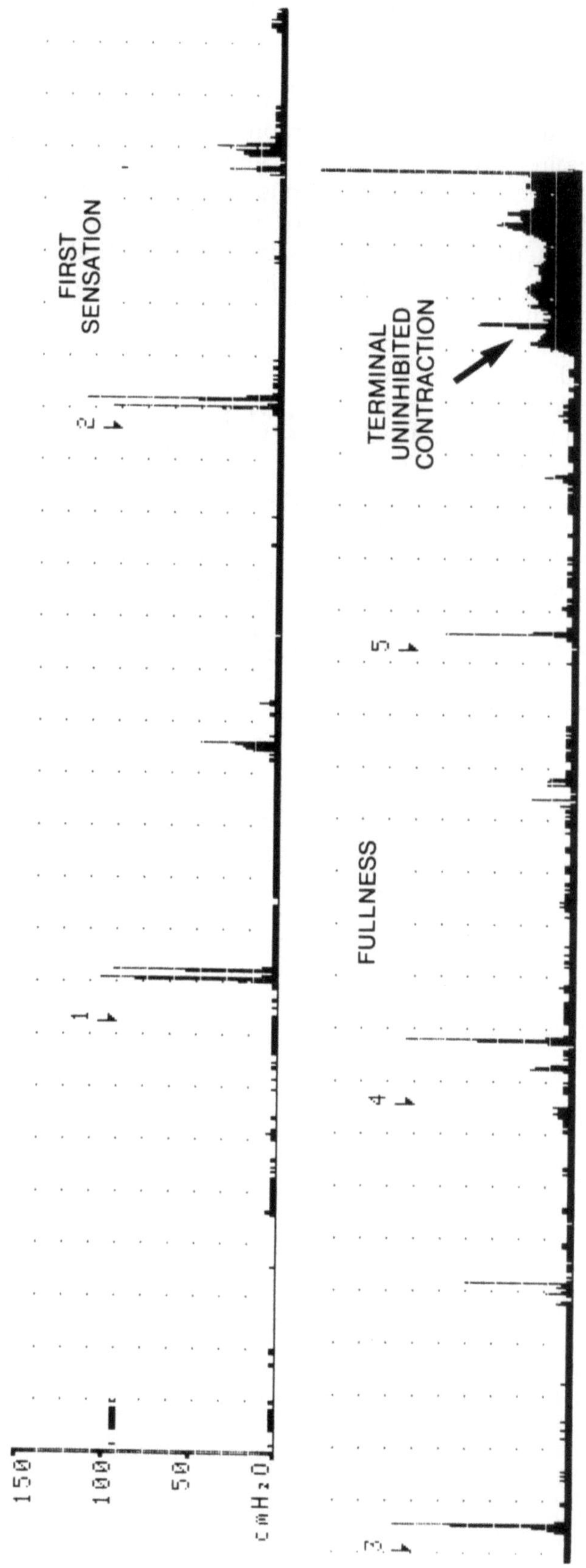


**Fig. 13.1.** Single channel electronic cystometrogram.

maximum cystometric capacity was reached, when the patient could stand no further fluid due to pain or autonomic symptoms. However, before this point was reached, the patient began to have an involuntary uninhibited detrusor contraction. The patient's bladder pressure rose to 18 $cmH_2O$ which was associated with a strong urge. The patient was asked to deeply inspire at this point to rule out an increase in intra-abdominal pressure which might mimic a detrusor contraction. However, with inspiration there was little decrease in detrusor pressure, which rose even further with time. Throughout this process, the patient was asked to attempt to inhibit this contraction. However, even after 20 s, the patient was unable to inhibit the detrusor contraction. Filling was stopped at this point, with the patient reaching a maximum cystometric capacity of 580 ml. This patient was found to have an unstable detrusor as the underlying cause of her urinary incontinence. This was later confirmed on multichannel urethrocystometry. If this were a normal study, the patient would have been able to tolerate this volume of fluid without having an uninhibited involuntary detrusor contraction. At maximum cystometric capacity, the patient would have been asked to initiate a detrusor contraction and then to inhibit it. The patient should be able to begin to inhibit a detrusor contraction quite rapidly. During the course of the cystometry study the bladder pressure should rise no more than 15 cm $H_2O$. Gradual rises greater than this usually represent decreased bladder compliance.

Single channel cystometry can easily be accomplished in the physician's office in a short period of time (5–10 min). It should be considered necessary in the evaluation of all incontinent women who are to undergo corrective surgery.

## Bibliography

Cucchi A: Screening tests for detrusor instability in clinical urodynamics. Int Urogynecol J 2:101, 1991.

Ouslander J, Leach G, Abelson S et al: Simple versus multichannel cystometry in the evaluation of bladder function in an incontinent geriatric population. J Urol 140: 1483, 1988.

Sand PK, Brubaker LT, Novak T: Simple standing incremental cystometry as a screening method for detrusor instability. Obstet Gynecol 77:453, 1991.

Section III

# Multichannel Urodynamics: Normal Studies

## Chapter 14

# Who Needs Urodynamics?

Multichannel urodynamic evaluation of urinary incontinence involves the recording of urethrocystometry, sphincter EMG, urethral closure pressure profiles and voiding pressure studies. Integrating these tests and performing them at various states of bladder fullness as well as in different positions can allow the urodynamicist to obtain a great deal of useful information. However, this testing is costly and time consuming. Therefore, it is not appropriate for every patient who suffers from lower urinary tract dysfunction to undergo multichannel urodynamics. Various laboratories across the country have their exact criteria for who needs urodynamics and who does not. It is safe to say that most researchers would enjoy the opportunity to study all their patients if possible. Where to draw the line between who undergoes multichannel studies and who undergoes single channel standing cystometry, stress testing and other simple clinical tests is difficult. The performance of EMG testing with voiding pressure studies is essential in the patient who has urinary retention. However, it also provides useful information in those patients about to undergo incontinence surgery. In the former case it is a necessity in order to establish the diagnosis of the underlying cause of urinary retention. In the latter case it is helpful in order to establish the voiding mechanism and the risk of urinary retention or dysfunction following incontinence surgery. Performance of urethrocystometry with or without EMG is very useful in establishing the diagnosis of overactive detrusor function whether it be due to an underlying neurologic problem (detrusor hyperreflexia) or in the absence of an underlying neurologic abnormality (detrusor instability). But overactive detrusor function may also be established on a simple standing single channel cystometrogram. These simple studies are not as sensitive as urethrocystometry and may also produce many false positive diagnoses of overactive detrusor function because of the effect of increased intra-abdominal pressure during cystometry. Urethrocystometry avoids this by providing the true detrusor pressure or the pressure in the bladder in the absence of any intra-abdominal pressure artifact. It is for this reason that we usually perform urethrocystometry in surgical candidates who have a suspicious or positive single channel cystometrogram. The presence of detrusor overactivity will independently reduce the chances of successfully curing genuine stress incontinence in surgical patients with mixed incontinence as opposed to pure genuine stress incontinence. For the non-surgical candidate it is probably not as crucial to avoid overdiagnosing detrusor instability or detrusor hyperreflexia. However, because standing single channel cystometrograms may have sensitivities as low as 60% when compared to urethrocystometry, one must question whether all patients could benefit from the more complicated studies. This is especially important in older populations where the prevalence of detrusor instability may be as high as 60%.

Contrary to this, some investigators have shown that premenopausal women with complaints of stress incontinence in the absence of urgency, frequency, nocturia and urge incontinence have a very low risk of detrusor instability and may not need any assessment of their detrusor prior to contemplated anti-incontinence surgery. Results from our lab and others do not confirm this conclusion. Although there is some controversy most investigators feel that as a minimum, any patient who is to undergo an anti-incontinence operation, regardless of her history or age, should at least undergo standing single channel cystometry.

The performance of urethral closure pressure profiles either at rest or with Valsalva or repetitive coughing has been found to be quite useful by some investigators but useless by others. We find the performance of urethral closure pressure profiles to be useful in the establishment of the diagnosis of genuine stress incontinence when pressure equalization is noted with Valsalva and repetitive coughing. In addition, static urethral closure pressure profiles may tell us about the integrity of the intrinsic sphincteric mechanism at various states of bladder fullness. It has been established that patients with low urethral closure pressure are at increased risk of failing retropubic urethropexies. For this reason all patients who are at risk of having low urethral closure pressure (postmenopausal patients and patients with prior periurethral surgery) may benefit from having urethral closure pressure profiles performed.

Determining who needs multichannel urodynamics remains controversial. It is clear that most investigators would agree that patients with previous incontinence surgery as well as those with mixed symptoms or mixed genuine stress incontinence and overactive detrusor function on simple evaluation who fail to respond to conservative therapy, as well as those with urinary retention should undergo multichannel urodynamics. In addition, many would add postmenopausal patients as well as those who had evidence on simple cystometry of overactive detrusor function to rule out false positive diagnoses of detrusor instability. But perhaps the most important indication for further testing is when a simple evaluation fails to explain completely the patient's symptoms.

## Bibliography

Farrar DJ, Whiteside CG, Osborne JL et al: A urodynamic analysis of micturition symptoms in the female. Surg Gynecol Obstet 141:875, 1975.

Hastie KJ, Masey CU: Are urodynamics necessary in female patients presenting with stress incontinence? Br J Urol 63:155, 1989.

Le Coutour X, Jung-Faerber S, Klein P et al: Female urinary incontinence: comparative value of history and urodynamic investigations. Eur J Obstet Gynecol Reprod Biol 37:279, 1990.

Sand PK, Bowen LW, Ostergard DR et al: The effect of retropubic urethropexy on detrusor stability. Obstet Gynecol 71:818, 1988.

Sand PK, Hill RC, Ostergard DR: Supine urethroscopic and standing cystometry as screening methods for the detection of detrusor instability. Obstet Gynecol 70:57, 1987.

Chapter 15

# Urethral Closure Pressure Profiles

Urethral closure pressure profiles are measurements of integrated pressure curves from the entire length of the urethra and are measured by the slow withdrawal of a pressure-measuring catheter through the urethra at a constant rate. Urethral closure profiles may be static, done with the patient at rest either in the supine, sitting or standing position; or they may be dynamic, recorded while the patient is either coughing repetitively, performing a Valsalva maneuver or squeezing to prevent the passage of flatus or the passage of urine. Measurement of static urethral closure pressure profiles allows the investigator to make comparisons of preoperative and postoperative measurements or between different positions and states of bladder fullness in the same patient. Such static assessment, although not diagnostic for genuine stress incontinence may still provide the examiner with useful information. Comparisons of dynamic profiles during coughing and Valsalva allow the examiner to make the diagnosis of genuine stress incontinence when pressure equalization is noted in the absence of an increase in detrusor pressure.

Fig. 15.1 demonstrates a theoretical static urethral closure pressure profile. Measurements may be made of the total or anatomic urethral length, the functional length, the urethral pressure, the maximal urethral pressure, the bladder pressure, the urethral closure pressure, the maximal urethral closure pressure, the integrated area underneath the curve (representing total urethral closure pressure) and the length to maximal pressure as well as the length from maximal pressure to the external meatus. The total urethral length is a measurement made from the first rise in urethral closure pressure until the pressure reaches zero atmospheric pressure at the external urethral meatus. Normal anatomic length in the female ranges from 3 to 5 cm. The functional length is the length of the urethra that has a positive closure pressure. This is the portion of the urethra that is acting to maintain continence. The closure pressure represents the difference of urethral pressure minus bladder pressure. When this is positive along any or all of the urethra the patient will remain continent. If there is no positive closure pressure then the patient will be incontinent of urine. The bladder pressure is the pressure measured within the bladder. This differs from the true detrusor pressure which is the bladder pressure minus the intra-abdominal pressure. Measurement of the true detrusor pressure subtracts any artifactual increase in bladder pressure due to intra-abdominal pressure. The integrated area under the curve or total closure pressure and measurements of partial urethral lengths are used primarily for research purposes.

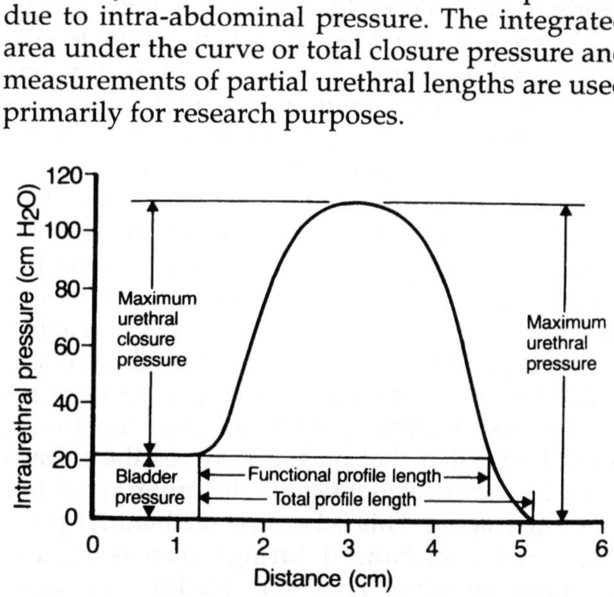


**Fig. 15.1.** Theoretical urethral closure pressure profile. Reprinted by permission of the author and Williams & Wilkins, Baltimore. From Ostergard, D.R., Bent, A.E. (Eds.) Urogynecology and Urodynamics: Theory and Practice, Third Edition, 1991

The actual measurement of these normal urethral closure pressure profiles in Fig. 15.2 involves the measurement of the EMG activity in the first line of the tracing, the measurement of intra-abdominal pressure (vaginal or rectal) in the second line of the tracing, the measurement of bladder pressure on the third line, intraurethral pressure on the fourth line of the tracing, true detrusor pressure (bladder pressure minus abdominal pressure) on the fifth line of the tracing and the urethral closure pressure (urethral pressure minus bladder pressure) on the sixth line of the tracing. These were all recorded simultaneously as the paper moved at a speed of 1 mm/s. During the measurement of urethral closure pressure profiles the withdrawal arm removing the pressure transducer catheter from the urethra is moving at a speed of 1 mm/s during resting profiles and 5 mm/s during augmented and Valsalva profiles. During these profiles the paper speed is also increased to 5 mm/s. Therefore along all tracings, each small box along the X-axis represents 1 mm or 1 s of elapsed time. Each small box along the Y-axis represents 5 $cmH_2O$ and each large box represents 25 $cmH_2O$.

Fig. 15.2 demonstrates the actual measurement of normal urethral closure pressure profiles in a postmenopausal woman in the sitting position. Resting or static profiles are measured a minimum of three times until a fairly consistent tracing is obtained. Measurement of these resting urethral closure pressure profiles demonstrate that this postmenopausal woman has a closure pressure of approximately 35 $cmH_2O$ with a functional length of 33 mm and a total length of 43 mm. The length to maximal pressure is approximately 18 mm and therefore the length from the maximal pressure to the urethral meatus is 25 mm. In between these three resting profiles the closure pressure is actually zero because the urethral pressure transducer is within the bladder and therefore actually measuring bladder pressure. The point where the pressure curve first starts to rise corresponds to the proximal urethra and the curve reaches maximal pressure in the mid urethra falling eventually to zero atmospheric pressure on the urethral pressure tracing at the urethral meatus. It should be noted that on these curves the intraurethral pressure is identical to the urethral closure pressure tracing. This is because the bladder pressure remains unchanged during the measurement of these profiles. Had the bladder pressure increased during the measurement of these tracings or had a bladder contraction occurred these two tracings would be different.

Augmenting profiles during rectal squeeze and urethral squeeze are measured at speeds of 5 mm/s as the patient is asked to squeeze the rectum tightly closed and then to squeeze the muscles around the urethra tightly closed as if she were trying to prevent the passage of flatus or the passage of urine respectively. Both accomplish the same thing in asking the patient voluntarily to contract the levator muscles. The normal expected response includes an elevation of closure pressure and an increase in functional length. Absence of this augmentation may signal partial denervation of these muscles or rigidity of the urethral wall which does not allow an increase in intraurethral pressure from outside forces. However, these augmenting profiles are difficult to obtain and reproduce reliably. When these profiles are performed properly we note that there is an increase in the EMG activity while the patient is asked to squeeze the muscles around the rectum and squeeze the muscles around the urethra. This is properly accomplished with no increase in intra-abdominal pressure. However, in these profiles there is also no augmentation. That means that there is no significant increase in closure pressure nor functional length during augmenting maneuvers.

The next tracing is a Valsalva urethral closure pressure profile. This is obtained while the patient is asked to bear down as it she were trying to move her bowels. It is accompanied by an increase in EMG activity as well as an increase in intra-abdominal pressure. Here we see little change in closure pressure and functional length suggesting equal transmission of pressure to the urethra and bladder and no evidence of genuine stress incontinence.

The final urethral closure pressure profile is the cough profile which is performed during repetitive coughing. Here the patient is asked to cough repetitively approximately every two to three seconds while the pressure transducer is withdrawn at a rate of 1 mm/s through the urethra. With each cough an assessment can be made of pressure transmission to the urethra. Positive spikes on the urethral closure pressure tracing indicate positive pressure transmission greater than 100% (Chapter 23). This patient is noted to have positive urethral closure pressure transmission throughout most of the mid urethra. Negative pressure transmission and pressure equalization (closure pressure $\leq 0$ with each cough) are not seen here but would signal the presence of genuine stress incontinence.

Urethral closure pressure profiles both in the static and dynamic states, when carefully

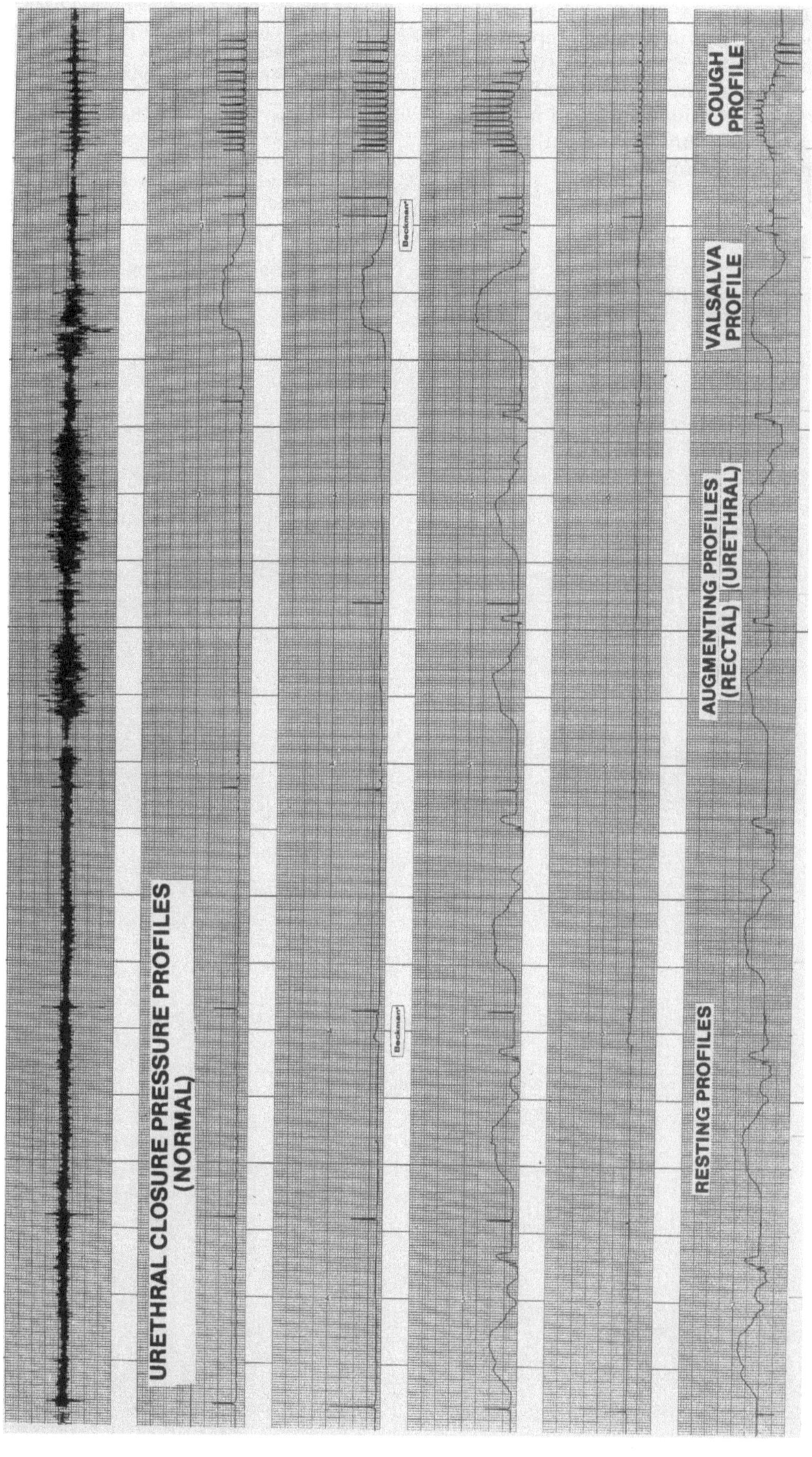


**Fig. 15.2.** Normal urethral closure pressure profiles in a postmenopausal woman.

performed, can provide a great deal of useful information. Their clinical usefulness, reproduceability and reliability are frequently questioned in the literature. However, in clinical practice we have found them to be quite useful and informative in understanding the underlying pathophysiology of genuine stress incontinence.

## Bibliography

Constantinou CE: Resting and stress urethral pressures as a clinical guide to the mechanism of continence in the female patient. Urol Clin North Am 12:247, 1985.

Hilton P, Stanton SL: Urethral pressure measurement by microtransducer: the results in symptom-free women and in those with genuine stress incontinence. Br J Obstet Gynaecol 90:919, 1983.

Sand PK, Bowen LW, Panganiban R et al: The low pressure urethra as a factor in failed retropubic urethropexy. Obstet Gynecol 69:399, 1987.

Versi E, Cardozo L. Studd J et al: Evaluation of urethral pressure profilometry for the diagnosis of genuine stress incontinence. World J Urol 4:6, 1986.

Weil A. Reyes H, Bischof P et al: Clinical relevance of urethral stress profile using microtransducers after surgery for stress incontinence in females. Urol Int 38:363, 1983.

Chapter 16

# Augmenting Urethral Closure Pressure Profiles

Augmenting urethral closure pressure profiles are used to identify the voluntary ability of the patient to contract her periurethral and pelvic striated musculature around the urethra to effect an increase in intraurethral pressure. This effort is identical to that of progressive resistance exercise or Kegel's maneuver and represents the urodynamic measure of this activity. In the prior chapter in Figure 15.2 we noted that the patient was not able to augment her urethral closure pressure nor functional length by contracting the pelvic floor. The absence of an increase in closure pressure and functional length during these profiles may represent a failure of the patient to understand the maneuver, partial or total denervation of the pelvic skeletal muscles, or a rigid fibrotic urethra which cannot respond to extrinsic efforts to increase intraurethral pressure. Usually the lack of augmentation represents the patient's inability to understand and perform the maneuver properly. Frequently patients will Valsalva or lift their body cephalad in relation to the urethral pressure catheter.

Fig. 16.1 demonstrates the measurement of augmenting urethral closure pressure profiles in relationship to a resting profile. At rest this patient has a urethral closure pressure of 77 $cmH_2O$ and a functional length of 33 mm. With squeezing of the rectal muscles the maximal urethral closure pressure increases to 113 $cmH_2O$. The functional length also increases to 36 mm. Similarly with the patient squeezing the muscles around the urethra to try to prevent urinary leakage there is augmentation of the urethral closure pressure to 118 $cmH_2O$ and an increase in functional length to 40 mm. The artifact noted on the tracing is a subtraction artifact where increases in intra-abdominal pressure are not registered as completely on the vaginal pressure transducer as they are on the bladder transducer. This leads to an increase in true detrusor pressure with any increase in intra-abdominal pressure such as coughing and Valsalva. These augmenting profiles, although interesting in some patients, are very difficult to perform without relative movement of the catheter, Valsalva or other artifact. They have not been found to have any prognostic value for women undergoing surgery and are rarely used by most centers.

## Bibliography

Sand PK, Bowen LW, Ostergard DR: The prognostic significance of augmentation of urethral closure pressure and functional length. Int J Gynecol Obstet 33:135, 1990.

Tanagho EA, Stoller ML: Urodynamics: cystometry and urethral closure pressure profile. In Ostergard DR, Bent AE (eds) Urogynecology and urodynamics, 3rd edn. Baltimore, Williams & Wilkins, 1991, pp. 122–142.

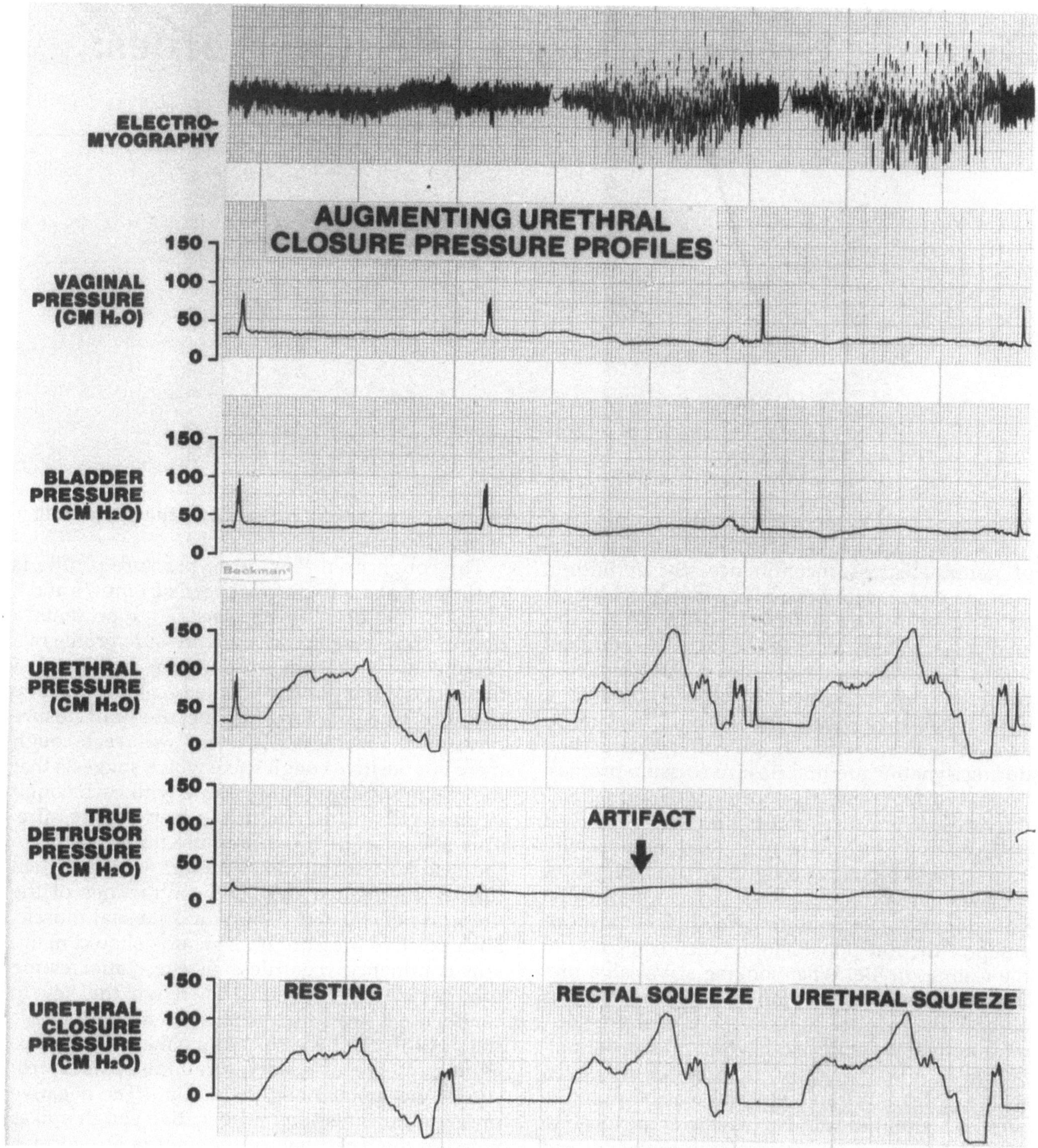


**Fig. 16.1.** Augmenting urethral closure pressure profiles.

Chapter 17

# Dynamic Urethral Closure Pressure Profiles: Valsalva and Cough Profiles

Dynamic urethral closure pressure profiles are useful tests in the establishment of the diagnosis of genuine stress incontinence. By definition, genuine stress incontinence is a condition where an increase in intra-abdominal pressure leads to an increase in bladder pressure that is greater than urethral pressure in the absence of a bladder contraction. This condition is represented by a dynamic change in urethral closure pressure to zero or below known as pressure equalization during dynamic urethral closure pressure profiles.

Fig. 17.1 represents the recording of normal urethral closure pressure profiles first at rest and then with augmenting maneuvers and finally with Valsalva and repetitive coughing. These pressures measured in a postmenopausal woman show equal pressure transmission during Valsalva but a shortening of the functional length when compared to the resting profile. When looking at Valsalva urethral closure pressure profiles, it is important to observe the increase in intra-abdominal pressure, intraurethral pressure and bladder pressure simultaneously. A poor Valsalva effort may be associated with a normal Valsalva urethral closure pressure profile. A stronger Valsalva maneuver may lead to further descent of the urethrovesical junction and negative pressure transmission associated with urinary loss. Therefore it is important when doing these profiles to ask for a maximal Valsalva effort. If one is suspicious that there is a poor Valsalva maneuver, then the profile should be repeated. As mentioned previously, this profile is obtained with a catheter withdrawal speed of 5 mm/s as the chart speed is also increased to 5 mm/s in an analog system. Computerized systems will rectify recorder speed to correspond to the profilometer speed automatically.

The cough urethral closure pressure profile is performed at a withdrawal speed of 1 mm/s and a paper speed of 1 mm/s. Fig 17.1 represents a normal cough urethral closure pressure profile in a postmenopausal woman. Along the first 2 cm of the urethra, the patient is noted to have positive pressure transmission. On the urethral closure pressure channel it is noted that with each cough there is a positive cough spike which suggests that the rise in intraurethral pressure with each cough is greater than the rise in the bladder pressure. This results from equal pressure transmission to the bladder and proximal urethra which is then further augmented by reflex contractions of the urethral skeletal and periurethral skeletal muscle. Such positive pressure transmission should maintain continence regardless of the static resting urethral closure pressure. Therefore the key to continence is pressure transmission in the dynamic state. All that is necessary to maintain continence is the presence of positive urethral closure pressure at any point along the urethra. The negative pressure transmission and negative cough spikes noted in the distal half of the urethra are normal. The distal half of the urethra lies below the genital hiatus and therefore is not well augmented by increases in intra-abdominal pressure.

Fig. 17.2 demonstrates abnormal dynamic urethral closure pressure profiles during Valsalva and coughing. In the first profile done during Valsalva, in the supine position with a relatively empty bladder, there is a positive closure pressure of 9 $cmH_2O$ associated with a functional length of

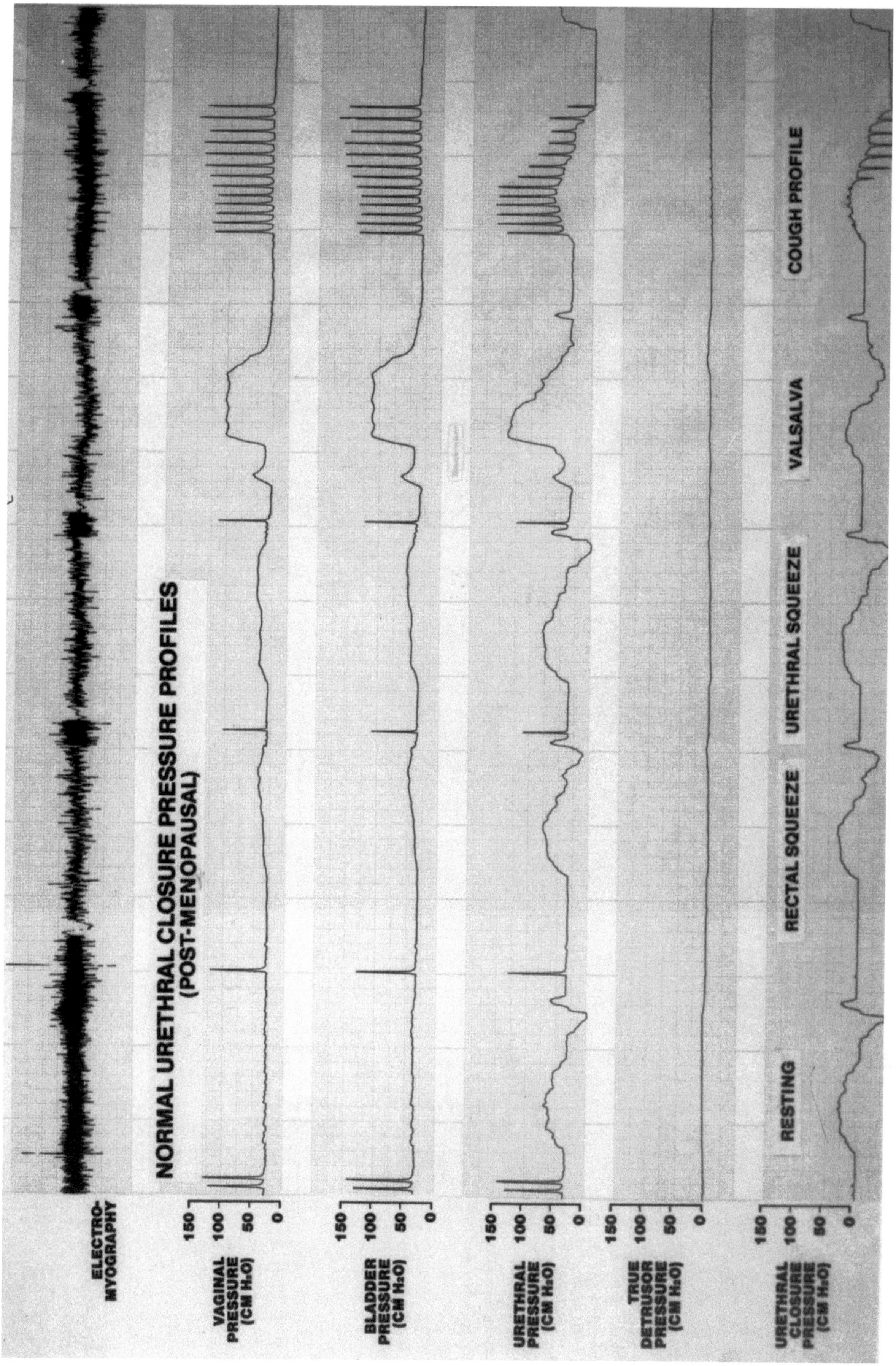


**Fig. 17.1.** Normal urethral closure pressure profiles demonstrating dynamic and augmenting changes.

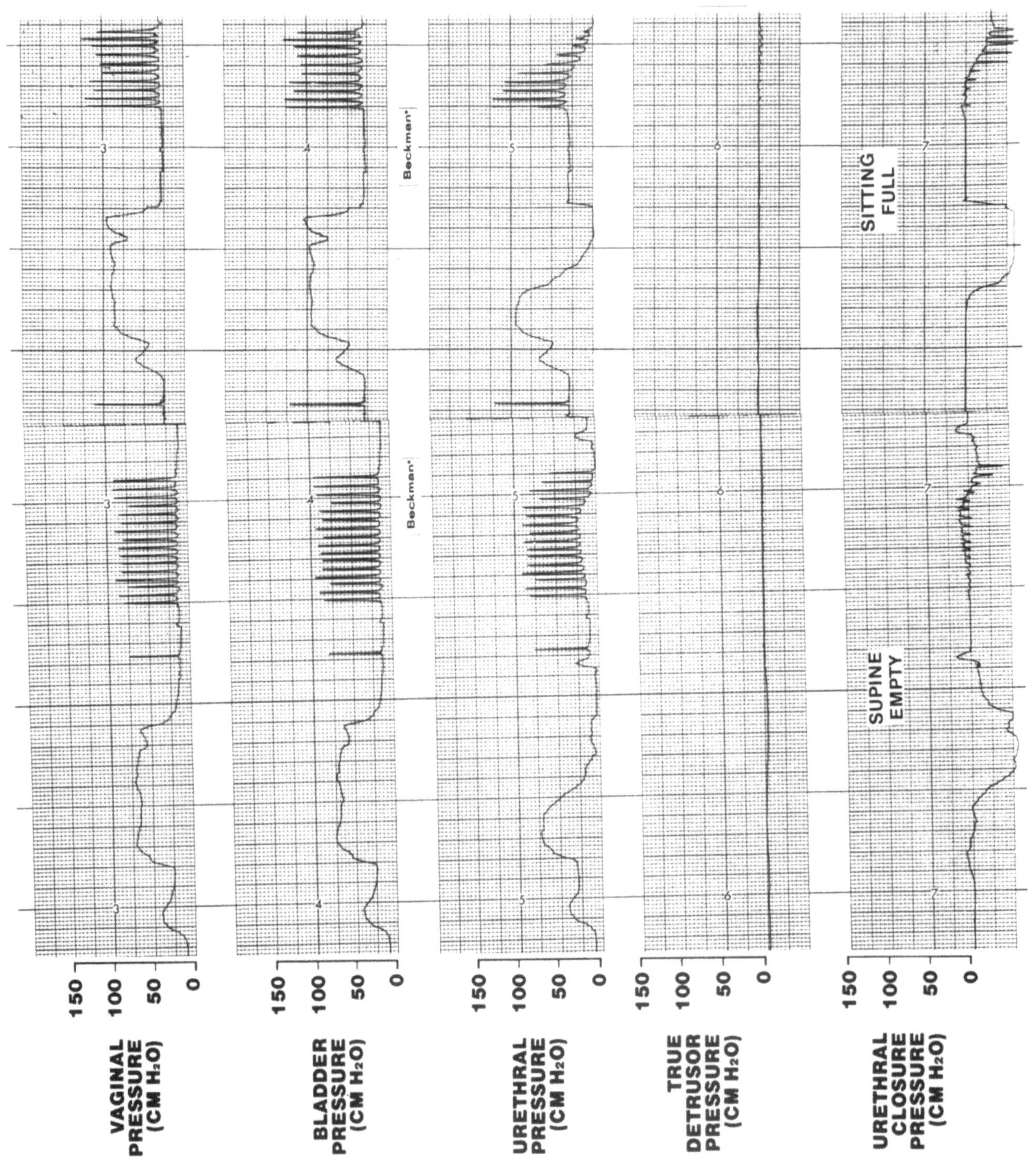


**Fig. 17.2.** Valsalva and cough urethral closure pressure profiles demonstrating urinary incontinence with pressure equalization.

12 mm. However, the repeat profile, done sitting upright with a full bladder at maximum cystometric capacity, shows absolutely no measurable closure pressure nor functional length. This is associated with urinary incontinence throughout the entire Valsalva urethral closure pressure profile. Similarly, the cough profiles are positive in both the supine empty and supine full position. We notice that along the entire length of the urethra there is negative pressure transmission with the cough spikes going negatively to the zero closure pressure line or below. Therefore with each cough there is negative pressure transmission and a negative closure pressure is reached along the entire length of the urethra. Urine is lost with each cough. This pressure equalization is the hallmark of genuine stress incontinence. It is important to notice that half the Valsalva profiles have been done in the supine position. With a relatively empty bladder, the diagnosis of genuine stress incontinence could have theoretically been missed. However, when the patient is studied in a sitting upright position at maximum cystometric capacity, the diagnosis of genuine stress incontinence due to pressure equalization is unmistakable. Secondarily, throughout these pressure profiles, the true detrusor pressure remains unchanged. Therefore we cannot blame the urine loss on any rise in detrusor pressure, thus establishing conclusively the diagnosis of genuine stress incontinence.

# Bibliography

Hilton P: The urethral pressure profile under stress: a comparison of profiles on coughing and straining. Neurourol Urodynam 2:55, 1983.

Richardson DA: Value of the cough pressure profile in the evaluation of patients with stress incontinence. Am J Obstet Gynecol 155:808, 1986.

Thind P, Lose G, Jorgensen L et al: Urethral pressure increment preceding and following bladder pressure elevation during stress episodes in healthy and stress incontinent women. Neurourol Urodyn 10:177, 1991.

# Chapter 18
# Urethral Responses to Position Changes

Urethral closure pressure will be affected by position changes in both the normal, continent woman and the woman suffering from genuine stress incontinence. Typically, as shown in Fig. 18.1, the continent woman will respond to the increasing stress of a more upright position by increasing skeletal muscle activity within the wall of the urethra as well as within the pelvic floor musculature to lead to an increase in urethral closure pressure. In Fig. 18.1, this is demonstrated by an increased urethral pressure and urethral closure pressure in the sitting position when compared to the supine position. This recruitment of skeletal muscle is a normal compensating response reflected in the periurethral EMG activity.

This increasing stress of movement to a more upright position will be met with an increase in skeletal muscle activity and urethral pressure in the normal continent patient, but will lead to decompensation of urethral pressure in the genuine stress incontinent woman who is unable to augment closure pressure in response to increasing stress. Because of the relative changes in urethral pressure in different positions, it is important to standardize the position of the patient during the measurement of urethral closure pressure profiles.

In this figure the patient is noted to have a urethral closure pressure averaging about 50 $cmH_2O$ in the supine position and a functional length of 34 mm. When she moves to the sitting position the urethral closure pressure increases to about 73 $cmH_2O$ with a functional length of about 32 mm. Surface EMG changes do not clearly increase in this example as we would ordinarily see with recruitment of skeletal muscle activity to compensate for the "stress" of a more upright position.

## Bibliography

Cadogan M, Awad S, Field C et al: A comparison of the cough and standing urethral pressure profile in the diagnosis of stress incontinence. Neurourol Urodynam 7:327, 1988.

Henrikson L. Ulmsten U, Anderson KE: The effect of changes of posture on the urethral closure pressure in stress-incontinent women. Scand J Urol Nephrol 11:207, 1977.

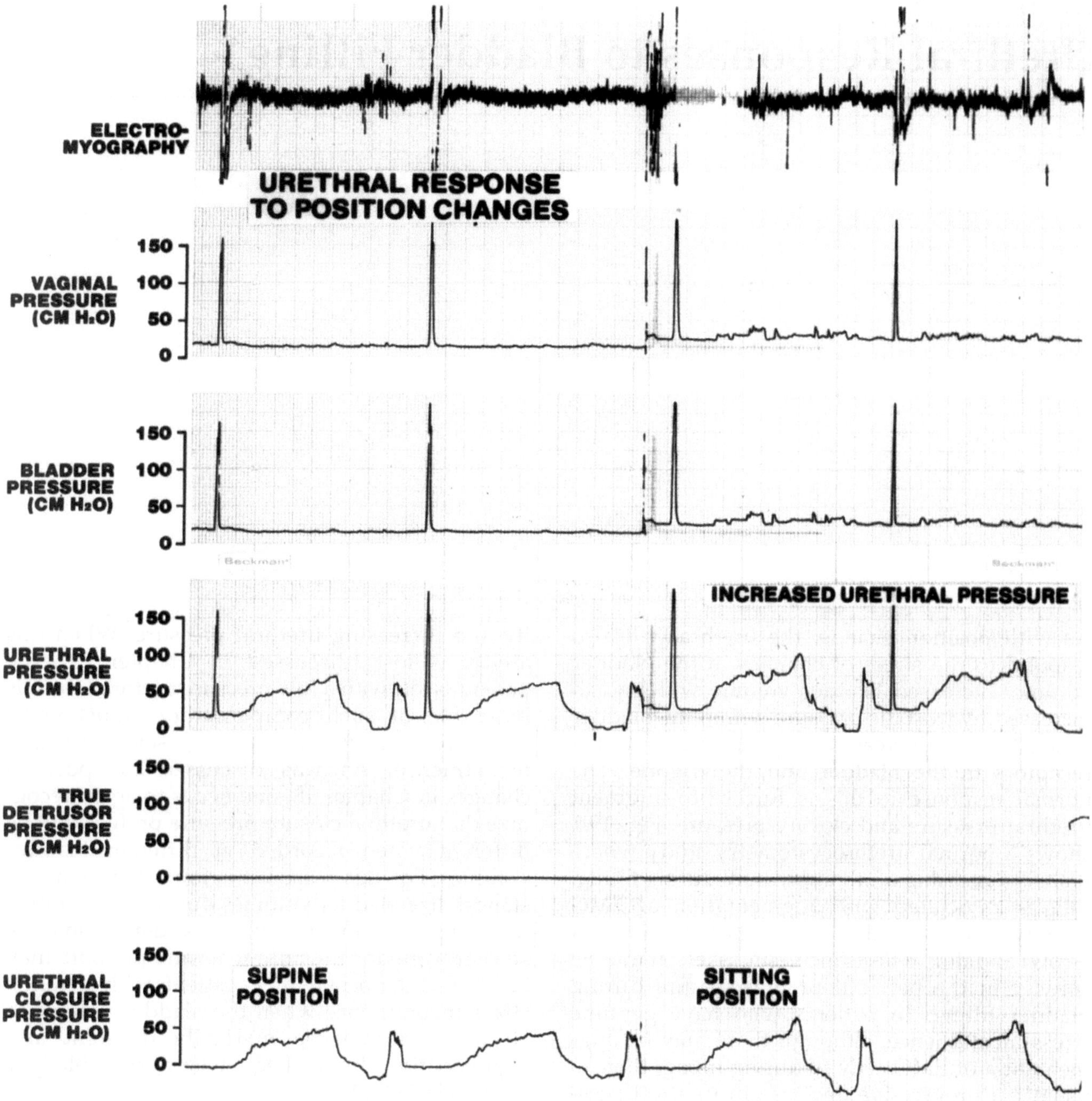


**Fig. 18.1.** Urethral responses to position changes.

# Chapter 19
# Urethral Responses to Bladder Filling

As with position change, the urethra will also respond to the stress of changes in the bladder volume. Increased bladder volume will lead to increased hydrostatic pressure within the bladder as well as an increased response from stretch receptors in the bladder and the trigone. The normal response to this is further to augment urethral pressure and closure pressure. Fig. 19.1 shows a normal urethrocystometry study where there is increasing urethral pressure during filling. This is associated with augmentation of EMG activity near the end of the study (curved open arrow) and thus reflects increasing skeletal muscle activity in the pelvic floor musculature during bladder filling. In patients who have genuine stress incontinence, although there may be augmentation of EMG activity during filling, there is usually a progressive decrease in urethral pressure and urethral closure pressure which facilitates eventual urinary leakage with increased intra-abdominal pressure. It is this normal compensatory response of the voluntary striated muscle within the urethra and pelvic floor that helps to prevent urinary incontinence in young and middle-aged women who have urethral hypermobility. Many of these patients may have urethral hypermobility on Q-tip testing or bladder neck funneling on videocystourethrography but fail to leak urine because of their excellent urethral tone and skeletal muscle function. With increasing stress, the urethral musculature is able to respond by further augmenting muscular activity and increasing urethral pressure. When this ability is lost (discussed in Chapter 29), the patient is left with a low pressure urethra which is incapable of such compensatory adjustments. These patients frequently have severe urinary incontinence. As was discussed for position changes in Chapter 18, one needs to again recognize that urethral closure pressure profiles will be different when recorded at different bladder volumes. For this reason it is important either to standardize bladder volumes during comparative trials or to document at what bladder volume the studies were done. Urethral closure pressure may be perfectly normal in a patient with genuine stress incontinence when the bladder volume is 50 ml, but may be markedly different and significantly diminished when the bladder volume is 500 ml.

In addition to these normal findings, this urodynamic tracing shows some artifacts arising from rectal peristalsis as will be discussed in Chapter 44. Throughout the standing urethrocystometry study in Fig. 19.1 there is marked variation in the rectal pressure channel from intrinsic bowel activity rather than from increases in intra-abdominal pressure. This is apparent because these changes are not mirrored on the bladder pressure channel. Thus, the true detrusor pressure channel which represents the difference between bladder and rectal pressure reflects this peristalsis in artifactual pressure decreases especially in the latter half of the tracing. In addition, to compen-

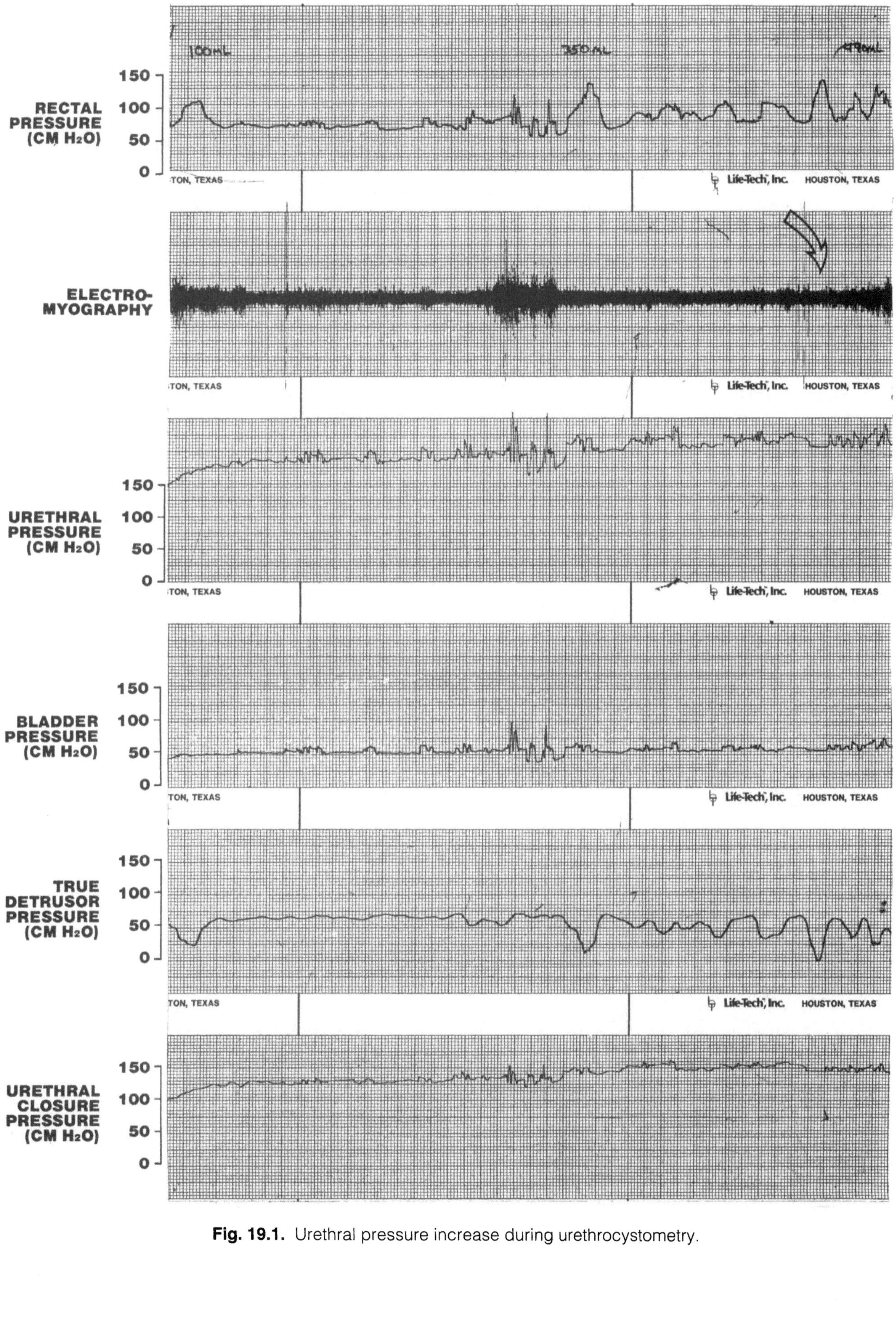


**Fig. 19.1.** Urethral pressure increase during urethrocystometry.

sate for the initially high peristaltic activity of the rectum, the true detrusor baseline pressure was initially set too high above its zero baseline leading to detrusor pressure measurements during the study of 65–70 $cmH_2O$; when the true detrusor pressure can actually only increase as much as the bladder pressure (5 $cmH_2O$).

# Bibliography

Tanagho EA, Stoller ML: Urodynamics: cystometry and urethral closure pressure profile. In Ostergard DR, Bent AE (eds): Urogynecology and Urodynamics, 3rd edn Baltimore, Williams & Wilkins, 1991, pp. 122–142.

# Chapter 20
# Multichannel Urethrocystometry

Multichannel urethrocystometry involves the measurement of abdominal pressure, urethral pressure, and bladder pressure during filling with or without the recording of electromyographic activity. The true detrusor pressure and urethral closure pressure may also be calculated and recorded. These multichannel studies allow us to better understand physiologic and pathophysiologic factors affecting the patient's ability to store urine. In some patients, the information obtained from multichannel studies may not add more than a simple single channel cystometry study, but in many patients it may be invaluable. The measurement of urethral pressure helps us to understand urethral compensatory responses to bladder filling during the storage phase, and may also help to elucidate urethral causes of urinary leakage, such as uninhibited urethral relaxation (Chapter 33), which will not be noted during simple measurement of bladder pressure with filling. Subtracted cystometry with the measurement of bladder pressure and abdominal pressure either through the vagina or rectum will allow the urodynamicist to avoid the false positive diagnosis of detrusor instability where an increase in bladder pressure might be assumed to represent an involuntary bladder contraction when it is merely a representation of increased intra-abdominal pressure. When the same pressure increase is seen on the abdominal pressure tracing, such as in Fig. 20.1 (arrow), this is not misconstrued as a bladder contraction, but instead correctly interpreted as increased intra-abdominal pressure. Measurement of the true detrusor pressure (bladder pressure minus abdominal pressure) allows us to recognize quickly that there is no evidence of an involuntary bladder contraction in this situation. In addition, urethrocystometry with small catheters enables us to avoid false negative studies when urinary leakage occurs in the absence of a rise in bladder pressure >15 $cmH_2O$. On multichannel urethrocystometry, even a small bladder contraction (<15 $cmH_2O$) can be identified to be significant enough to cause urinary leakage especially when it occurs in association with a significant reduction in urethral pressure. Numerous studies have shown that low pressure detrusor contractions can cause detrusor instability, and this has led to a recent change in the definition of detrusor instability by the International Continence Society (ICS) to reflect that any symptomatic involuntary detrusor contraction (not necessarily ≥15 $cmH_2O$) can be defined as an unstable detrusor contraction.

During a normal filling study, such as in Fig. 20.1, the patient is noted to have no increase in true detrusor pressure during the study despite increased intra-abdominal pressure and considerable variation in urethral pressure during bladder filling. The patient is also noted to have genuine stress incontinence on the tracing. If one merely looked at bladder pressure and observed for urinary leakage, then, at the end of the study where closure pressure is noted to drop to zero, we might assume that the patient had an involuntary bladder contraction to account for this leakage. However, because intra-abdominal pressure is also measured the investigator can see that this increase in bladder pressure is merely due to an increase in intra-abdominal pressure, thus resulting in genuine stress incontinence and urinary leakage. Multichannel urethrocystometric

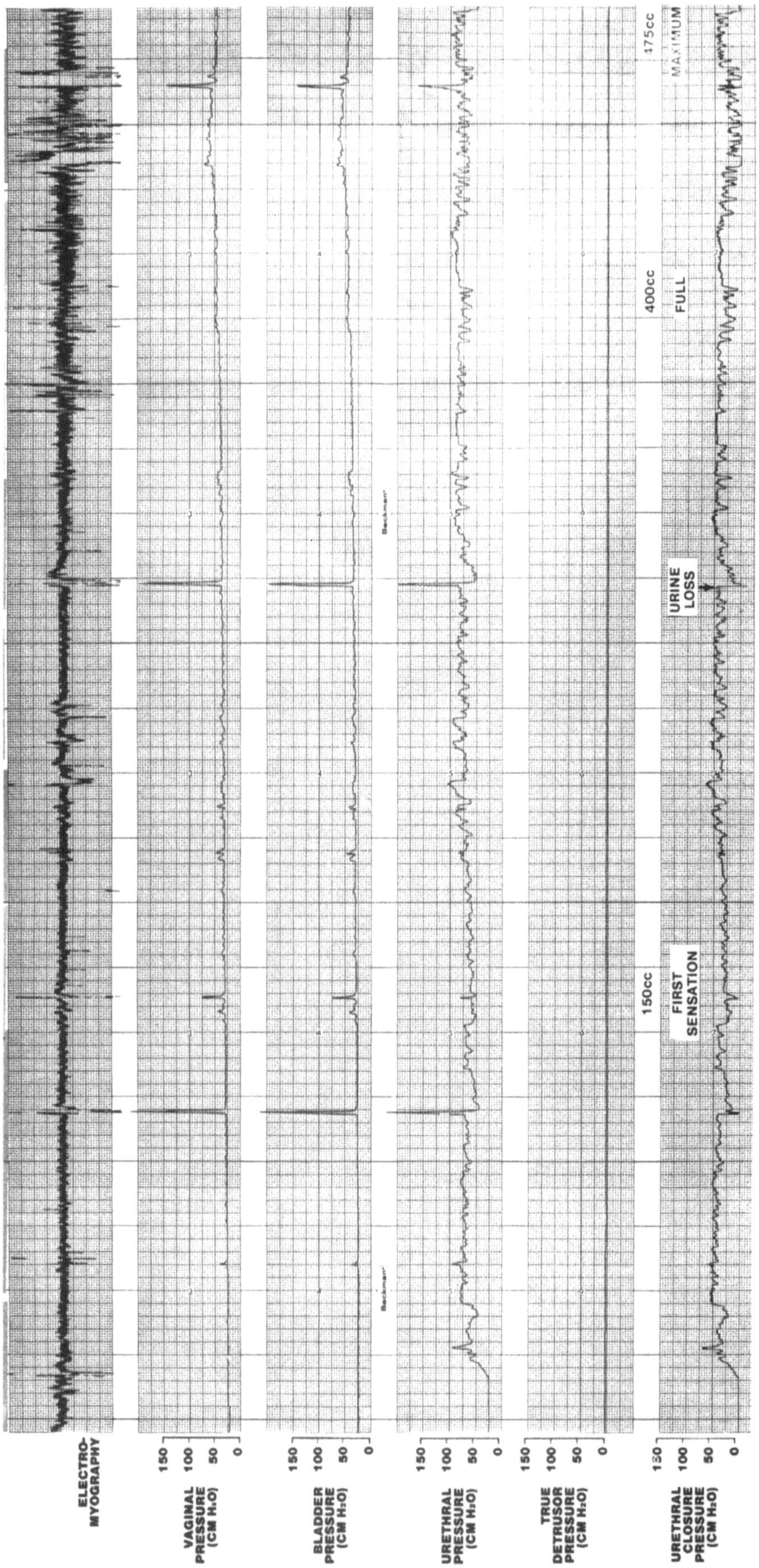


**Fig. 20.1.** Stable urethrocystometry study demonstrating genuine stress incontinence and urethral instability.

studies are perhaps our most valuable tool in diagnosing storage phase pathology. Patients noted to lose urine in the absence of involuntary bladder contractions usually have genuine stress incontinence whereas those who lose urine in response to involuntary detrusor contractions usually have detrusor instability or detrusor hyperreflexia. These studies, as will be seen in later chapters, also allow us to diagnose patients with other more unusual causes of urinary leakage such as low compliance bladders, uninhibited urethral relaxation, and overflow incontinence. Pharmacologic manipulation during bladder filling studies with multichannel urethrocystometry may also allow for expanded diagnostic and therapeutic conclusions. Performance of these studies on an ambulatory basis may dramatically extend their diagnostic sensitivity.

## Bibliography

Bhatia NN, Bradley WE, Haldeman S: Urodynamics: continuous monitoring. J Urol 128:963, 1982.

Coolsaet B: Bladder compliance and detrusor activity during the collection phase. Neurourol Urodynam 4:263, 1985.

Koonings PP, Bergman A: Urethral pressure changes in women with detrusor instability. Urology 37:540, 1991.

Wall LL: Diagnosis and management of urinary incontinence due to detrusor instability. Obstet Gynecol Surv Suppl 45:18, 1990.

# Chapter 21
# Voiding Pressure Studies

In much the same way that the urodynamacist can analyze storage phase defects by measuring urethral, abdominal and bladder pressure during bladder filling with multichannel urethrocystometry, one can use the same technique to analyze the emptying phase. Both normal micturition patterns and abnormal patterns such as detrusor sphincter dyssynergia (which will be discussed in Chapter 26) may be identified. In addition, analysis of voiding function will help to enable investigators to avoid postoperative voiding dysfunction as well as voiding dysfunction following non-surgical treatments of urinary incontinence.

The normal male voids by urethral relaxation followed within a few seconds by a detrusor contraction. Because the longitudinal muscle fibers of the detrusor continue on into the proximal urethra, contraction of the bladder results in elevation and opening of the urethrovesical junction. This normal activity is modulated by numerous reflex pathways which allow for the smooth initiation of voiding by urethral relaxation coordinated with a bladder contraction. These reflexes also allow for the normal cessation of voiding with termination of the detrusor contraction following contraction of the urethral and periurethral striated musculature. Although abnormal voiding in the male is almost always due to physical obstruction, this is rare in the female. Women, especially those with decreased urethral resistance may void normally on simple uroflowmetry studies by five different mechanisms including urethral relaxation alone, urethral relaxation with detrusor contraction, urethral relaxation with a detrusor contraction plus Valsalva, urethral relaxation and Valsalva in the absence of a detrusor contraction as well as Valsalva alone in women with markedly decreased urethral resistance. It is clear that women who void by either of the last two mechanisms might have voiding dysfunction following a surgery the purpose of which is to stop urinary leakage from increased intra-abdominal pressure. Thus, whereas these patients might be noted to void normally preoperatively they could have voiding dysfunction and retention postoperatively due to their attempted Valsalva voiding. If they are unable to change to another voiding pattern (urethral relaxation alone) they will either continue to suffer from voiding dysfunction or tear down their surgical repair. Accurate assessment of voiding function using voiding pressure studies with or without additional special tests, as will be discussed in Section V, allows for early diagnosis of potential problems.

Three different voiding patterns are shown here. All three patterns are fully capable of achieving normal uroflowmetric parameters. These studies are accomplished by placing the urethral pressure transducer in the mid urethra, approximately at the point of maximal urethral pressure while the bladder pressure transducer remains in the bladder and either a vaginal or rectal transducer catheter is used to assess intra-abdominal pressure. At the same time, a uroflowmeter is used to assess voiding velocity and surface, wire or needle electrodes may be used to measure EMG activity, especially where voiding dysfunction is anticipated. Perianal surface electrodes if not properly protected will become moist and produce poor tracings with electrical noise from the loss of contact with the skin. These may appear to be pathologic or uninterpretable.

Therefore, when using these, it is necessary to take great care to cover them and insulate them from urine dripping down over the perineum.

## 21.1 Detrusor Contraction and Urethral Relaxation

Fig. 21.1, shows, at the arrow, that urethral pressure drops from around 150 $cmH_2O$ to around 75 $cmH_2O$. Meanwhile the bladder pressure rises approximately 1 s after this initial urethral relaxation and urine flow begins approximately 5 s later. (Each large box along the $x$ axis on the tracing = 1 s.) Voiding by detrusor contraction and urethral relaxation as shown here is a very normal and efficient pattern which can result in very high flow rates. During this study, however, a maximum flow rate of only 15 ml/s is reached. As marked on this tracing, when the bladder emptied substantially, the end of the microtransducer catheter hit the bladder wall resulting in a marked increase in bladder and true detrusor pressure. As the catheter reorients and the bladder stops contracting the pressure is seen to go down gradually in the bladder. Bladder pressure decreases occur reflexively by vesicoinhibitory reflexes triggered by contraction of the urethral and pelvic floor musculature resulting in increased urethral pressure. If there were not this feedback from urethra to bladder, the bladder would continue to contract following cessation of voiding resulting in considerable discomfort. Although the maximum flow rate achieved during the study was borderline, it must be remembered that this study was done with a bladder volume of only 180 ml. The maximal flow rate would have been proportionally larger if a greater volume of fluid had been voided because flow rates are volume dependent. Because this patient voids normally by urethral relaxation associated with a detrusor contraction of considerable magnitude, concern regarding voiding dysfunction following surgery would be minimal in this patient. This would be in direct contrast to the patient who voids by Valsalva (Fig. 21.2).

## 21.2 Detrusor Contraction and Valsalva Voiding

The patient in Fig. 21.2 appears to initiate voiding by a small amount of urethral relaxation immediately followed by Valsalva and a detrusor contraction. One must be careful, because a similar pattern can be achieved by Valsalva voiding alone when the artifact of poor transmission of intra-abdominal pressure to the vagina or rectum compared to abdominal pressure transmission to the bladder, exists. In this study, however, careful observation reveals that the pattern of pressure increase on the bladder pressure tracing is different from that on the vaginal pressure tracing and therefore we are reassured that the bladder contraction registered on the true detrusor pressure channel is indeed real and not an artifact. Although initially, this patient relaxes her urethra there is reflex contraction of the skeletal muscle of the pelvic floor in response to her Valsalva effort. With funneling of the bladder neck, the urethral pressure transducer is now also reflecting bladder pressure because of the common cavity effect in the urethra created by bladder neck funneling. This patient voids by initial urethral relaxation followed by a detrusor contraction with Valsalva. Although the uroflow channel is not shown on this tracing, the patient was able to generate normal maximum flow rates without any evidence of urinary retention. Should this patient then undergo a retropubic urethropexy and persist in her attempts to Valsalva void she might incur some degree of voiding dysfunction. However, if she is able to stop these Valsalva efforts and merely void by urethral relaxation associated with the bladder contraction she should have no difficulty in voiding whatsoever. If her detrusor contraction were of very small magnitude, one might be concerned about retention due to an underactive detrusor following surgery with an inadequate bladder contraction of decreased magnitude or duration.

## 21.3 Detrusor Contraction and Urethral Relaxation with a Common Cavity

Fig. 21.3 also shows a voiding study done at the end of multichannel urethrocystometry where the patient initiates voiding by urethral relaxation followed 7 s later by a weak bladder contraction. It is difficult to tell in this tracing what is happening to urethral pressure, again because of a common cavity artifact. Both urethral pressure and bladder pressure channels are measuring the same bladder contraction. They also both reflect any increase in intra-abdominal pressure such as a short Valsalva effort. This tracing also demonstrates artifact in the electromyography channel

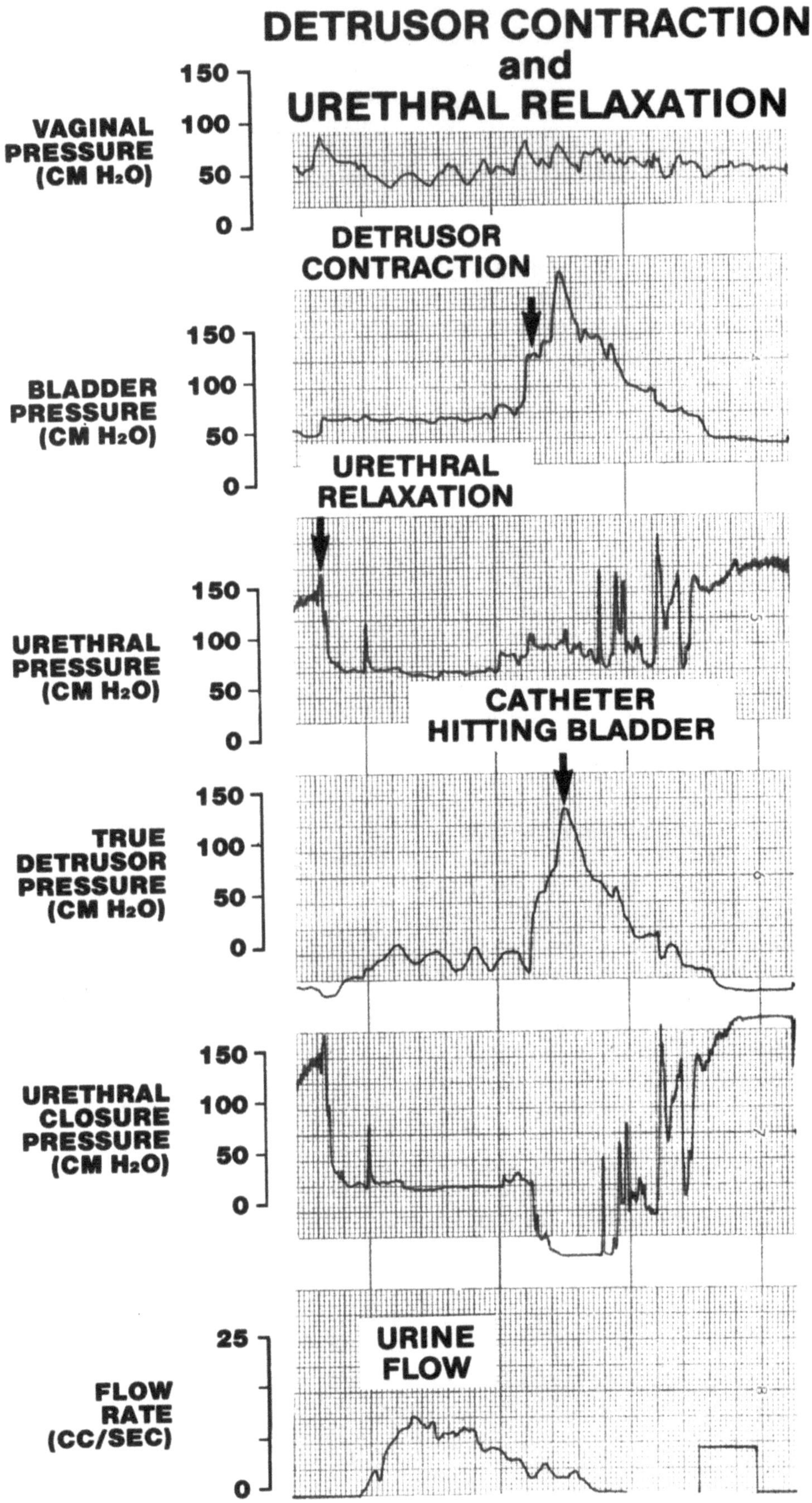


**Fig. 21.1.** Pressure voiding study demonstrating micturition by urethral relaxation with a detrusor contraction.

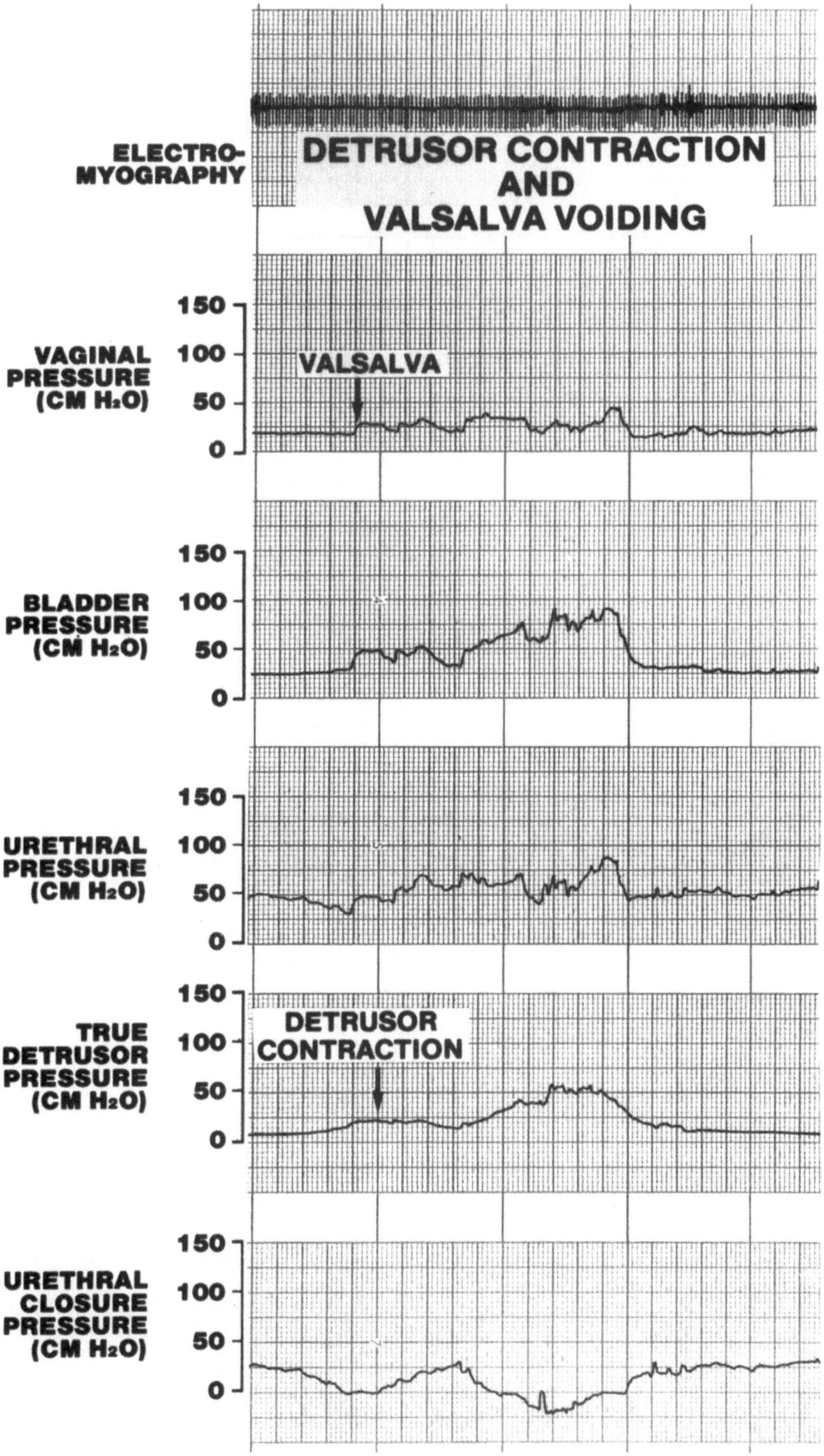


**Fig. 21.2.** Pressure voiding study demonstrating micturition by urethral relaxation with a detrusor contraction and Valsalva.

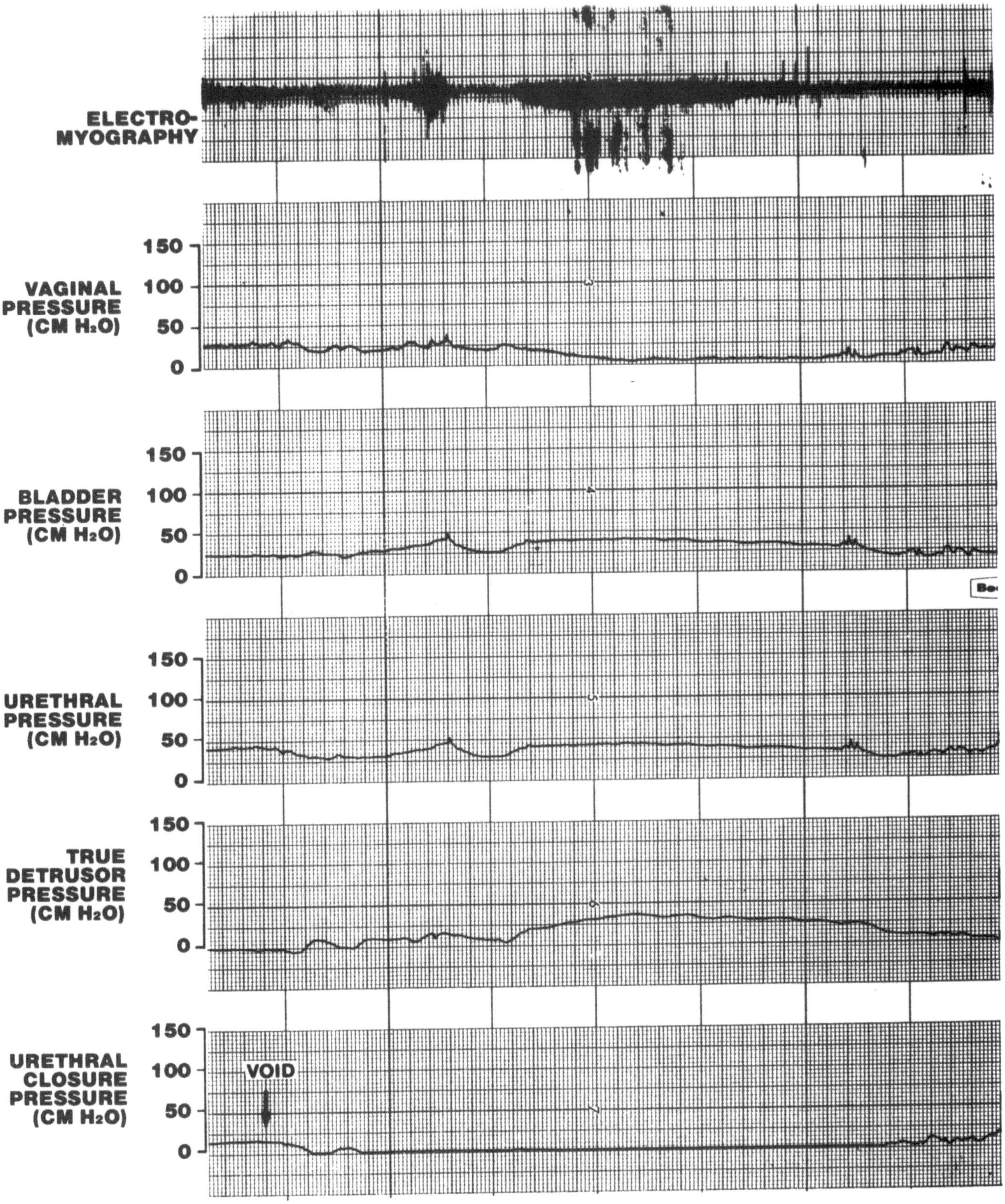


**Fig. 21.3.** Pressure voiding study demonstrating micturition by urethral relaxation with a detrusor contraction confounded by a common cavity effect.

when the perianal surface electrodes become wet. This may lead to a dramatic increase in activity suggesting the presence of detrusor sphincter dyssynergia when instead it is clear from the tracing that urethral closure pressure remains at 0 $cmH_2O$ or below and voiding continues uninterrupted. Such artifact may be avoided by better protection of these superficial electrodes with tape or an occlusive dressing or by the use of periurethral wires or needles.

## Bibliography

Bhatia NN, Bergman A: Use of preoperative uroflowmetry and simultaneous urethrocystometry for predicting risk of prolonged postoperative bladder drainage. J Urol 28:440, 1986.

Lose G, Jorgensen L, Mattensen SO et al: Voiding difficulties after colposuspension. Obstet Gynecol 69:33, 1987.

Mahoney DT, Lafert RO, Blais DJ: Integral storage and voiding reflexes. Urology 9:95, 1977.

Rud T, Ulmsten U, Anderson KE: Initiation of voiding in healthy women and in those with stress incontinence. Acta Obstet Gynecol Scand 57:457, 1978.

Rud T, Ulmsten U, Westby M: Initiation of micturition: a study of combined urethrocystometry and urethrocystography in healthy and stress incontinent females. Scand J Urol Nephrol 13:259, 1979.

Sjoberg B, Nyman CR: Hydrodynamics of micturition in healthy females: pressure and flow at different micturition volumes. Urol Int 36:23, 1981.

Sjoberg B, Nyman CR: Hydrodynamics of micturition in stress-incontinent women. Scand J Urol Nephrol 16:1, 1984.

Section IV

# Multichannel Urodynamics: Pathologic Studies

# Chapter 22
# Genuine Stress Incontinence

## 22.1 Cough Urethral Closure Pressure Profiles

Urodynamic studies are necessary by definition to establish the diagnosis of genuine stress incontinence with certainty. The classical study performed for this purpose is the cough urethral closure pressure profile. This study is performed by asking the patient to cough at one second intervals with a maximum effort while withdrawing the pressure recording catheter through the urethra at a continuous rate, equal to the paper or recorder speed (i.e. 1 mm/s). While the profile is in progress the true detrusor pressure channel is constantly monitored to detect any increase in detrusor pressure due to a bladder contraction. In addition, the synchrony of urine loss with the individual coughs is noted on the tracing. To optimize sensitivity it is most advantageous to perform this test in an upright position at maximum cystometric capacity. However, standing profiles are difficult to perform and often lead to the early breakdown of profilometers due to water damage. It is for this reason that sitting profiles at maximum capacity are usually utilized. When it is established that urine loss occurs in synchrony with individual cough efforts in the absence of detrusor contractions the diagnosis of genuine stress incontinence is established with certainty. A major confounding variable is the patient with a functionless urethra and Type III stress incontinence that will not respond with any significant intrinsic pressure increase during voluntary effort. This diagnosis can be established with certainty through either urethroscopic visualization of a tubularized, immobile drainpipe urethra or radiographic imaging of an open bladder neck at rest. This urethra demonstrates all the clinical and urodynamic criteria necessary for the diagnosis of genuine stress incontinence and is accompanied by no urethral hypermobility on Q-tip testing. This functionless urethra will not respond well to standard medical or surgical anti-incontinence therapy (Chapter 53).

This urodynamic tracing (Fig. 22.1) shows three different profiles varying with the bladder volume and position of the patient: supine position with an empty bladder (150 ml), sitting with an empty bladder (150 ml), and sitting with a subjectively full bladder (maximum cystometric capacity). The electromyographic recording demonstrates reflex pelvic floor contraction with each cough as normally seen. The magnitude of the pressure generated by each cough is visible in the vaginal, bladder, and urethral pressure channels and in this example approximates 150–200 $cmH_2O$ consistently. The true detrusor pressure channel remains flat throughout the tracing indicating the absence of detrusor contractions in response to the continuous coughing. In the urethral closure pressure channel characteristic pressure equalization is seen with each cough demonstrating equalization of pressure between the urethra and the bladder. Although actual urine flow rates are not shown on this tracing, the small deflections made by the manually operated event marker at the very bottom of the tracing indicate each time urine was seen to exit from the urethra during the cough pressure profile. It is important to be sure the urine is exiting from the urethra and not from the vagina as would be expected in the case of a

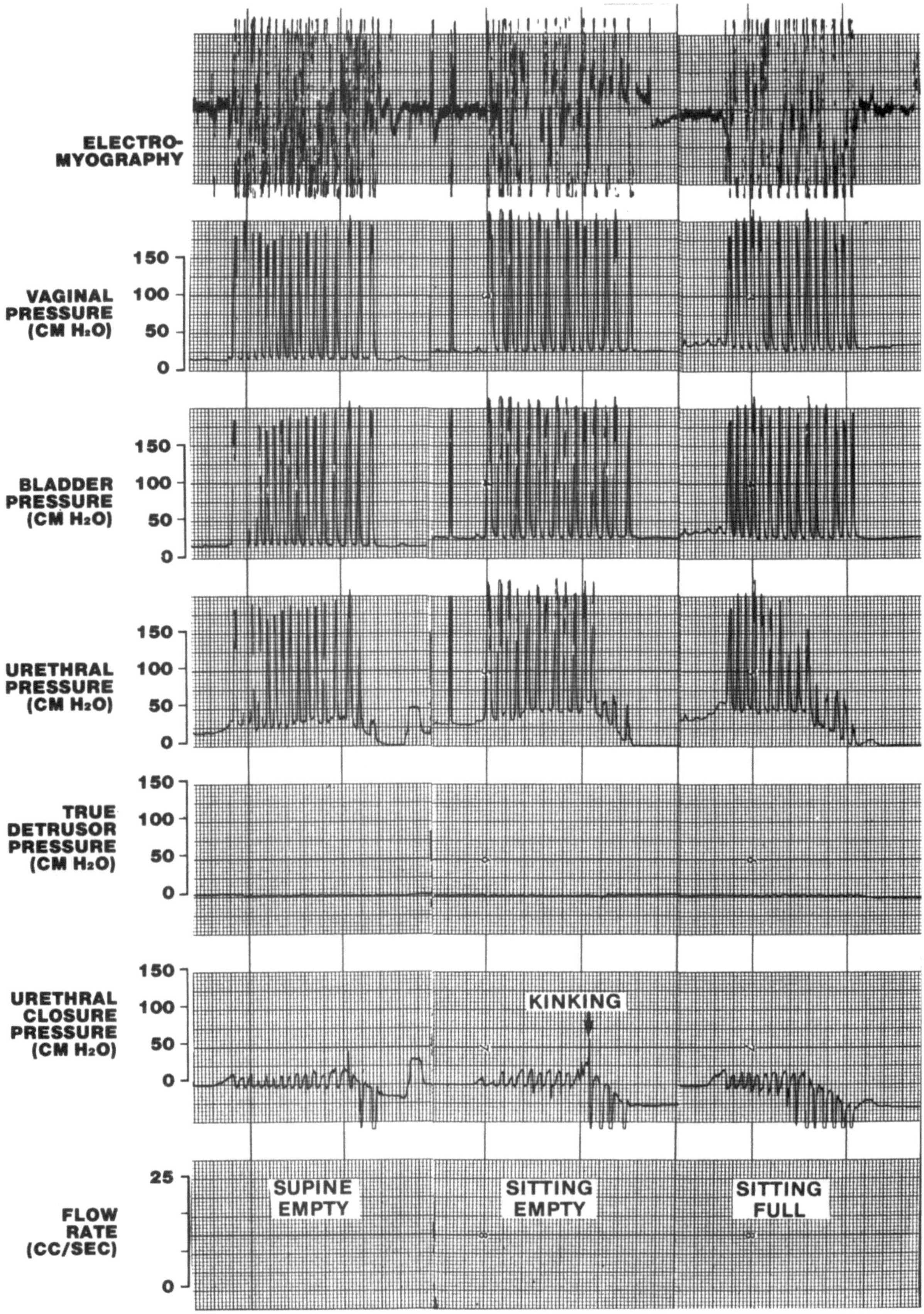


**Fig. 22.1.** Cough urethral closure pressure profiles in a woman with genuine stress incontinence (supine empty/sitting empty/sitting full).

urethrovaginal or vesicovaginal fistula. The tracing also demonstrates an example of a momentary kinking effect in the urethra as evidenced by a small area of positive pressure deflection in the cough pressure profile curve (arrow) associated with a single episode of positive pressure transmission (Chapter 23) in the sitting empty profile. Kinking is also seen in the supine empty profile. This was a momentary event that was repeated only once during the study and is of no significance in the establishment of the diagnosis of genuine stress incontinence but is one type of artifact that may compromise these studies. This study establishes the diagnosis of genuine stress incontinence as evidenced by the absence of detrusor contractions during continuous coughing associated with pressure equalization and synchronous urine loss.

## 22.2 Valsalva Urethral Closure Pressure Profiles

Valsalva pressure profiles are an adjunctive test in the establishment of the diagnosis of genuine stress incontinence. The test is also performed in varying positions with different bladder volumes. The patient is asked to strain with maximal effort while a pressure profile is obtained in the usual manner except that the withdrawal rate is accelerated as is the speed of the chart paper or urodynamic recorder (5 mm/s). The equalization of the paper and withdrawal speeds facilitates the measurement of profile parameters when indicated. This profile is usually used in a qualitative sense to compare detrusor activity during the profile with pressure equalization during a maximal straining effort. Fig. 22.2 demonstrates Valsalva profiles in the supine position with an empty bladder (150 ml) and in the sitting position with a subjectively full bladder (maximum cystometric capacity). Cough profiles are also shown which are characteristic of genuine stress incontinence with negative pressure transmission and pressure equalization with simultaneous urine loss. In the supine empty profile positive pressure remains under the curve (closed arrow) and urine is not lost. In the sitting full profile pressure equalization is found (open arrow) and is associated with coincident urine loss. This occurs in the absence of detrusor activity as indicated by the flat true detrusor pressure curve. The pressure equalization in the Valsalva sitting full profile, in the objective absence of detrusor contractions, further substantiates the diagnosis of genuine stress incontinence.

## Bibliography


Cadogan M, Awad S, Field C et al: A comparison of the cough and standing urethral pressure profile in the diagnosis of stress incontinence. Neurourol Urodynam 7:327, 1988.

Hilton P: The urethral pressure profile under stress: a comparison of profiles on coughing and straining. Neurourol Urodynam 2:55, 1983.

Richardson DA: Value of the cough pressure profile in the evaluation of patients with stress incontinence. Am J Obstet Gynecol 155:808; 1986.

Constantinou CE: Resting and stress urethral pressures as a clinical guide to the mechanism of continence in the female patient. Urol Clin North Am 12:247, 1985.

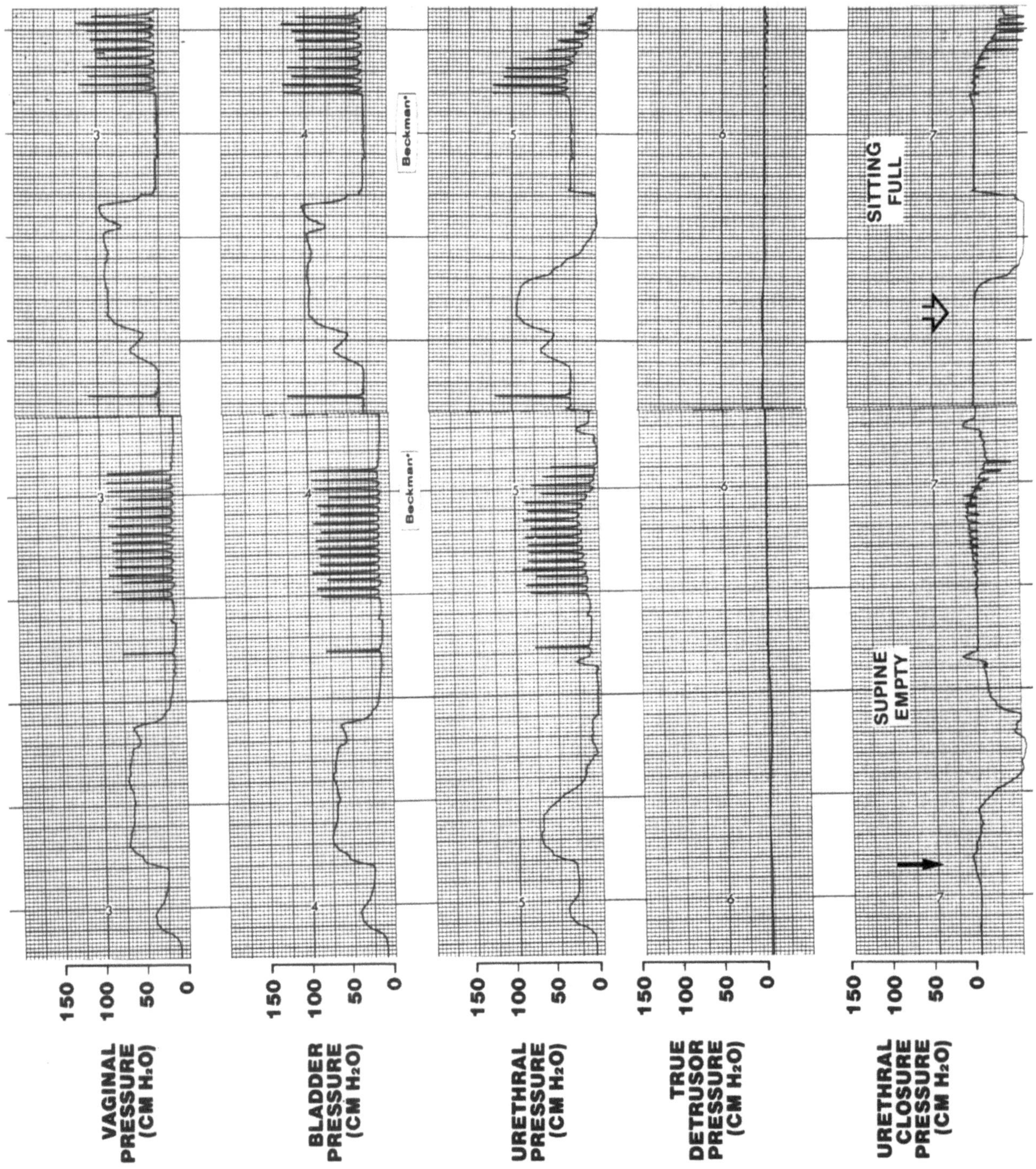


**Fig. 22.2.** Valsalva and cough urethral closure pressure profiles in a woman with genuine stress incontinence (supine empty/sitting full).

# Chapter 23
# Pressure Transmission Ratios

Pressure transmission ratios are designed to study objectively the relative transmission of pressure to the bladder and the urethra during stress. Characteristically the stress is continuous coughing during the measurement of the cough urethral closure pressure profile. The magnitude of the pressure transmitted to these two organs is determined in Fig. 23.1 by measuring the amount of pressure transmitted to the bladder (b) in a particular cough compared to that transmitted to a particular part of the urethra (u) during withdrawal of the urethral pressure transducer catheter. The pressure transmitted is measured as the bladder pressure increment and the urethral pressure increment above the urethral pressure profile curve caused by withdrawal of the urethral pressure transducer through the urethra during repetitive coughing. The ratio of these pressures is then calculated and multiplied by 100% ($u/b \times 100\%$) and termed the pressure transmission ratio. Inadequate transmission of intra-abdominal pressure to the urethra compared to that transmitted to the bladder is felt to be the primary pathologic process in genuine stress incontinence. Single or multiple sites for the measurement of pressure transmission ratios may be chosen. Positive pressure transmission is the hallmark of continence, whereas negative pressure transmission (characteristically expressed as a percentage less than 100%) is indicative of failure of the extrinsic continence mechanism and associated with genuine stress incontinence unless the intrinsic continence mechanism represented by the resting closure pressure is able to compensate for this negative pressure gradient. In the example in Fig. 23.2 both Valsalva and cough pressure profiles are illustrated. The Valsalva pressure profile on the left indicates the lack of pressure equalization and maintenance of positive pressure during a maximal straining effort. The cough pressure profile demonstrates positive pressure transmission as indicated by the small positive pressure spikes over the surface of the basic urethral closure pressure profile. The area under the curve of the pressure profile is referred to as "margin to leakage" since this is the pressure which must be overcome to cause pressure equalization and

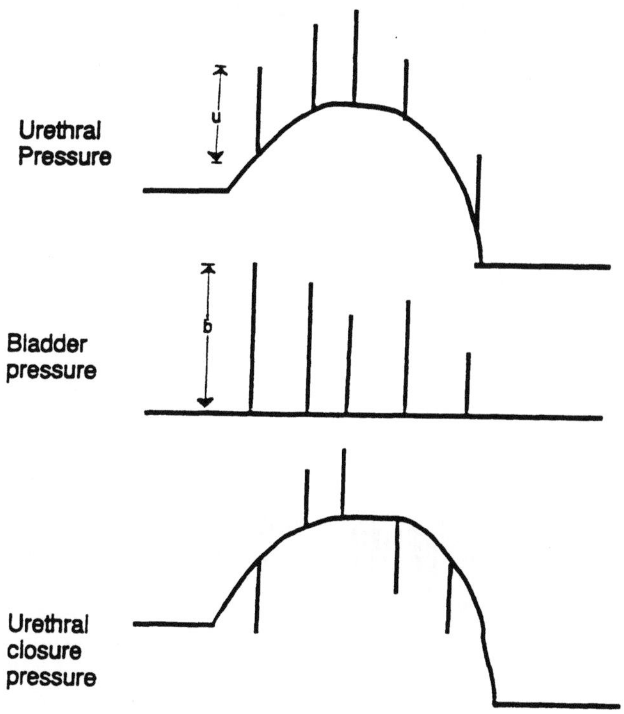


**Fig. 23.1.** Calculation of pressure transmission ratios during cough urethral closure pressure profiles.

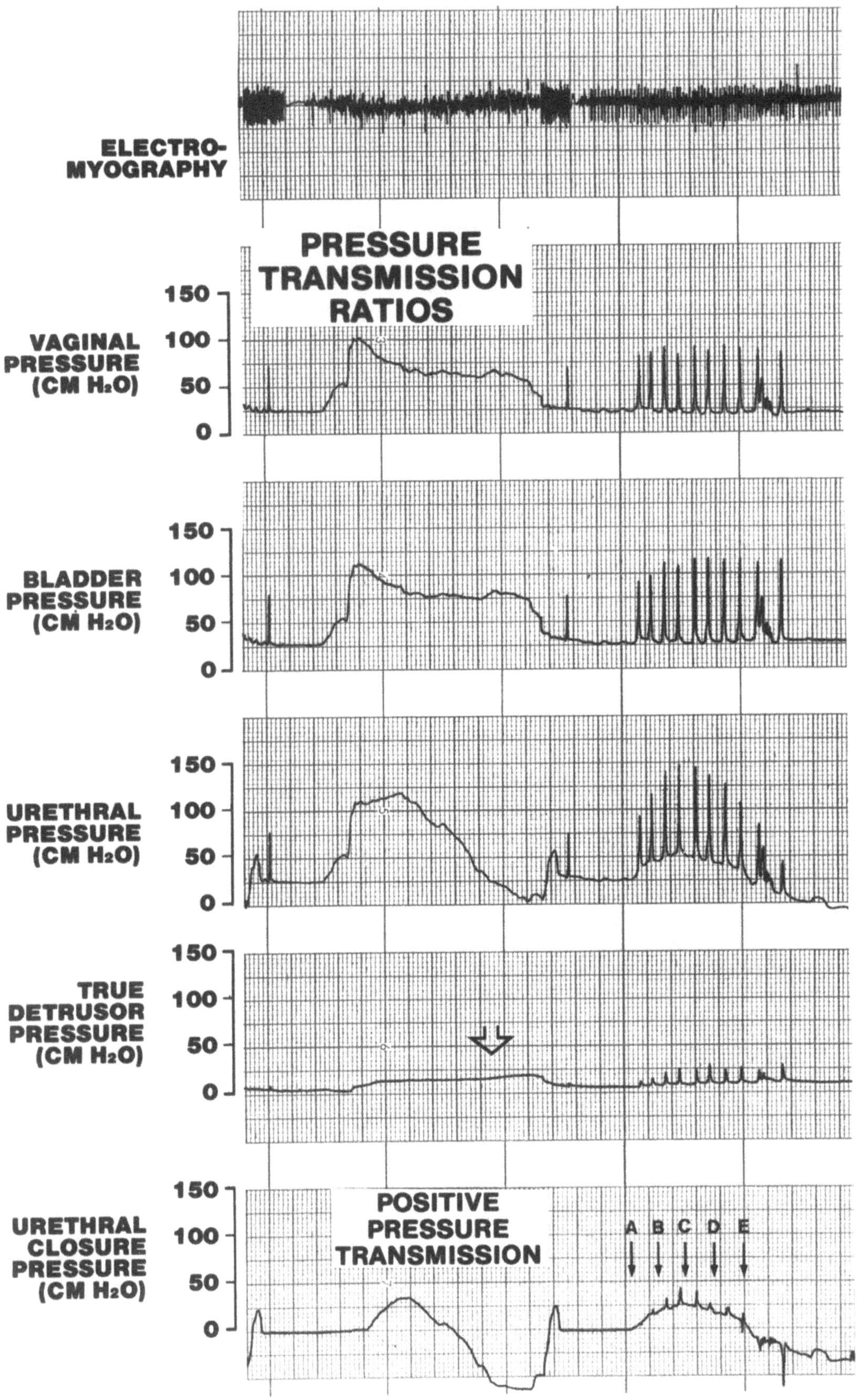


**Fig. 23.2.** Pressure transmission ratios measured during an actual cough urethral closure pressure profile.

urine loss. The margin to leakage is representative of the intrinsic sphincteric mechanism and is augmented in the normal continent woman by a healthy extrinsic continence mechanism with positive pressure transmission. The lettered arrows indicate possible choices for sites to measure pressure transmission ratios. For example, choosing the cough spike at arrow C the pressure produced by that cough in the bladder is 85 $cmH_2O$ and in the urethra is 98 $cmH_2O$. The ratio is calculated to be 115%. An artifact exists in the tracing since there is a calibration, measurement and/or transducer placement error evidenced in the true detrusor pressure channel. A pressure increase is found at the open arrow during Valsalva and a series of pressure increases during coughing. These pressure increases represent unequal pressure transmission between the bladder and vagina exactly coincidental with the pressures generated by Valsalva or coughing. This helps the urodynamicist conclude that this is artifactual, due to better transmission of pressure to the bladder than to the abdominal pressure transducer in the vagina rather than representing involuntary detrusor contractions which would persist after the increase in abdominal pressure ceased. This indicates that this is probably more related to placement of the measuring transducer than to other possible sources of error. This might be rectified by placing the abdominal pressure transducer in the rectum instead of the vagina.

Pressure transmission ratios are designed to provide objective measurements of pressure transmission to the bladder and urethra for the precise study of the function of these organs under stress. These profiles were done at 1 mm/s and cannot demonstrate timing differences in the urethral and bladder pressure increment, but faster studies would show that normally the urethral pressure spike is not only larger but occurs earlier than the bladder pressure spike. This timing increment appears to be lost with stress incontinence even if corrected by surgery. Current research in this field relies heavily on these studies, especially for understanding the effects of medical or surgical management on urethrovesical function.

## Bibliography


Bump RC, Copeland WE Hurt WG et al: Dynamic urethral pressure/profilometry pressure transmission ratio determinations in stress incontinent and stress continent subjects. Am J Obstet Gynecol 159:749, 1988.

Constantinou CE, Govan DE: Contribution and timing of transmitted and generated pressure components in the female urethra. Prog Clin Biol Res 78:113, 1981.

Rosenzweig BA, Bhatia NN, Nelson AL: Dynamic urethral pressure profilometry pressure transmission: ratio what do the numbers really mean? Obstet Gynecol 77:586, 1991.

Rosenzweig BA, Bhatia NN: Temporal separation of cough-induced urethral and bladder pressure spikes in women with urinary incontinence. Urology 39:165, 1992.

Thind P, Lose G, Jorgensen L et al: Urethral pressure increment preceding and following bladder pressure elevation during stress episodes in healthy and stress incontinent women. Neurourol Urodynam 10:177, 1991.

# Chapter 24
# Detrusor Instability

## 24.1 Stress Induced Detrusor Instability Without Leakage

Detrusor instability is defined as the presence of spontaneous or provoked involuntary contractions during filling which cannot be suppressed. This term is used when the condition is idiopathic, that is, without known cause. When the cause is known to be a lesion of the brain or spinal cord affecting the upper motor neurons involved with bladder control, the term detrusor hyperreflexia is used to distinguish these two entities from the standpoint of causation. These abnormal bladder contractions are detected by the cystometrogram as described in Chapters 13 and 20. The best method of detection is by urethrocystometry and will be illustrated in the following examples. Detrusor instability is frequently induced by various activating procedures. Examples of such activating events include the upright posture, heel bouncing, coughing, handwashing, hearing running water and the use of carbon dioxide as the infusing medium. Handwashing appears to be the most provocative of these maneuvers. A cystometrogram is incomplete if the appropriate detrusor activating procedures have been omitted. Simulation in the urodynamic laboratory of whatever events trigger possible detrusor activity is necessary in order to arrive at an appropriate diagnosis.

In the first example (Fig. 24.1) detrusor contractions (open arrow) are induced by coughing. The initial transducer localization cough (arrow) results in a low pressure detrusor contraction of 13 $cmH_2O$ followed by a series of such contractions during the cough profile (curved arrow) with no evidence of pressure equalization. Although urine leakage did not occur in this example due to the maintenance of adequate closure pressure in the urethra during continuous coughing, it is easy to see that in the absence of adequate urethral closure pressure, without urodynamic testing, urine loss would erroneously be attributed to pressure equalization rather than the presence of detrusor contractions. With such low level detrusor contractions there might not be enough reflex urethral relaxation to cause incontinence thereby hiding the true cause of the patient's urine loss to the casual observer. Usually the effect of these contractions, if they are clinically important, will be seen with the use of the detrusor activating procedures discussed above. It is important to recognize that some patients may effectively hide their detrusor instability by their remarkably well-trained pelvic floor musculature which maintains adequate closure pressure in the urethra and prevents urine loss. These patients often present with urinary urgency in the absence of urge incontinence. In this example the EMG activity is appropriate and increases with each cough.

## 24.2 Cough and Valsalva Induced Contractions

Fig. 24.2 shows both cough and Valsalva induced contractions. The initial transducer localization cough (arrow) is accompanied by a detrusor contraction which is either the result of the cough alone or the transducer physically contacting the

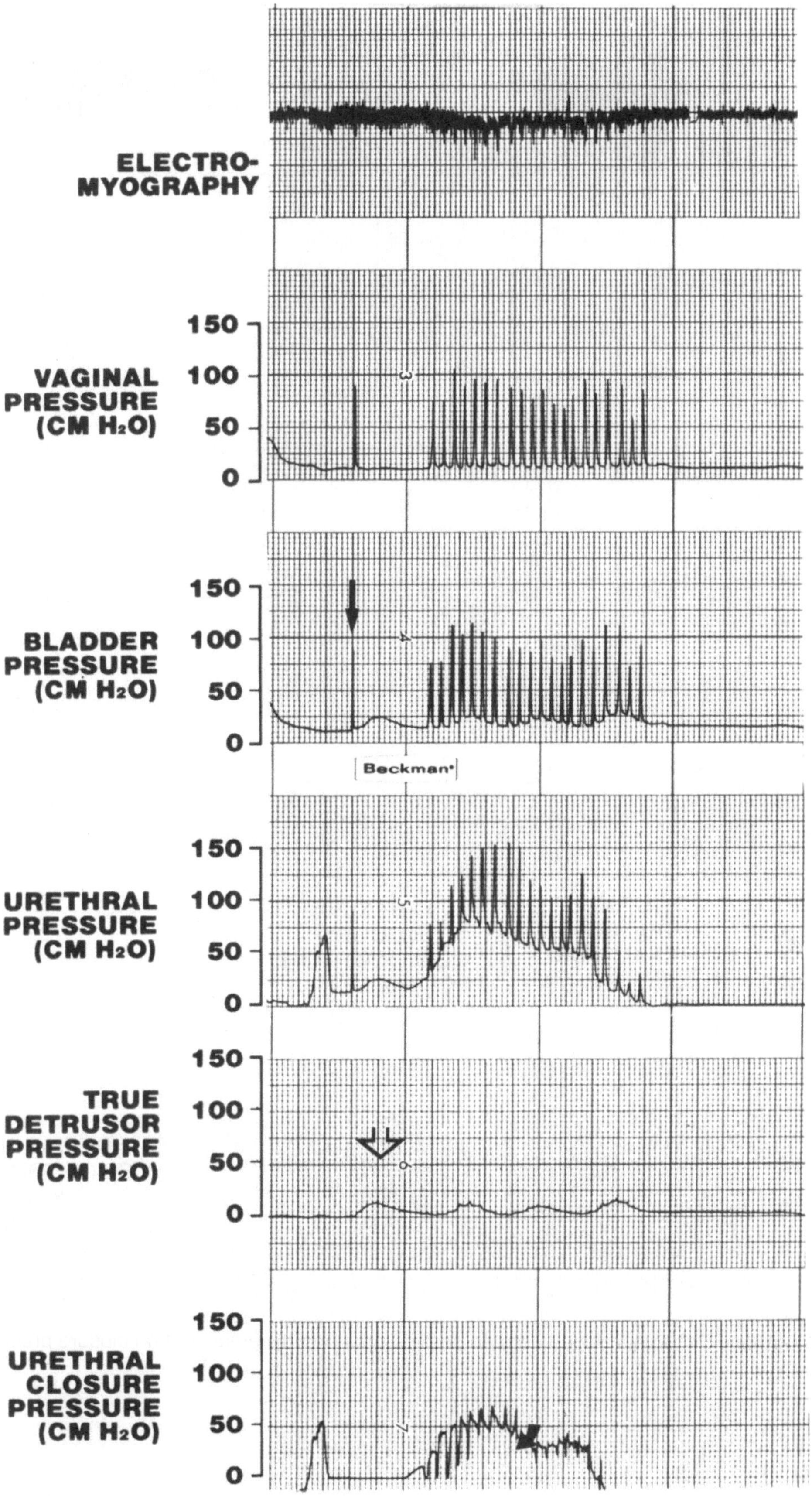


**Fig. 24.1.** Cough-induced detrusor instability during a cough urethral closure pressure profile.

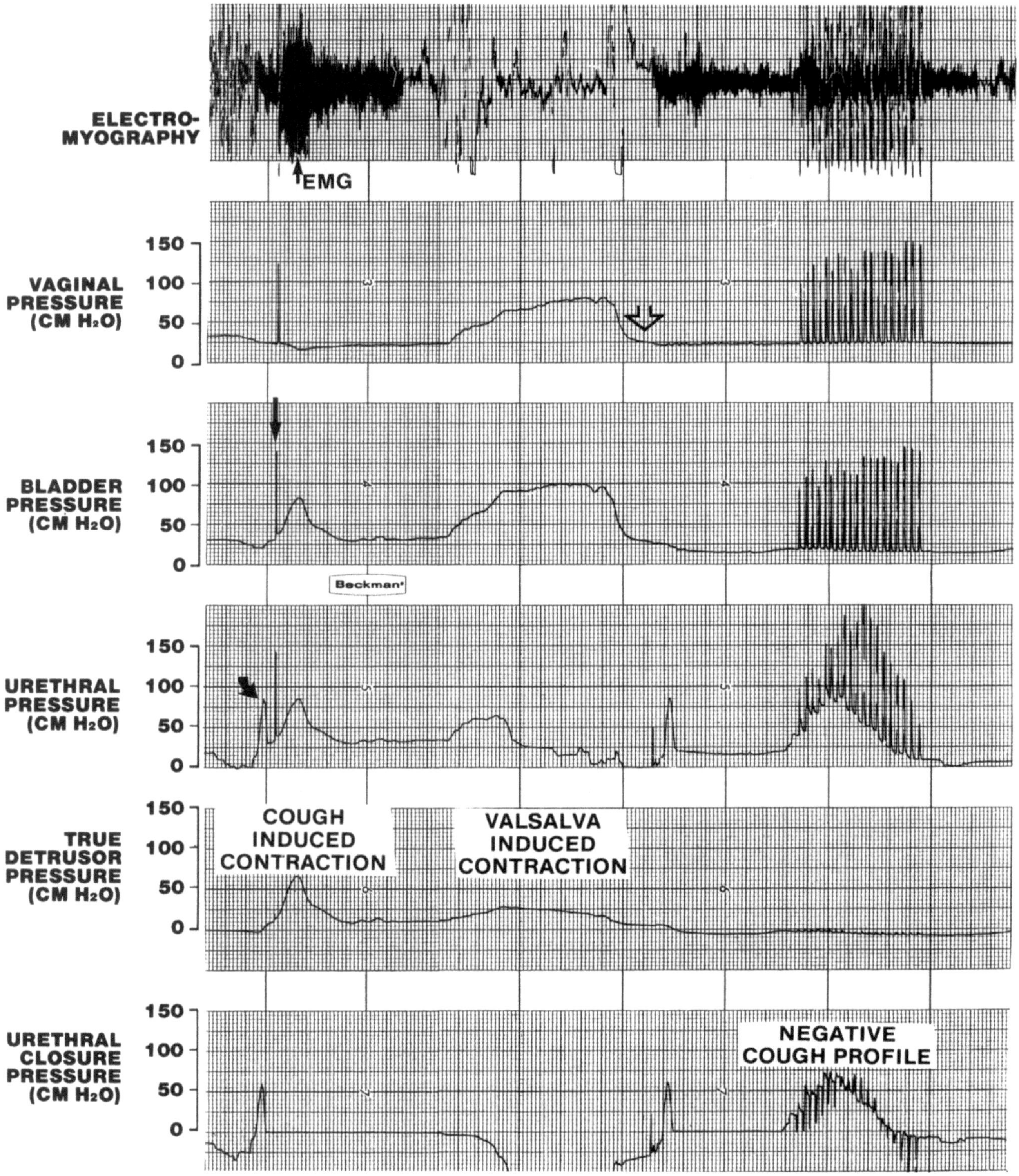


**Fig. 24.2.** Cough-and Valsalva-induced detrusor instability during dynamic urethral closure pressure profiles.

bladder wall during its introduction into the bladder as illustrated by the pressure curve generated during reintroduction of the transducer into the bladder (curved arrow) or a combination of the two. It is important to note that the contraction immediately follows the cough. To the casual observer without urodynamics the urine loss associated with this cough would be attributed to pressure equalization and stress incontinence. The EMG channel demonstrates the patient's natural defense against urine loss as the pelvic floor voluntarily contracts during the detrusor contraction (EMG arrow). This could also suggest detrusor sphincter dyssynergia (Chapter 26) and further studies might be necessary to evaluate the patient for this diagnosis. The Valsalva effort results in an increase of true detrusor pressure which begins coincident with the onset of the Valsalva maneuver. This might be confused with the artifact associated with an electronic subtraction error except that its duration is longer than the Valsalva effort which ends at the open arrow. The contraction continues for an additional 8 s with urine leakage. The subsequent cough profile does not demonstrate pressure equalization and maintains a positive margin to leakage, confirming that this patient has stress-induced detrusor instability rather than genuine stress incontinence.

## 24.3 Giggle Incontinence

Fig. 24.3 illustrates a series of detrusor contractions (closed arrow) resulting from an episode of laughing. These contractions are each associated with concomitant urethral relaxation (open arrow). Note the absence of increased EMG activity indicating that detrusor sphincter dyssynergia is not present.

## 24.4 The Effect of Bladder Filling

Filling of the bladder is one of the common stimulants of detrusor activity. In Fig. 24.4 simultaneous urethrocystometry is performed in the sitting position. The urethral pressure measuring transducer is situated at peak urethral pressure and closure pressure is indicated in that channel. The true detrusor pressure tracing is flat until 180 ml has been instilled into the bladder. Since the rectal pressure is slightly greater than the bladder pressure throughout, the true detrusor pressure is artifactually placed below the zero line. The detrusor pressure is recorded and gradually the pressure increases (arrow). The patient is asked to inhibit the contraction but this is not possible. She can, however, increase pelvic floor activity as seen in the EMG tracing (curved arrow). This voluntary urethral contraction is insufficient to overcome the reflex urethral relaxation accompanying this involuntary detrusor contraction. Gradually the detrusor contraction diminishes as the bladder empties. A cough (open arrow) does not affect the outcome of this event and does not result in pressure equalization.

These examples of detrusor instability induced by a variety of different events demonstrates the multitude of diverse stimuli capable of influencing detrusor activity. Detrusor instability is diagnosed when involuntary detrusor activity cannot be suppressed by the patient. This definition presupposes that the physician performing the urethrocystometry always requests that the patient inhibit any detrusor contraction. Lack of inhibition can only be determined after the patient fails to inhibit the detrusor activity. One of the major goals of the urodynamicist is to differentiate detrusor instability from genuine stress incontinence. The close temporal association of coughing with detrusor activity emphasizes the difficulties encountered by the clinician in trying to make this distinction. Significant errors will be made in the absence of the objective evidence provided by a urodynamic study.

## Bibliography

Coolsaet B: Bladder compliance and detrusor activity during the collection phase. Neurourol Urodynam 4:263, 1985.

Kadar N: The value of bladder filling in the clinical detection of urine loss and selection of patients for urodynamic testing. Br J Obstet Gynaecol 95:698, 1988.

Mayer R, Wells T, Brink C et al: Handwashing in the cystometric evaluation of detrusor instability. Neurourol Urodynam 10:563, 1991.

Ostergard DR, McCarthy TA: Diagnostic procedures in female urology. Am J Obstet Gynecol 137:401, 1980.

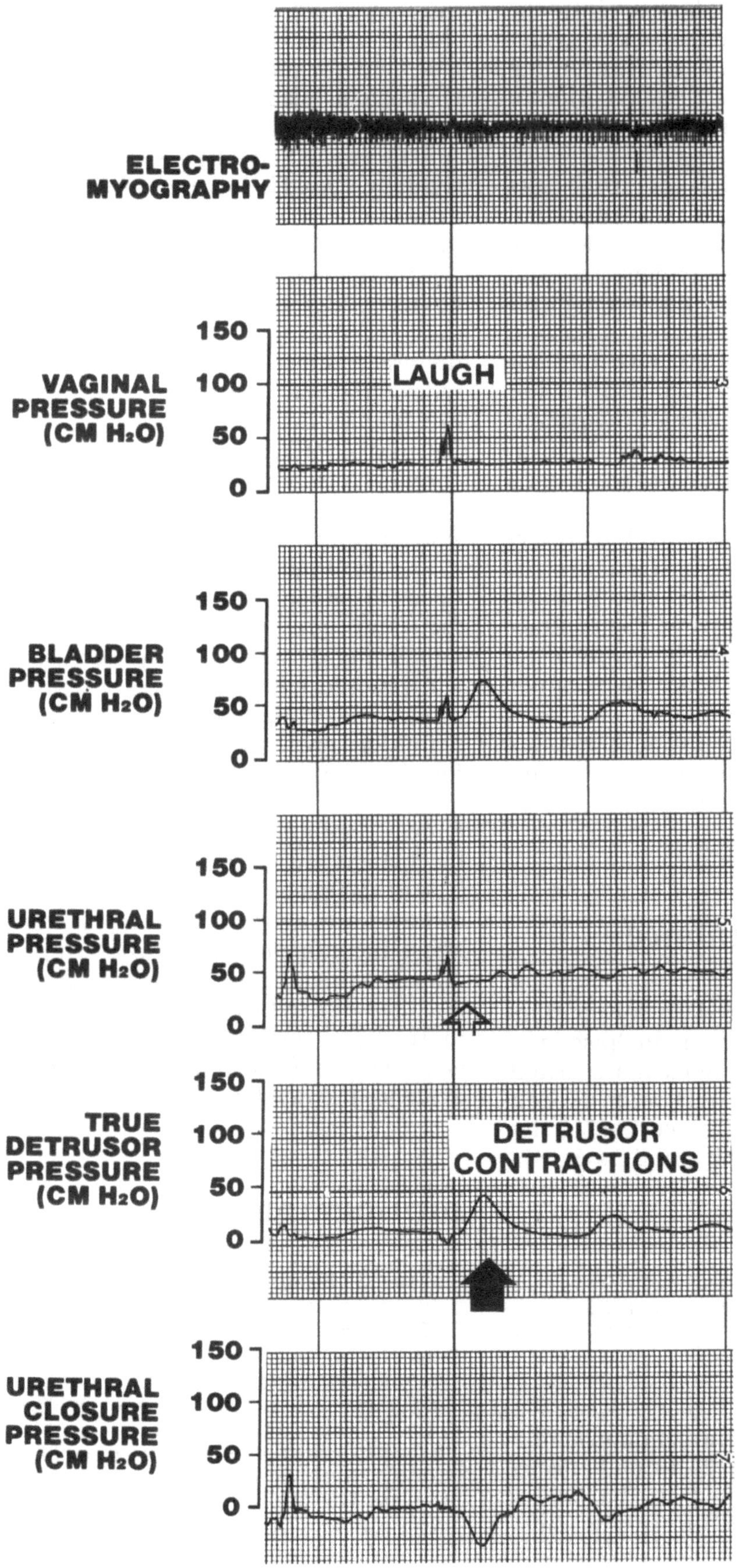


**Fig. 24.3.** Laugh-induced detrusor instability during urethrocystometry.

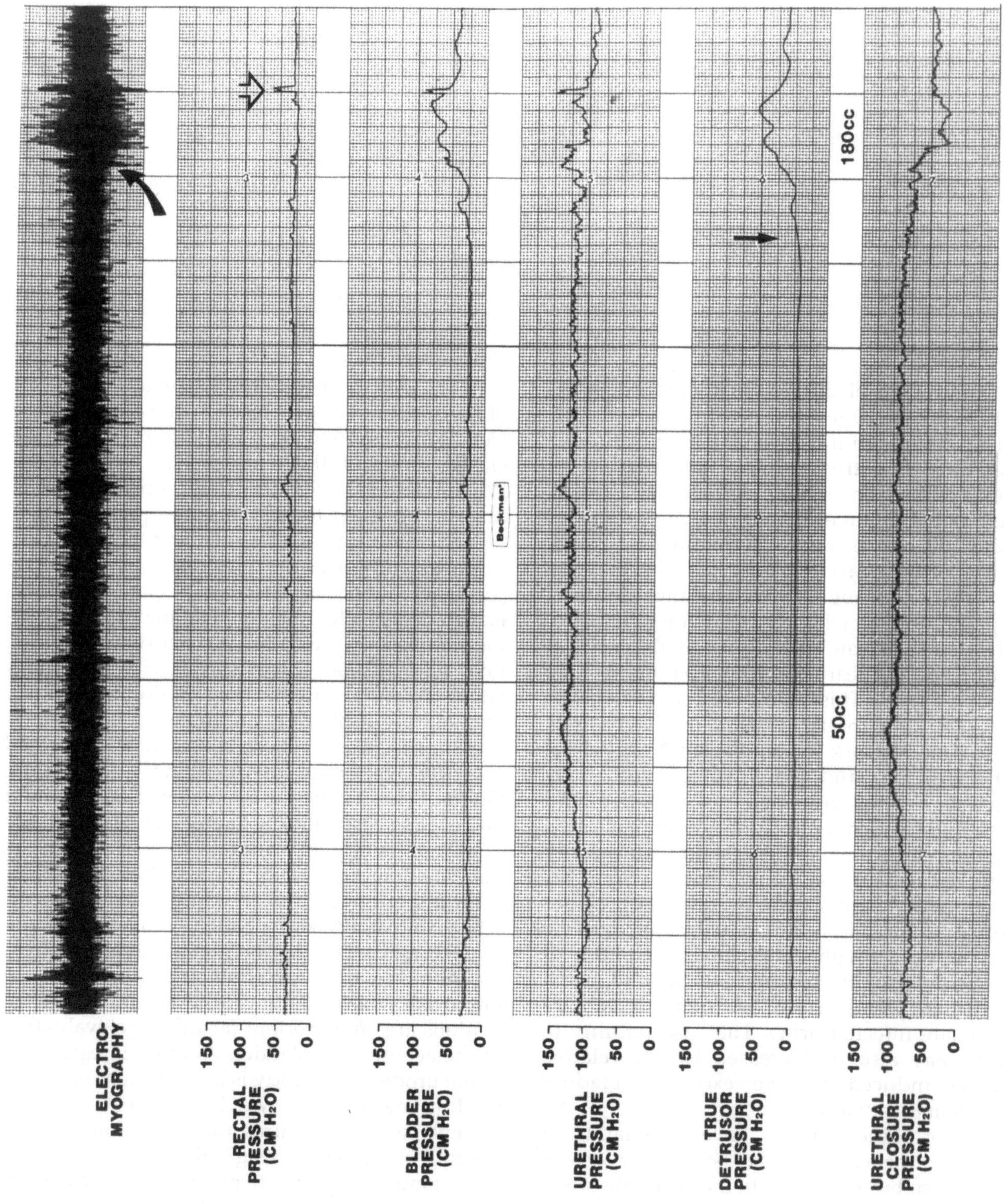


**Fig. 24.4.** Detrusor instability during urethrocystometry.

Chapter 25
# The Acontractile Bladder

The acontractile bladder is characterized by its ability to accept large volumes of fluid with little or no increase in intravesical pressure. Although the absence of detrusor contractions may be an unmistakable sign of normal detrusor control, large bladder volumes may be a sign of detrusor muscle decompensation. Retention of large volumes of urine may be a learned phenomenon in some women, taught by well-meaning mothers and grandmothers who tell their little girls not to void in an "unclean" place such as the toilet at school. The child learns to delay voiding for long periods of time. This may be carried over into adult years as a matter of habit reinforced by a lack of time at work for regular voiding. School teachers, nurses and other women with busy occupations characterize this type of patient. All is well until evidence of bladder decompensation occurs at which time detrusor contractile activity is lost. The patient may still be able to empty her bladder completely simply by relaxation of her urethra. When this is not possible, incomplete emptying results with accompanying retention of large volumes of residual urine. Repeated episodes of cystitis may result from the inability to evacuate infected urine. The susceptibility to cystitis may also be increased by the relative ischemia induced by the excessive bladder volumes in these patients.

Many of these patients have complaints of stress incontinence which may be due to overflow incontinence but the distinction of genuine stress incontinence from overflow incontinence is difficult by clinical examination alone. This differentiation is made possible by objective urodynamic testing with electromyography.

In Fig. 25.1 this bladder is able to accept 1200 ml of fluid without any increase in detrusor pressure. Detrusor pressure will be found to increase as the elastic limits of the bladder wall are reached. When filling is started the urethral pressure transducer is adjusted to peak urethral pressure. First sensation occurs at 450 ml. This is a delayed response and raises the question of partial detrusor denervation. The sensation of bladder fullness is also delayed to 1000 ml. The maximum cystometric capacity was 1200 ml. Periodic coughing does not cause any detrusor activity or demonstrate pressure equalization. Periodic rhythmic fluctuations of pressure are found in the primary pressure channels. These represent exaggerated pressure responses to breathing and talking. Urethral closure pressure remains steady without evidence of instability (Chapter 32). The detrusor does not contract voluntarily even when the patient attempts to void. The acontractile bladder is an important part of the differential diagnosis when confronted with a patient with stress incontinence since the distinction of genuine stress incontinence from overflow incontinence is an important consideration. Residual urine determinations are an important factor in the evaluation of the acontractile bladder. Another integral part of the urodynamic study is a determination of the voiding mechanism which for most of these patients will be by urethral relaxation with or without an accompanying Valsalva maneuver. In long-standing cases, patients may adapt by using Credé maneuvers to empty their bladders. Self-catheterization is used as a primary treatment for these patients and usually will resolve the incontinence and prevent recurrent infections.

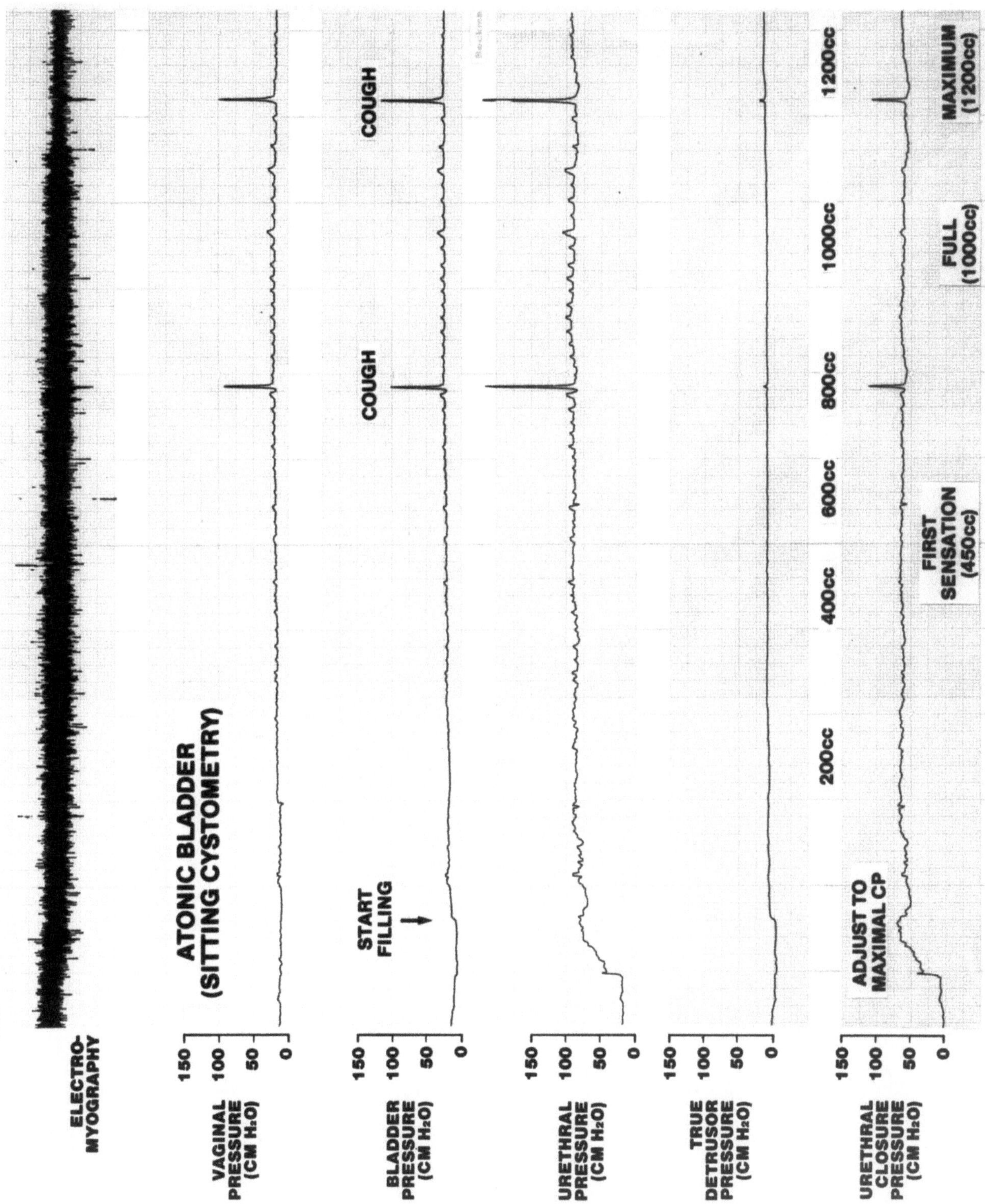


**Fig. 25.1.** Acontractile bladder during sitting urethrocystometry.

## Bibliography

De Luce FG, Swenson O, Fisher JH et al: The dysfunctional lazy bladder syndrome in children. Arch Dis Child 37:117, 1962.

Firlit CF, Cook WA: Voiding pattern abnormalities in children. Urology 10:25, 1977.

Koff SA: Non-neuropathic vesico-urethral dysfunction in children. In Mundy AR, Stevenson TP, Wein AJ (eds) Urodynamics: principles, practice and application. Edinburgh, Churchill Livingstone, 1984, pp. 311–325.

Park YC, Kaneko S, Yachiku S et al: Accurate diagnosis of detrusor areflexia using combined uroflowmetry and abdominal wall electromyography. Urology 26:423, 1985.

# Chapter 26
# Detrusor Sphincter Dyssynergia

Detrusor sphincter dyssynergia is defined as the lack of external sphincter relaxation during voluntary voiding. This should not be confused with the term "detrusor dyssynergia" which has been applied to the unstable bladder. Detrusor sphincter dyssynergia frequently results in an incomplete voiding effort with elevated residual urine volumes. This condition commonly accompanies detrusor hyperreflexia and may occur in some patients without neurologic disease as a habituation to using a "guarding" reflex to prevent urinary leakage with detrusor instability. The first defense against urine loss is the voluntary contraction of the external striated sphincter of the urethra when an unstable bladder contraction occurs. With time this voluntary contraction becomes almost involuntary (habituation) and occurs automatically every time a detrusor contraction occurs. The end result is evidenced by the trabeculation found in the bladder on cystoscopic examination, the increased EMG activity of the pelvic floor during attempted voiding, and the seemingly paradoxical increased residual urine volumes resulting from this involuntary obstruction to urine flow.

In this example (Fig. 26.1), the patient with detrusor hyperreflexia secondary to a cerebral vascular accident is asked to void (arrow). Increased EMG activity of the pelvic floor is recorded through the perianal patch electrodes. This occurs immediately with the request to initiate micturition. Intermittently increased EMG activity occurs with detrusor contractions until it becomes virtually constant. Intermittent episodes of urethral relaxation occur but are quickly aborted by contraction of the urethral skeletal musculature as is evidenced by the increased EMG activity (open arrows). Voiding remains ineffectual and incomplete due to continued external sphincter activity as evidenced in the EMG recording. This occurs despite strong initial detrusor contractions (up to 98 $cmH_2O$) followed by abortive contractions of decreasing strength. A 350 ml residual was found at the end of the study after the patient voids only 100 ml (uroflow not pictured).

Detrusor sphincter dyssynergic voiding patterns may accompany detrusor hyperreflexia where it accounts for the paradoxical elevated residual urine volumes frequently seen with this condition. It may also occur without incontinence. The knowledge that a patient voids dyssynergically is prognostically important when incontinence surgery is contemplated since this type of obstruction during voiding may lead to prolonged catheter drainage and retention postoperatively. Treatment for detrusor sphincter dyssynergia is crucial to prevent recurrent urinary tract infection, vesicoureteral reflux and renal damage. The mainstay of treatment is the establishment of safe effective emptying through intermittent self-catheterization. This may be augmented by pharmacologic attempts to relax the striated and smooth muscle of the urethra. Alpha blockers, smooth muscle relaxants and diazepam have been used to block urethral spasm and decrease urethral resistance. Baclofen may also be used to block skeletal muscle activity. Biofeedback has also been used successfully. Where the condition is believed to be non-neurogenic, treatment of the underlying detrusor instability or urethral spasm may remove the need for intermittent catheterization.

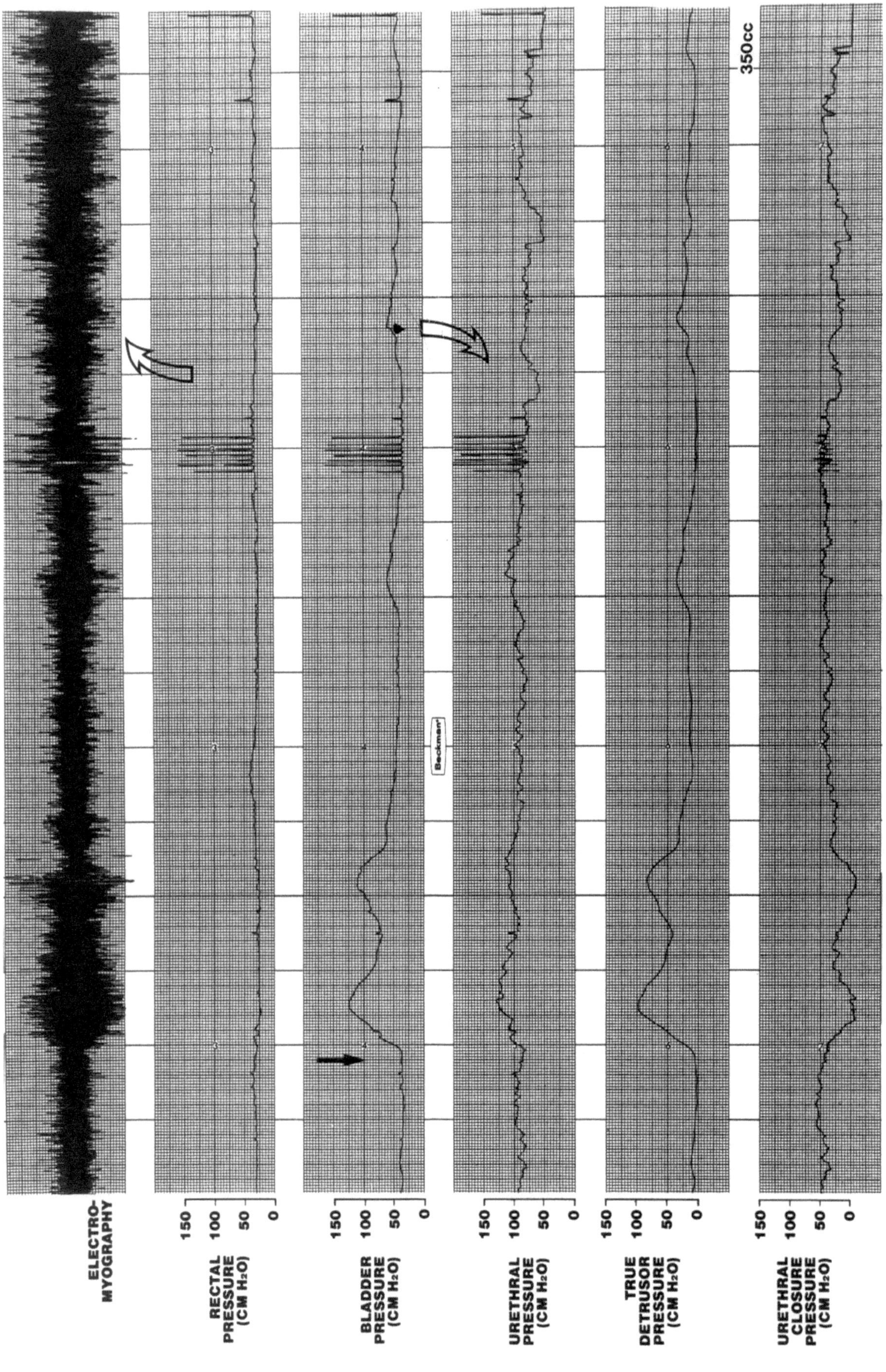


**Fig. 26.1.** Detrusor sphincter dyssynergia during a pressure voiding study.

# Bibliography


Allen TD: The non-neurogenic neurogenic bladder. J Urol 117:232, 1977.

Allen TD, Bright TC: Urodynamic patterns in children with dysfunctional voiding problems. J Urol 119:247, 1978.

Koff SA: Bladder-sphincter dysfunction in childhood. Urology 19:457, 1982.

Koff SA, Murtagh DS: The uninhibited bladder in children: effect of treatment on recurrence of urinary infection and on vesicoureteral reflux resolution. J Urol 130:1138, 1983.

Norgaard JP, Djurhuus JC: Treatment of detrusor sphincter dyssynergia by biofeedback. Urol Int 37:236, 1982.

Rudy DS, Awad SA, Downie JW: External sphincter dyssynergia: an abnormal continence reflex. J Urol 140:105, 1988.

Siroky MB, Krane RJ: Neurologic aspects of detrusor-sphincter dyssynergia with reference to the guarding reflex. J Urol 127:953, 1982.

Smey P, King LR, Firlit CF: Dysfunctional voiding in children secondary to internal sphincter dyssynergia: treatment with phenoxybenzamine. Urol Clin North Am 7:337, 1980.

Vereecken RL, Poppel HV, Boeckx G et al: Long term alpha-adrenergic-blocking therapy in detrusor-urethra dyssynergia. Eur Urol 9:167, 1983.

Chapter 27

# The Low Compliance Bladder

Compliance is defined as the increase in pressure per unit of volume ($V/P$). Normally the bladder is very compliant and may be filled to large volumes with very little increase in detrusor pressure. The low compliance bladder results from intrinsic disease processes within the bladder wall which result in fibrosis and decreased elasticity. This decreased elasticity of the bladder wall is reflected in the urodynamic tracing as a loss of accommodation with a gradual pressure increase during filling. This is frequently associated with a diminished bladder capacity in conditions such as radiation cystitis. When the lack of bladder wall compliance results in bladder pressure equalization with the urethra, incontinence results in a pattern similar to the atonic bladder when the bladder can distend no longer but at much smaller volumes.

In Fig. 27.1 a patient with prior pelvic irradiation undergoes bladder filling during the cystometrogram until at a bladder volume of 400 ml the intravesical pressure gradually begins to increase and eventually reaches 25 $cmH_2O$ at 500 ml (arrow). In this cystometrogram there is also a decrease in proximal urethral resistance with a decrease in urethral pressure associated with some funneling at the bladder neck despite a slight increase in EMG activity beginning at the curved arrow. When pressure equalization is reached (open arrow) this event is associated with urine loss. This patient's low compliance bladder and incontinence is also associated with genuine stress incontinence as evidenced by the pressure equalization and urine loss with the cough at the beginning of the study (curved open arrow).

Incontinence associated with the low compliance bladder is another condition to be considered in the differential diagnosis of genuine stress incontinence. When a low compliance bladder is found without a history of prior bladder irradiation, other conditions such as interstitial cystitis should be sought as a possible etiology. This may be discovered by filling and refilling the bladder to its maximal volume either in the office or in the operating room under anesthesia in order to produce the characteristic cystoscopic abnormalities. Treatment of the low compliance bladder is difficult when the condition is severe. For this patient with a very mild loss of compliance, continence can be maintained by regular voiding or prompted voiding. However, in severe conditions where the functional bladder capacity is under 100 ml, conservative interventions such as antispasmodics and anticholinergics are of little use and patients require continent diversion or bladder augmentation.

## Bibliography


Aron BS, Schlesinger A: Complications of radiation therapy: the genitourinary tract. Semin Roentgenol 9:65, 1974.

Coolsaet B: Bladder compliance and detrusor activity during the collection phase. Neurourol Urodynam 4:263, 1985.

Farguharson DIM, Shingleton H, Sanford SP et al: The short-term effect of pelvic irradiation for gynecologic malignancies on bladder function. Obstet Gynecol 70:81, 1987.

Ram MD: Complications of radiotherapy for carcinoma of the bladder. Proc Soc Med 63:93, 1970.

Susset JG: Cystometry. In Krause RJ, Siroky MB (eds) Clinical neurourology. Boston, Little, Brawn 1991, pp. 163–184.

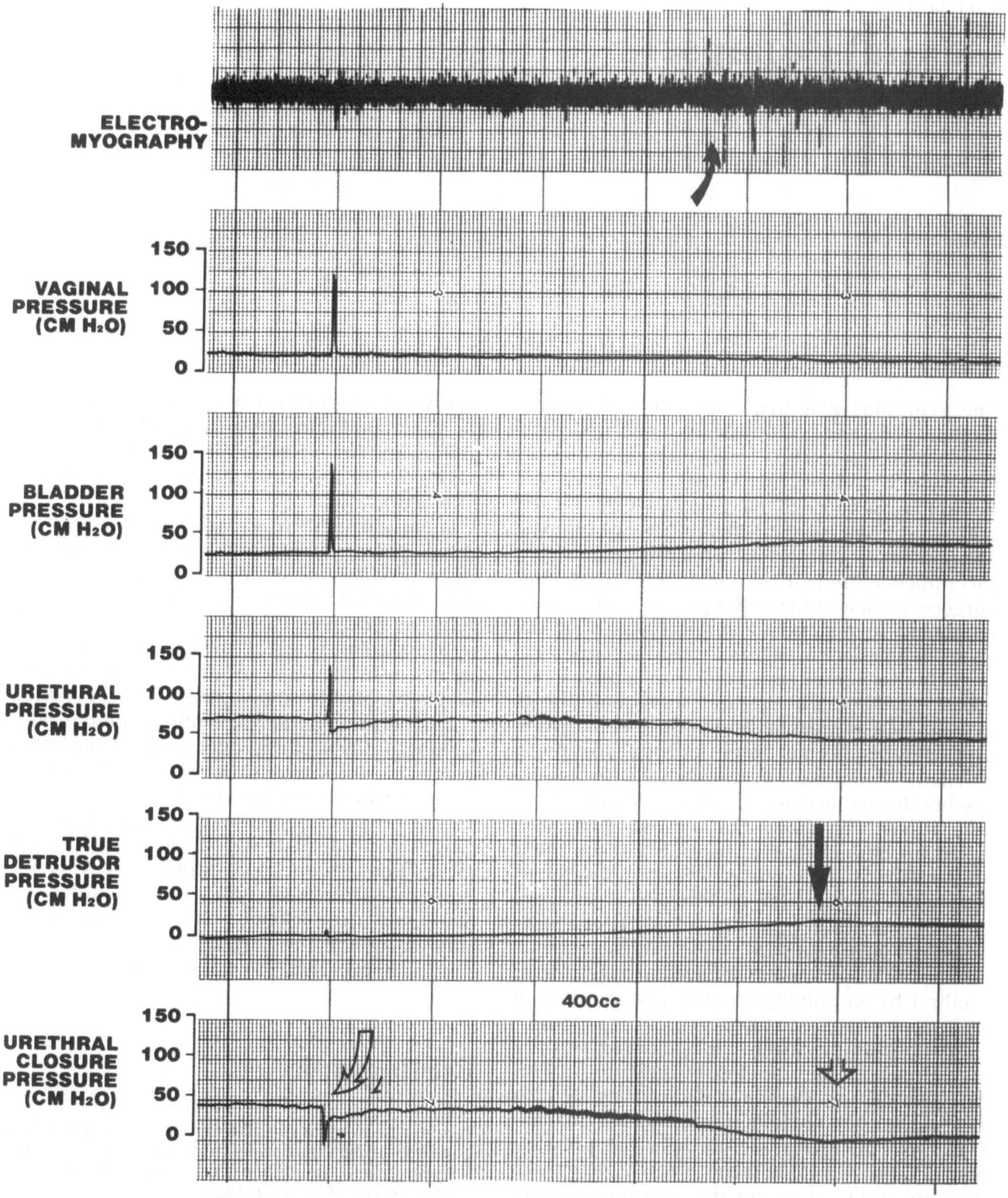


**Fig. 27.1.** Reduced bladder compliance during urethrocystometry.

# Chapter 28
# Genital Prolapse

The gynecologist is frequently confronted with patients who have incontinence associated with pelvic floor relaxation and uterine prolapse. Standard clinical and urodynamic evaluation will determine the cause of that patient's incontinence and appropriate surgical therapy can be offered. Many patients with genital prolapse do not have incontinence and it is incumbent upon the surgeon to determine if the patient will remain continent after standard surgical repair procedures. If a patient has normal urethral supports it is likely that genuine stress incontinence will not result. However, if urethral hypermobility is present there is great likelihood that the patient is artificially protected from incontinence by a mechanical kinking effect which occurs in the urethra during increases in intra-abdominal pressure. It has been shown that these patients have up to an 80% chance of becoming incontinent after surgery if appropriate steps are not taken to adequately support the urethrovesical junction. By using a pessary, barrier or proctoswabs as described in Chapter 34, these patients can be detected and appropriate surgical management of urethral hypermobility instituted at the time of their reconstructive surgery.

In the example in Fig 28.1, characteristically high pressure urethral closure pressure profiles (>150 $cmH_2O$) are evident in the resting state with even further accentuation during Valsalva maneuvers. Note the increased "off the scale" pressure of the Valsalva profile (solid arrow). The cough pressure profile does not demonstrate pressure equalization and there is a very large margin to leakage with positive pressure transmission (open curved arrow). If this patient is destined to become incontinent with surgical reduction of her genital prolapse, the insertion of a pessary to resupport the prolapse in the urodynamic laboratory would result in marked loss of pressure in the urethral closure pressure profiles. The cough profile and/or Valsalva profile would become positive with pressure equalization and demonstrable urine loss.

In this tracing there are two artifacts. The first is at the open arrow where the recorder was turned off to produce the indicated markings. In addition, there is a subtraction artifact in the true detrusor pressure channel as indicated by the series of small pressure deflections at the small arrows resulting from unequal pressure transmission to the bladder and vagina (bladder > vagina).

Genital prolapse is frequently accompanied by kinking in the urethra which protects the patient from urine loss during stress. Should this mechanical obstruction be relieved by surgical reduction of the genital prolapse, without due attention to the provision of adequate support to the urethrovesical junction, postoperative incontinence will result. Properly performed urodynamic studies will determine if the patient will become incontinent and will guide the surgeon to choose the best surgical approach to prevent incontinence.

## Bibliography


Bergman A, Koonings PP, Ballard CA: Predicting postoperative urinary incontinence development in women undergoing operation for genitourinary prolapse. Am J Obstet Gynecol 158:1171, 1988.

Bump RC, Fantl JA, Hurt WG: The mechanism of urinary continence in women with severe uterovaginal prolapse: results of barrier studies. Obstet Gynecol 3:291, 1988.

Fianu S, Kjaeldgaard A, Larson B: Preoperative screen for latent stress incontinence in women with cystocele. Neurourol Urodynam 4:3, 1985.

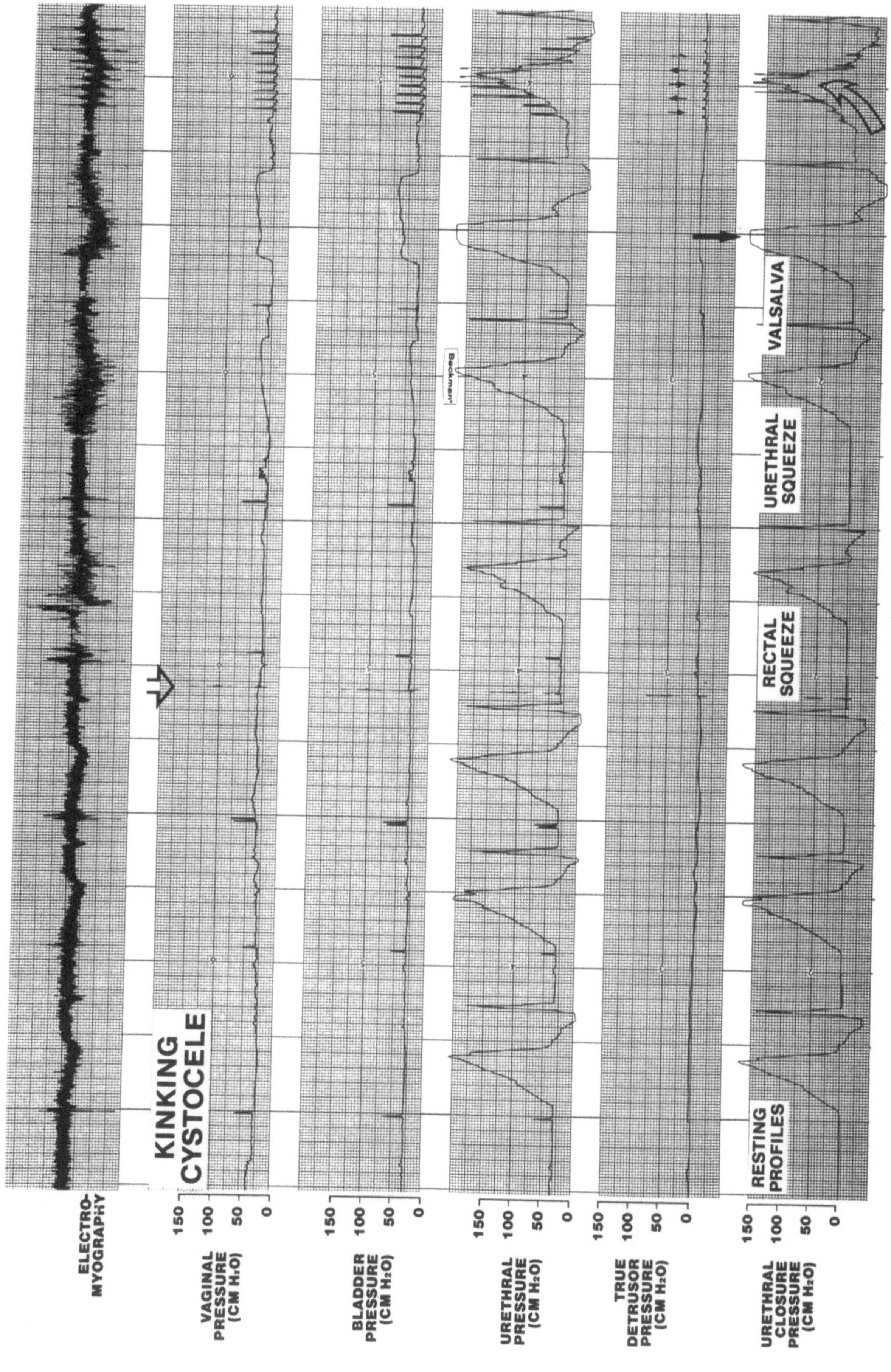


**Fig. 28.1.** The effect of a large cystocele on urethral closure pressure profiles.

Chapter 29

# The Low Pressure Urethra

Patients maintain urinary continence by having adequate intrinsic sphincteric activity and tone, as well as, equal or positive pressure transmission to the proximal urethra during increases in intra-abdominal pressure. Most patients with genuine stress incontinence have a condition where there is urethral hypermobility which results in decreased pressure transmission to the proximal urethra. This deficit in the extrinsic continence mechanism may be corrected by surgery and compensated for by some non-surgical treatments. However, deficits in the intrinsic urethral resistance and sphincteric function are not usually corrected by routine, anti-incontinence operations. The intrinsic urethral resistance or sphincteric function is maintained by a number of different factors. Intrinsic skeletal muscle, smooth muscle, elastic and collagenous tissues contribute to the resting intraurethral pressure and tone. In addition, the periurethral vasculature and periurethral skeletal muscle add to the intrinsic urethral resistance. Mucosal coaptation also appears to play a role in the intrinsic sphincteric function. If these intrinsic factors are compromised, then resting urethral pressure or resistance will be decreased. It has been demonstrated that loss of resting urethral resistance or pressure may cause urinary incontinence, even when the proximal urethra is well-supported. This is described as Type III stress incontinence and will be discussed in Chapter 53. Where urethral hypermobility and decreased urethral resistance co-exist, the condition is called the low pressure urethra. This condition is the single largest risk factor for failure of routine anti-incontinence operations. The low pressure urethra has been defined as a resting urethral closure pressure of less than or equal to 20 $cmH_2O$ in the sitting position at maximum cystometric capacity. Various authors have shown that patients who have a low pressure urethra may have up to a 54% risk of failing anti-incontinence operations, such as the retropubic urethropexies and needle suspensions. It has been suggested that these patients need not only support and elevation of the proximal urethra, but also something to compensate for their lost intrinsic sphincteric function. Obstructive procedures such as slings and artificial urinary sphincters have been used in these patients. Therefore, determination of which patients have low urethral closure pressure in the sitting position, while at maximum cystometric capacity, is vital to the preoperative evaluation of the incontinent female.

In Fig. 29.1, a 72-year-old female who had undergone a prior Stamey bladder neck suspension is now found to have a low pressure urethra. Her bladder has been filled to 300 ml which is her maximum cystometric capacity. At this bladder volume, resting urethral closure pressure profiles reveal a marked decrease in urethral closure pressure. The points of maximum urethral closure pressure for both of these profiles are demonstrated by the two arrows. The first, smaller arrow, points to the closure pressure for the first profile which is 12 $cmH_2O$. The second profile (larger arrow) demonstrates a closure pressure of 14 $cmH_2O$. The functional length of the first profile is 18 mm and the functional length of the second profile is 20 mm. This patient, either because of her advanced age, prior periurethral procedure (Stamey procedure) hypoestrogenism or a combination of these factors now has dramati-

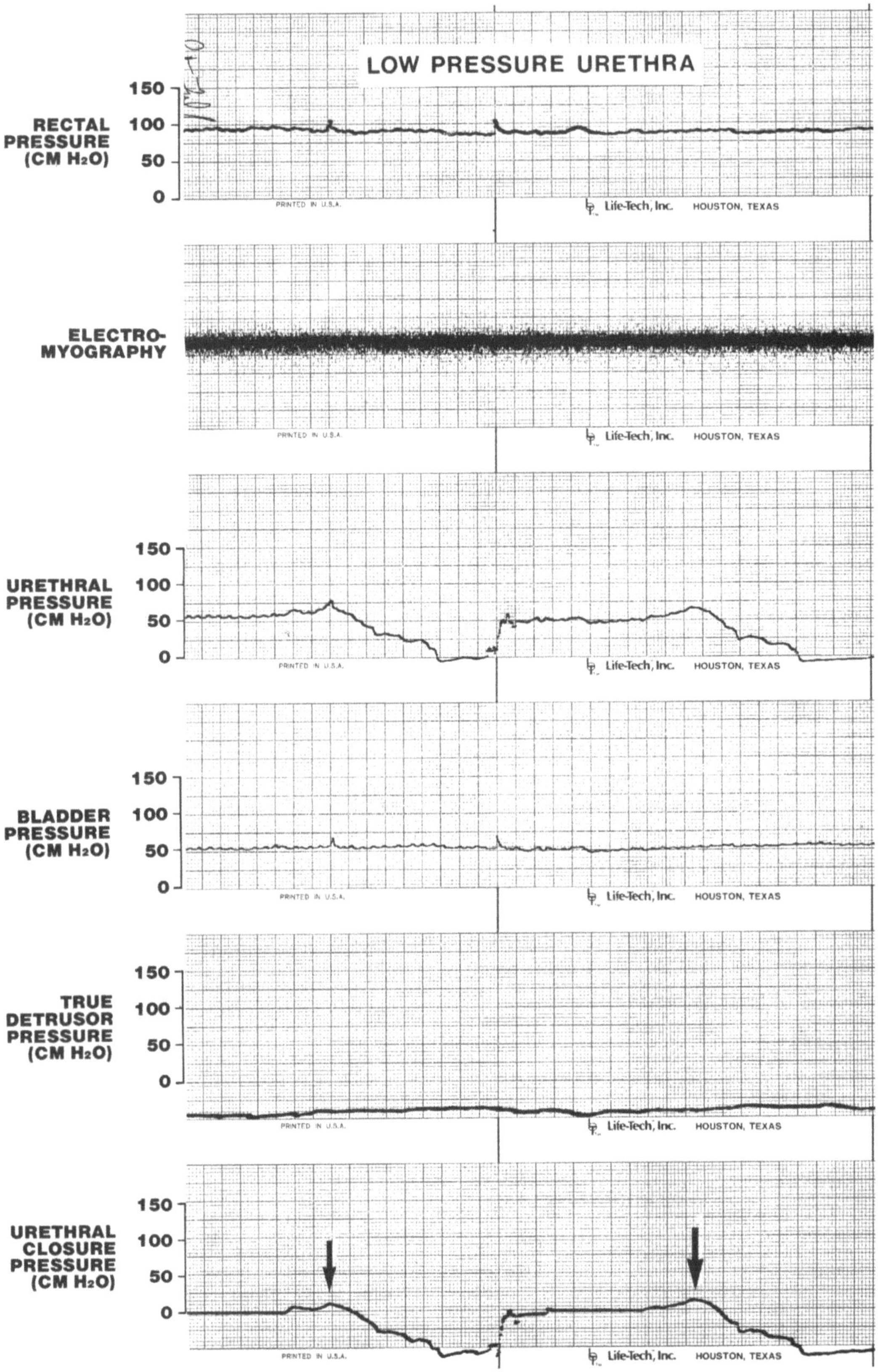


**Fig. 29.1.** Detection of the low pressure urethra during resting urethral closure pressure profiles.

cally decreased urethral resistance which accounts for her marked urinary incontinence. The patient wears an adult diaper and needs to change this several times a day. Whereas a second needle suspension procedure, such as a Stamey, Gittes, modified Pereyra or Raz procedure might only have a 50%–60% chance of curing her urinary incontinence, a suburethral sling procedure should have an 80%–90% chance of curing her urinary leakage. In fact, this patient was successfully treated with a Gore-Tex® suburethral sling procedure with resolution of her incontinence.

This patient is also noted to have a negative true detrusor pressure which goes off the scale. This is due to the elevated rectal pressure during these urethral closure pressure profiles. Initially, the rectal pressure was calibrated to be equal to the bladder pressure at the beginning of this study. This made the true detrusor pressure zero at the beginning of the urodynamic study. However, during the preceding urethrocystometry study, the rectal pressure was noted to increase from where it had been at baseline. This would account for the subtraction artifact, leading to a negative true detrusor pressure shown throughout this Figure. Since true detrusor pressure is a relative measure, the absolute baseline pressure measurement is not crucial.

## Bibliography

Bergman A, Ballard CA, Koonings PP: Comparison of three different surgical procedures for genuine stress incontinence: prospective randomized study. Am J Obstet Gynecol 160:1102, 1989.

Hilton P: A clinical and urodynamic study comparing the Stamey bladder neck suspension and suburethral sling procedures in the treatment of genuine stress incontinence. Br J Obstet Gynaecol 96:213, 1989.

Horbach NS, Blanco JS, Ostergard DR et al: A suburethral sling procedure with polytetrafluoroethylene for the treatment of genuine stress incontinence in patients with low urethral closure pressure. Obstet Gynecol 71:648, 1988.

McGuire EJ: Urodynamic findings in patients after failure of stress incontinence operations. Prog Clin Biol Res 78:351, 1981.

Sand PK, Bowen LW, Panganiban R, Ostergard DR: The low pressure urethra as a factor in failed retropubic urethropexy. Obstet Gynecol 69:399, 1987.

Summit RL, Bent AE, Ostergard DR et al: Suburethral sling procedure for genuine stress incontinence and low urethral closure pressure. A continued experience. Int Urogynecol J 3:18, 1992.

Chapter 30
# Urethrovaginal Fistulas

Urethrovaginal fistulas characteristically result in inactive pressure segments that are apparent during urethral closure pressure profilometry. The fistula usually destroys a segment of the urethral wall leaving a void which reduces urethral pressure at that area of the urethra. Inflammation and scarring around the fistula site may also reduce urethral pressure around the hole in the urethra.

In Fig. 30.1 urethral closure pressure profilometry is shown in both the preoperative and postoperative periods. In the preoperative tracing the pressure profile begins at the curved solid arrow. Positive pressure is seen initially in the proximal urethral segment which rapidly decreases as the fistula site is approached (solid arrow). Urethral pressure then gradually increases in the distal urethral segment beyond the fistula (open arrow). In addition to the fistula the patient also has a low pressure urethra.

Postoperatively a similar sequence of events is observed with the repaired fistula site still evident. The proximal urethral closure pressure is more than doubled when compared to that found preoperatively (open curved arrow). The pressure profile is also longer than that seen preoperatively due to the effects of the repair and specifically from the interposition of a bulbocavernosus fat pad graft which was used because of the compromised blood supply to this area. Continence was restored.

When a defect in the urethral wall exists either in the form of a fistula or a diverticular orifice (Chapter 31), that segment of the urethra becomes inactive with diminished or no pressure present in that location. If this is found unexpectedly during a pressure profile, specific causes of that localized loss of pressure must be determined. The urodynamicist should always document that urine loss is coming from the urethral meatus and not from the vagina during increases in intra-abdominal pressure as may occur in a urethrovaginal fistula.

## Bibliography


Webster GD, Sihelnik SA, Stone AR: Urethrovaginal fistula: a review of the surgical management. J Urol 132:460, 1984.

Lee RA, Symmonds RE, Williams TJ: Current status of genitourinary fistula. Obstet Gynecol 72:313, 1988.

Gray LA: Urethrovaginal fistulas and fistulas of the urethrovesical junction. In Slate WG (ed) Disorders of the female urethra and urinary incontinence. Baltimore, Williams & Wilkins, 1978, pp. 178–186.

Guerriero WG: Gynecologic injuries to the ureter, bladder and urethra. In Raz S (ed) Female Urology. Philadelphia, WB Saunders, 1983, pp. 357–371.

Blaivas JG: Vaginal flap urethral reconstruction: an alternative to the bladder flap neourethra. J Urol 141:542, 1989.

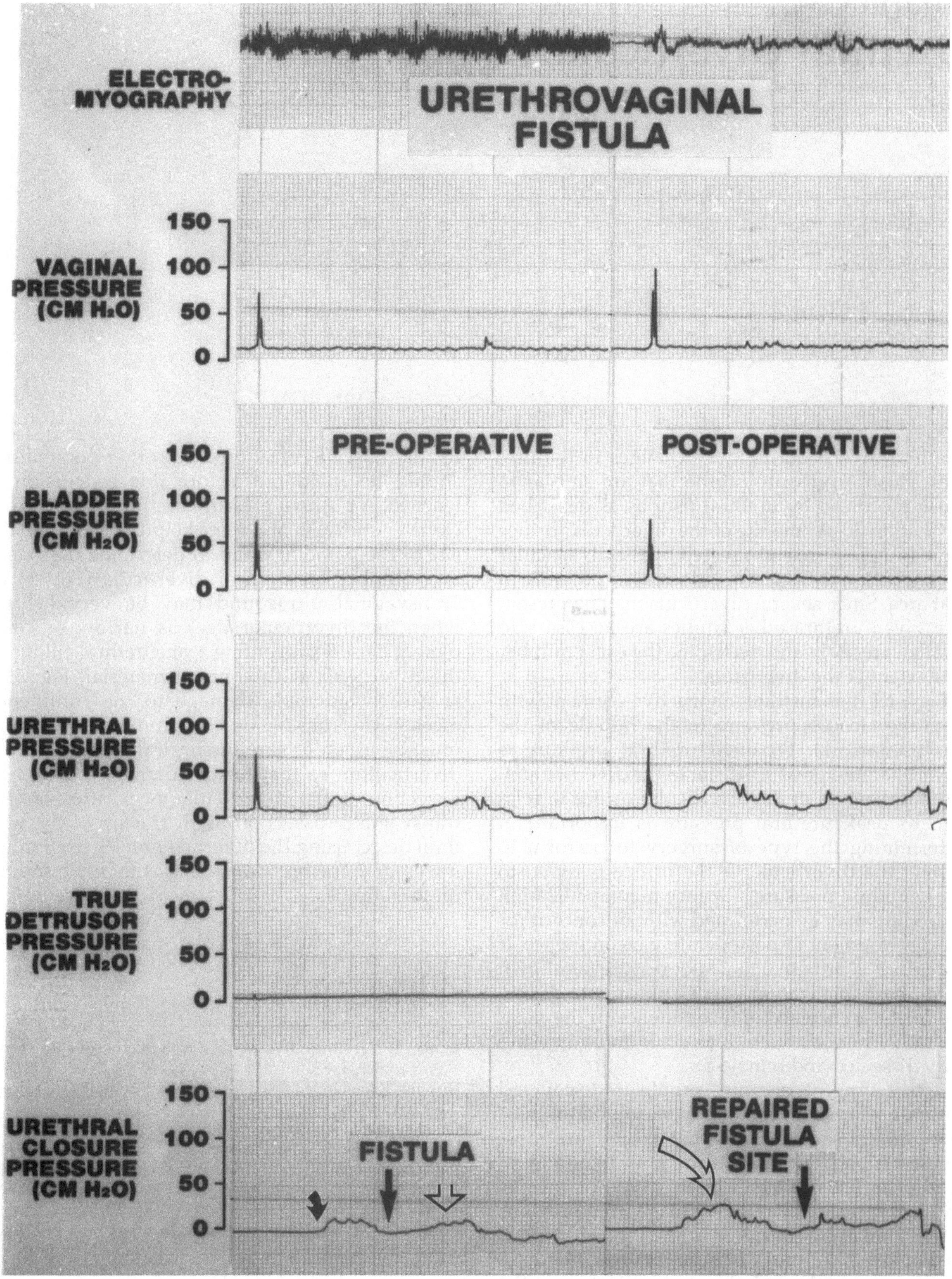


**Fig. 30.1.** Urethral closure pressure profiles before and after closure of a urethrovaginal fistula.

# Chapter 31
# Urethral Diverticula

Urethral diverticula produce changes in the urethral closure pressure profile that are similar to those produced by urethral fistulas as described in Chapter 30. At the site of the diverticular orifice there is a pressure sink created by the diverticular neck which is reflected in a decreased pressure in that area. Since several diverticula may be present in a given urethra other studies are necessary to localize precisely and determine the exact number and extent of the diverticula.

Fig. 31.1 demonstrates an inactive segment with negative closure pressure in the middle of the urethra (arrow). Proximal urethral pressure is lower than the pressure distal to the diverticulum. The localization of the diverticular orifice in relation to peak urethral pressure is important in determining the type of surgery to perform to correct the diverticula. If the orifice is distal to peak urethral pressure a Spence marsupialization procedure may be performed without concern for the development of postoperative incontinence. If the orifice is proximal to peak pressure (as shown here) marsupialization is not appropriate due to the likely occurrence of incontinence in the postoperative period. Such diverticula must be carefully dissected and removed.

If this type of pressure profile is discovered without prior suspicion of any reason for an inactive urethral segment, then the exact cause must be ascertained. Although a urethral diverticulum heads the list of causes of this type of profile, urethrovaginal fistulas and damage from previous surgery must be considered. The urethroscope is particularly helpful in distinguishing these various causes through direct visualization of the fistula or diverticular orifice. When previous surgery has been performed near the urethra, a fistula must be considered but other possibilities should be ruled out before this conclusion is reached. A positive pressure urethrogram (Tratner catheter study) is also very helpful to localize the site of the pathology and to determine the extent and number of urethral diverticula (Fig. 31.2). Transvaginal ultrasound may be very helpful when the diverticular neck is narrow or completely closed preventing transurethral filling of the diverticula with contrast material. Fig. 31.1 shows considerable damage to the continence mechanism from the diverticulum and great care must be given to careful surgical excision of the diverticulum so that further damage is avoided. Resection at the diverticular neck after careful transvaginal dissection, with closure of the urethral defect using the diverticular neck itself minimizes any further damage to the surrounding urethral tissues.

## Bibliography


Drutz HP: Urethral diverticula. Obstet Gynecol Clin North Am 16:923, 1989.

Downs RA: Urethral diverticula in females. Urology 29:201, 1987.

Ginsberg DS, Genadry R: Suburethral diverticulum in the female. Obstet Gynecol Surv 39:1, 1984.

Lee RA: Diverticulum of the urethra: clinical presentation, diagnosis and management. Clin Obstet Gynecol 27:490, 1984.

Robertson JR: Urethral divertula. In Ostergard DR, Bent AE (eds) Urogynecology and urodynamics. Baltimore, Williams & Wilkins, 1991, pp. 283–291.

Tancer ML, Moopan MMU, Pierre-Louis C et al: Suburethral diverticulum: treatment by partial ablation. Obstet Gynecol 62:511, 1983.

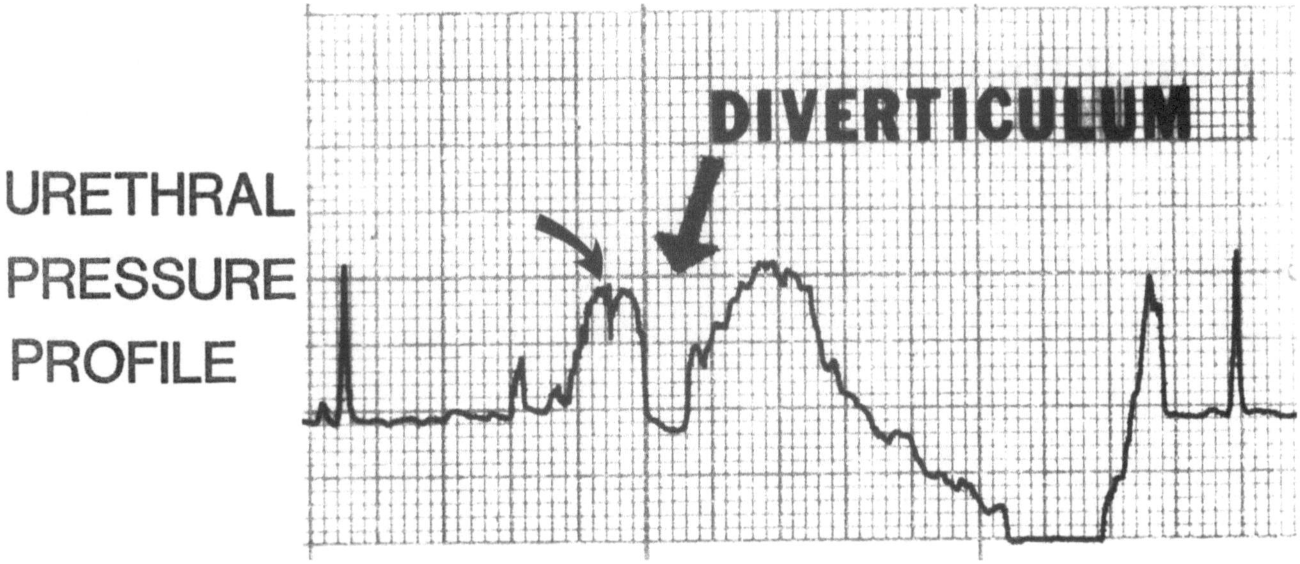


**Fig. 31.1.** Urethral closure pressure profile demonstration of the urethral diverticulum seen in Fig. 31.2.

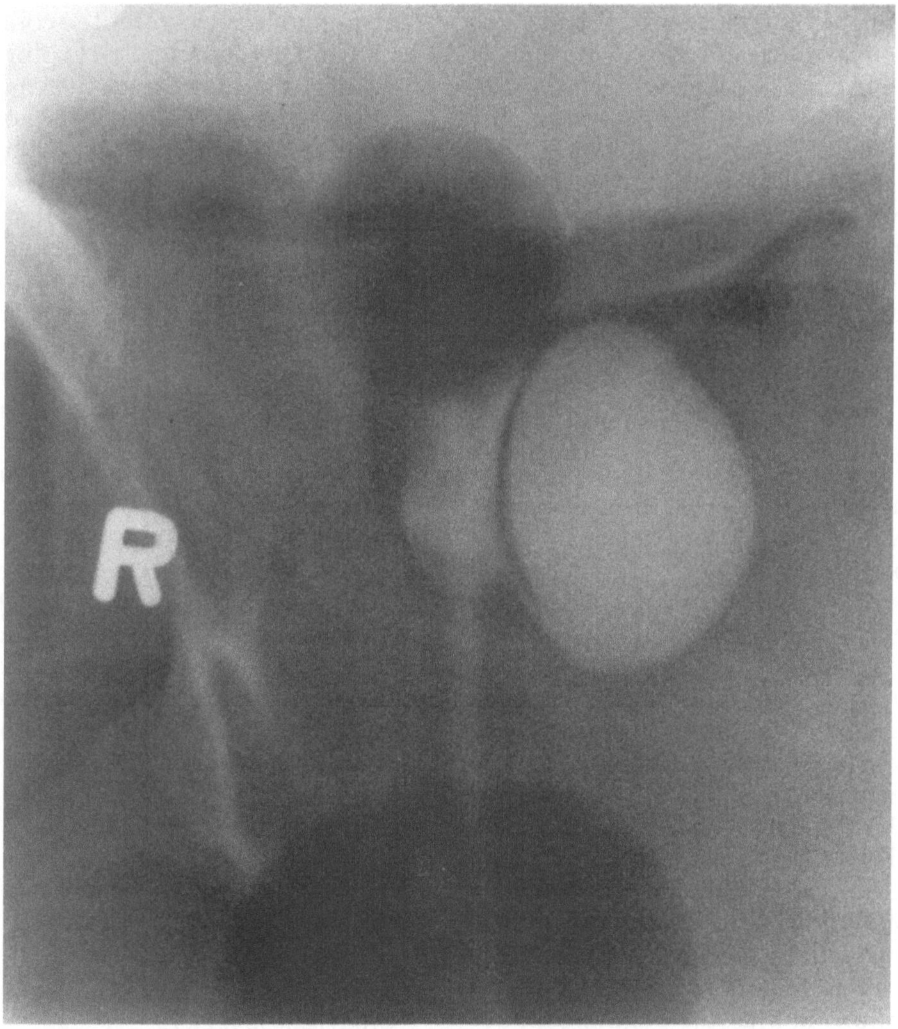


**Fig. 31.2.** Tratner catheter urethrogram showing urethral diverticulum.

# Chapter 32
# Urethral Instability

Urethral instability is defined by most investigators as oscillations in the continuously measured urethral pressure of greater than 15 $cmH_2O$ with or without associated incontinence. Some have defined it statistically in a normal population finding that pressure variation above one-third of the resting maximum urethral pressure should be viewed as abnormal. This definition would raise the pressure threshold to variation greater than 25 $cmH_2O$ before urethral instability was diagnosed. Urethral pressure oscillations must be measured without other confounding variables such as bladder filling, catheter or transducer movement and changes in intra-abdominal pressure. Several investigators have shown that these pressure oscillations come from changes in skeletal muscle activity, smooth muscle activity or a combination of the two. Urethral instability has been associated with symptoms of urgency and frequency as well as with detrusor instability. Where urine loss is due only to urethral relaxation, we prefer to use the term uninhibited urethral relaxation to describe the condition (Chapter 33). Ambulatory urodynamic studies suggest that urethral instability may just be a harbinger of detrusor instability with involuntary bladder contractions eventually being found in almost all of these patients.

In Fig. 32.1 the patient is initially voluntarily squeezing the skeletal component of her urethral sphincteric mechanism during the early filling stages of the cystometrogram. She then voluntarily relaxes the activity of her skeletal sphincter for a short period of time (open arrow). Shortly thereafter, wide variations in pressure begin again but are involuntary. Many of these pressure oscillations are greater than 50 $cmH_2O$. Intermittent leakage results when pressure equalization occurs (curved arrow). These rapid excursions of pressure are no longer under the control of the patient and are now completely involuntary. No concurrent intravesical pressure increases are seen in the true detrusor pressure channel. EMG activity concomitantly increases in a fashion consistent with increased skeletal muscle activity of the pelvic floor. There is an artifactually depressed true detrusor pressure recording which is due to gradually increasing rectal pressure in the presence of stable bladder pressure (arrow).

The true significance of urethral instability is still being debated in the medical literature. The condition may be found in as many as 15% of asymptomatic women who are totally continent. Whether or not this is the beginning of a continuum is unknown. The asymptomatic women may develop urgency, frequency and urge incontinence in the future. The true significance of this condition will only be known as these women are followed longitudinally with urodynamic studies. Alpha blockers, alpha stimulators and central relaxants such as diazepam have been used to treat women who are symptomatic with varying degrees of success.

## Bibliography


Kulseng-Hanssen S: Urethral pressure variations in women with neurourological symptoms: II. Neurourol Urodynam 6:79, 1987.

Kulseng-Hanssen S, Stien R, Fonstelien E: Urethral pres-

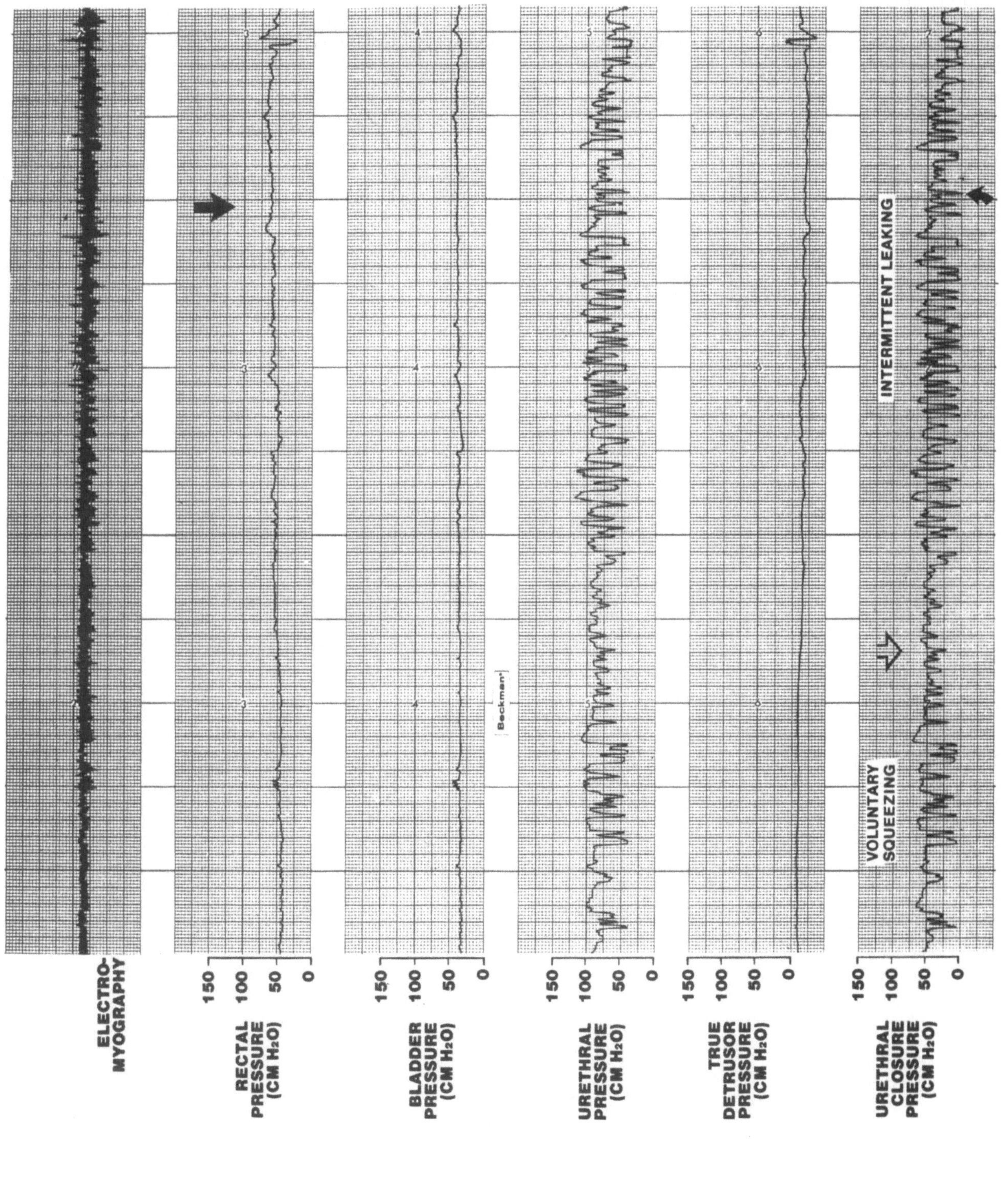


**Fig. 32.1.** Voluntary and involuntary urethral pressure variations in a patient with urethral instability.

sure variations in women with neurourological symptoms: I. Neurourol Urodynam 6:71, 1987.
Raz S, Smith RB: External sphincter spasticity syndrome in female patients. J Urol 115:443, 1976.
Tapp AJS, Cardozo LD, Versi E et al: The prevalence of variation of resting urethral pressure in women and its association with lower urinary tract function. Br J Urol 61:314, 1988.
Ulmsten U, Henriksson L, Iosif S: The unstable female urethra. Am J Obstet Gynecol 144:93, 1982.
Verecken RL, Das J: Urethral instability: related to stress and/or urge incontinence. J Urol 134:698,1985.
Versi E, Cardozo L: Urethral instability: diagnosis based on variation of the maximum urethral pressure in normal climacteric women. Neurourol Urodynam 5:535, 1986.
Weil A, Miege B, Rottenberg R et al: Clinical significance of urethral instability. Obstet Gynecol 68:106,1986.

# Chapter 33
# Uninhibited Urethral Relaxation

Uninhibited urethral relaxation is a rare form of incontinence which may complicate urethral instability. The International Continence Society defines this as a variant of urethral instability. In one large series it was found to be the sole cause of incontinence in 0.3% of cases. It is a condition where the urethra relaxes in the absence of a bladder contraction and results in urinary leakage.

In Fig. 33.1 an isolated episode of urethral instability occurs (arrow) which is followed rapidly by complete urethral relaxation (open arrow). This relaxation is involuntary and results in urine loss. There is no associated detrusor activity as indicated by the absence of pressure increases in the true detrusor pressure channel. There is an artifactually increased true detrusor pressure in this tracing which is consistent and resulting from the unequal recording of abdominal pressure between the rectal and bladder transducers.

Although this is a rare cause of incontinence it must be considered as part of the differential diagnosis of genuine stress incontinence. In order to diagnose uninhibited urethral relaxation definitively the investigator must be careful to rule out associated detrusor instability.

It is unclear whether or not this disorder represents an early stage in a continuum which may culminate in the development of detrusor instability. Treatment of uninhibited urethral relaxation has been successfully accomplished by alpha-adrenergic therapy or anti-incontinence operations.

## Bibliography

McGuire EJ: Reflex urethral instability. Br J Urol 50:200, 1978.

Sand PK, Bowen LW, Ostergard DR: Uninhibited urethral relaxation: an unusual cause of incontinence. Obstet Gynecol 68:645, 1986.

Vereecken RL, Das J: Urethral instability: related to stress and/or urge incontinence? J Urol 134: 698, 1985.

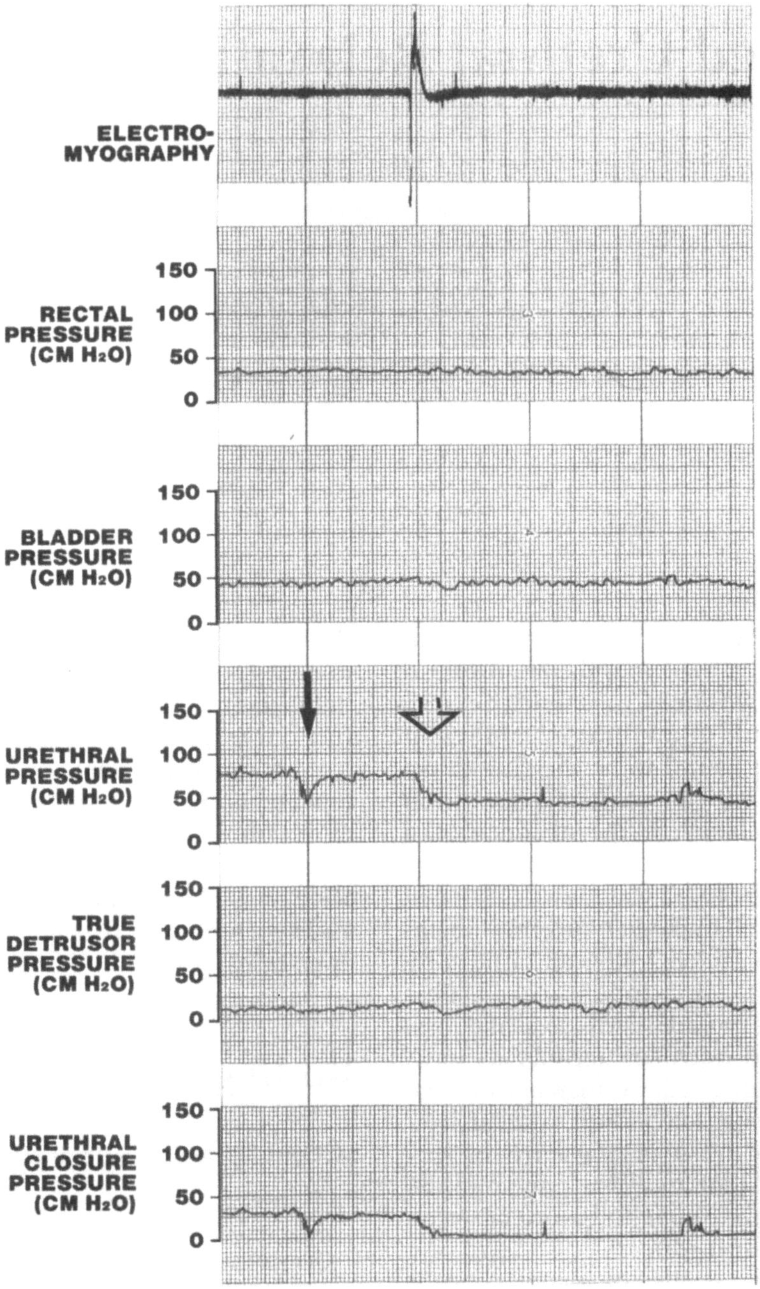


**Fig. 33.1.** Uninhibited urethral relaxation with urinary incontinence.

Section V

# Special Tests

# Chapter 34
# Prolapse Pessary Tests

Urodynamic testing with and without pessaries or other vaginal supports are necessary to evaluate patients who have genital prolapse and associated urethral hypermobility even if they do not complain of urinary stress incontinence. This is particularly important since the prolapse may protect the patient from stress incontinence by a mechanical kinking effect in the urethra during periods of elevated intra-abdominal pressure from coughing or other activities (Chapter 28). Certain patients may apparently develop stress incontinence following surgical repair of their genital prolapse if sufficient attention is not paid to providing permanent support to the urethrovesical junction. Urodynamics with a pessary or other vaginal support is designed to simulate, in the urodynamics laboratory, the surgical correction of genital prolapse without resupporting the bladder neck. Urodynamic evaluation of these patients with and without support of their genital prolapse provides information on urethrovesical function which may guide the surgeon in selecting the most appropriate surgical procedure for that particular patient.

## 34.1 Urodynamic Study Without Pessary

In the example in Fig. 34.1 urethral closure pressure profiles are performed at maximum cystometric capacity while at rest, during rectal squeeze, urethral squeeze, Valsalva and repetitive coughing as previously described (Chapters 15–17). This patient was a 54-year-old mother of two children who had never complained of urinary incontinence but for the past year had noted prolapse of her cervix and proximal anterior vaginal wall to the introitus. Q-tip testing on initial evaluation did not demonstrate hypermobility.

Of major importance is the recognition in the rectal and urethral squeeze profiles of a marked increase in pressure in the distal urethra (small arrows). This dramatic increase of urethral pressure most likely represents a mechanical kinking effect which is only apparent when these maneuvers are performed. Positive pressure transmission is also demonstrated in the Valsalva and cough profiles when compared to the resting profile. This occurs because of the accentuation of the kink from the descending cystocele during increases in intra-abdominal pressure. All maneuvers demonstrate continence.

There are some artifacts in the tracing. The closed curved arrows indicate vaginal pressure waves and the open arrows indicate a minimal Valsalva effort accompanying the urethral and rectal squeeze profiles. The open curved arrows demonstrate the inequality of pressure transmitted between the bladder and the vagina and the effect this has on the true detrusor pressure.

## 34.2 Urodynamic Study with Pessary Demonstrating Continence

Fig. 34.2 demonstrates the changes seen in the same patient as shown in Fig. 34.1 with genital prolapse when a pessary was inserted. The study is normal except for the absence of pressure

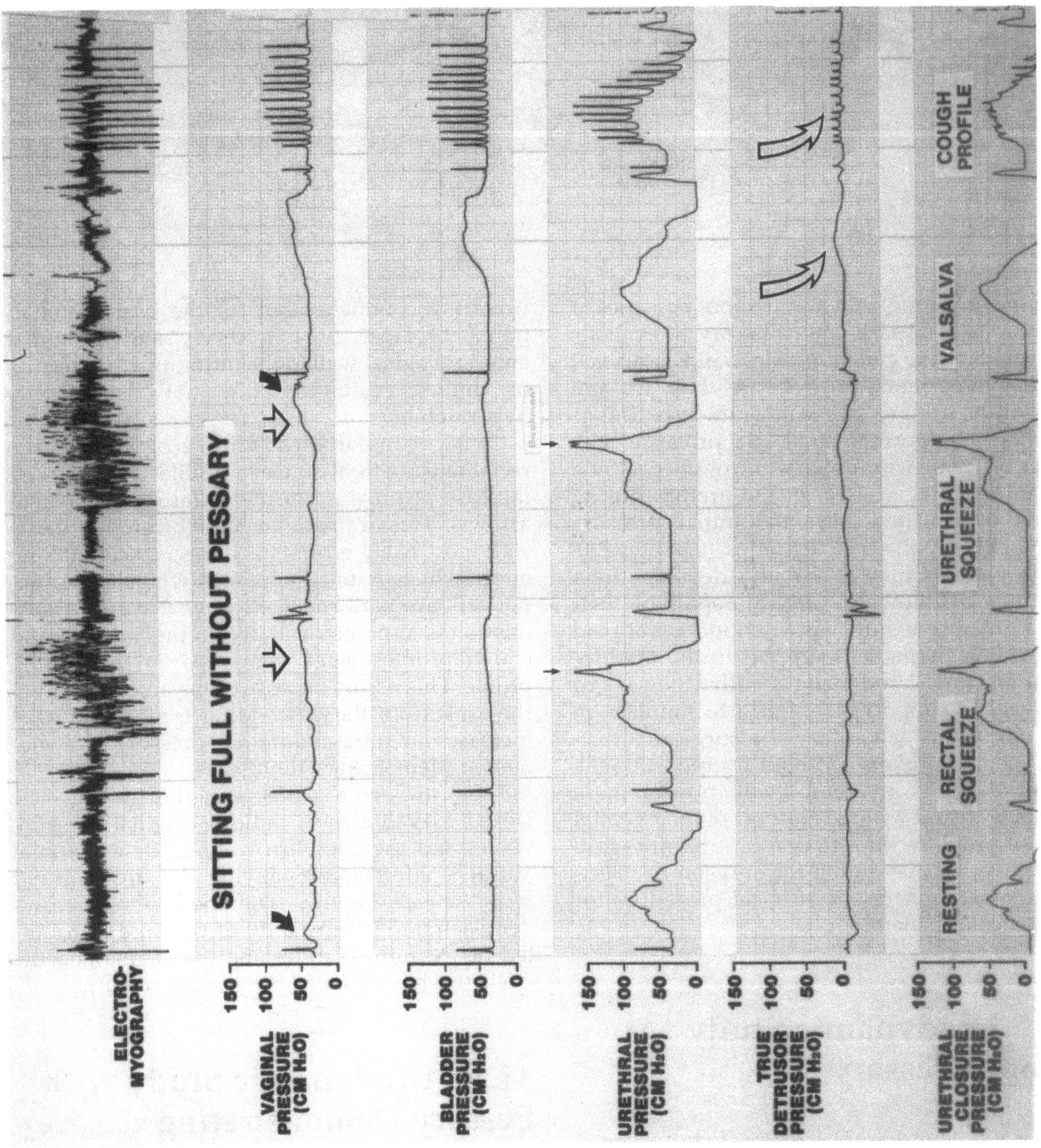


**Fig. 34.1.** Urethral closure pressure profiles in a patient with genital prolapse without a pessary supporting the prolapse.

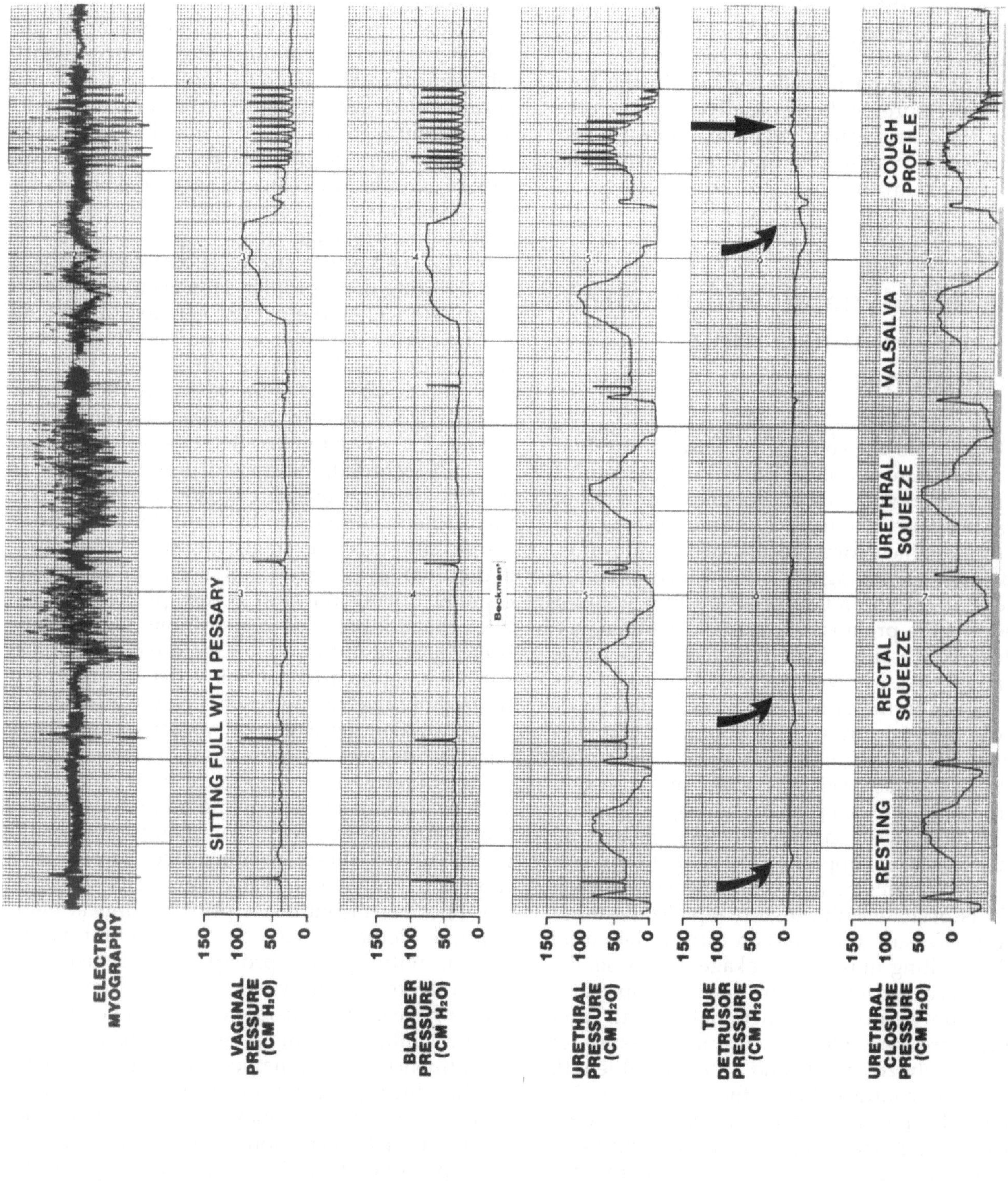


**Fig. 34.2.** Urethral closure pressure profiles in the same continent patient as in Fig. 34.1 with a pessary supporting the prolapse.

augmentation during coughing and Valsalva, but there is positive pressure transmission in the proximal urethra during coughing (small arrow). This might have been expected from her normal urethrovesical junction anatomy without evidence of urethral hypermobility on Q-tip testing.

One minor artifact exists at the arrow. This is a subtraction artifact resulting from the unequal pressure transmission between the bladder and the vagina with positive deflections in the true detrusor pressure. Multiple negative pressure artifacts in the true detrusor pressure are also noted due to small vaginal contractions during the study (curved arrows).

## 34.3 Urodynamic Study with Pessary Demonstrating Incontinence

Fig. 34.3 shows the cough and Valsalva urethral closure pressure profiles of a 42-year-old multiparous woman with and without reduction of her genital prolapse. She has uterine procidentia and a cystocele which comes to the vaginal introitus. She denies ever having any urinary incontinence.

The first cough and Valsalva profiles without support of the prolapse show good maintenance of closure pressure during increases in intra-abdominal pressure with no clear kinking effects such as seen in the previous figures. At the small arrow, a pressure transmission ratio of 98.6% is calculated from the midurethra during the cough profile. In contrast, the large arrow in the second cough profile shows a pressure transmission ratio calculation from the same point along the urethra when a pessary is supporting the genital prolapse. This ratio is calculated as 68.3% in comparison and is associated with pressure equalization and negative pressure transmission during the entire profile resulting in urinary leakage. Likewise, the first Valsalva profile shown here demonstrates good maintenance of functional length and urethral pressure with a closure pressure of approximately 28 $cmH_2O$ and a functional length of 22 mm. In contrast, during the second Valsalva profile with a pessary in place, the patient is noted to have a functional length and closure pressure of zero resulting in a large amount of urinary leakage. These profiles, with and without support of the genital prolapse, demonstrate the presence of potential genuine stress incontinence in this patient. Although she does not complain of urinary incontinence initially, testing with support of the prolapse to remove any potential mechanical obstruction at the bladder neck or along the urethra, reveals the presence of genuine stress incontinence due to negative pressure transmission with pressure equalization. Had such testing not been done, the patient may have undergone corrective surgery for her genital prolapse and had considerable genuine stress incontinence following this. However, the proper performance of urethral closure pressure profiles with support of the genital prolapse, either using a pessary, Sim's speculum or proctoswabs, reveals the presence of genuine stress incontinence and allows for simultaneous surgical correction of the problem to avoid urinary leakage.

In Fig. 34.3, there are no subtraction artifacts noted during these profiles. However, in the rectal pressure channel, the patient is noted to have no tracing during the first cough profile. This channel was inadvertently turned off during the first recorded urethral closure pressure profile and then switched on during the Valsalva profile that followed. Despite the fact that this rectal pressure was not recorded, subtracted pressures, such as the true detrusor pressure which is dependent on this value, continued to be accurately measured. Thus, although the registration of the intra-abdominal pressure is not seen on the rectal channel during the first cough profile, we can infer that its pressure registrations would have been identical to those found in the bladder pressure channel because there is a flat line recorded throughout the true detrusor pressure tracing.

The patient with genital prolapse may have varying degrees of prolapse of the bladder, rectum, uterus or the presence of an enterocele with or without accompanying urethral hypermobility. Any patient who complaints of incontinence under these circumstances deserves a thorough urodynamic evaluation to determine the nature of her incontinence prior to surgical intervention. Perhaps even more important is the patient with genital prolapse associated with urethral hypermobility who does not complain of incontinence. Due consideration must be given to the possibility that this patient is protected from incontinence by a mechanical kinking effect in her urethra during stress. If this is not recognized the urethrovesical junction may not be well supported by the surgical correction of her genital prolapse and postoperative incontinence may result. Urodynamics with and without support of the prolapse will determine whether or not the patient will develop incontinence (potential genuine stress incontinence) and will guide the

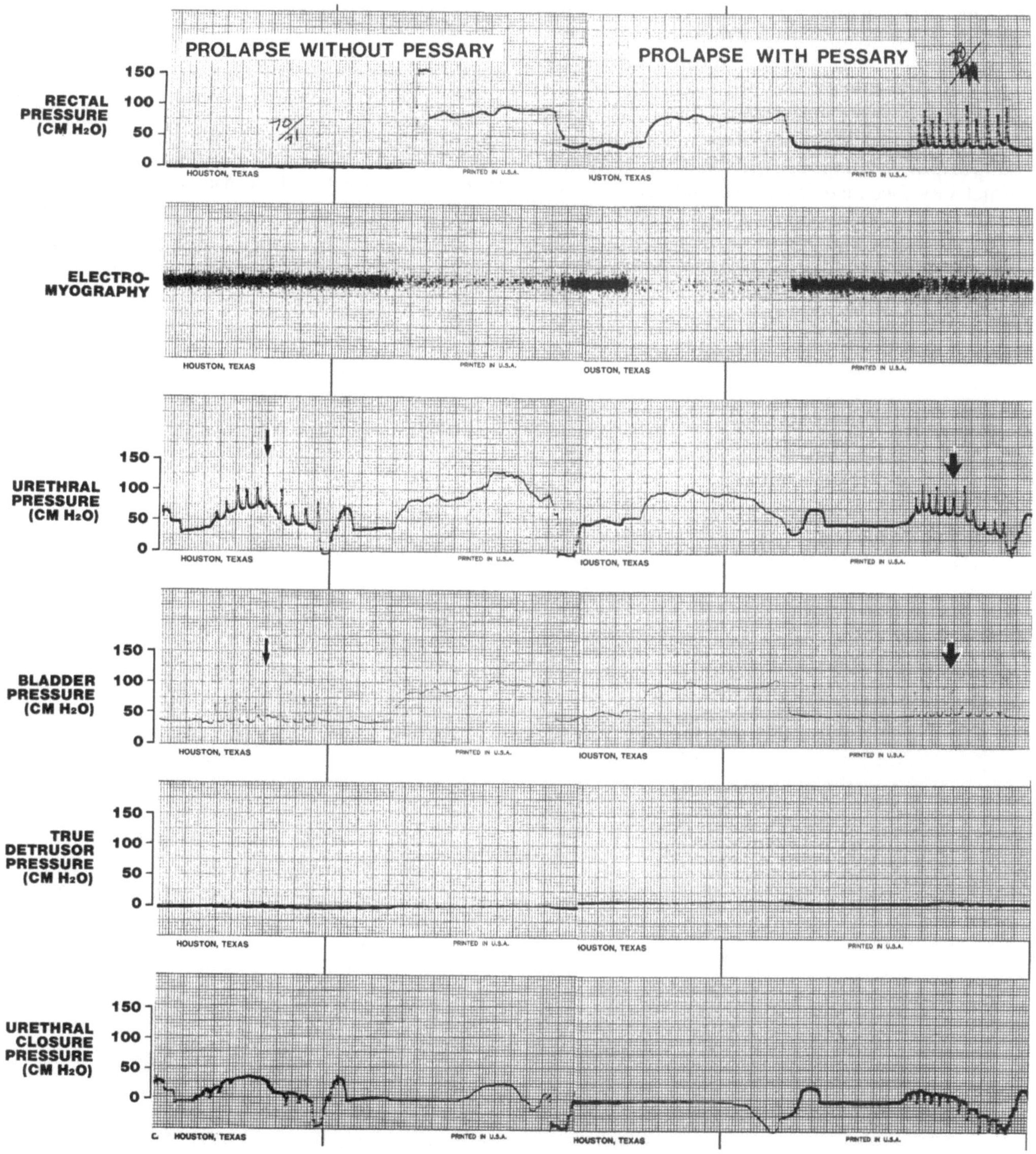


**Fig. 34.3.** Dynamic urethral closure pressure profiles in a patient with genital prolapse and potential genuine stress incontinence with and without pessary support.

surgeon to the performance of the most appropriate surgical procedure. Such urodynamic investigations may also reveal hidden detrusor instability in women with prolapse who do not complain of urge incontinence but may have symptoms of frequency, urgency and nocturia. It is important to diagnose this hidden detrusor overactivity because long-term neglect of this condition may lead to ureteral reflux or detrusor decompensation and retention due to repetitive high pressure involuntary bladder contractions against an obstructed bladder neck.

## Bibliography

Bowen LW, Sand PK, Ostergard DR: Urodynamic effects of a vaginal pessary in women with genital prolapse, paper presented at the Seventh Annual Meeting of the Gynecologic Urology Society, Montreal, Canada, October, 1986.

Hertogs K, Stanton SL: Mechanism of urinary continence after colposuspension: barrier studies. Br J Obstet Gynaecol 92:1184,1985.

Richardson DA, Bent AE, Ostergard DR: The effect of uterovaginal prolapse on urethral pressure dynamics. Am J Obstet Gynecol 146:901, 1983.

Chapter 35

# Urethral Denervation Testing

This test relies on Cannon's hypothesis that a denervated organ becomes hypersensitive to its neurotransmitter. Since the urethra is primarily an alpha-adrenergic organ, its denervation should produce a hypersensitivity to alpha-adrenergic stimulants. This hypersensitivity should be reflected in a higher urethral pressure in the urethral closure pressure profile after administration of the drug compared to the baseline urethral pressure. The drug used in testing is ethylphenylephrine in a usual dosage of 4 mg IV. Urethral closure pressure profiles are obtained before and after its administration for comparison. An increase of 15 $cmH_2O$ is considered positive and evidence of denervation of the urethra.

## 35.1 Baseline Profiles

In Fig. 35.1 the urethral closure pressure before the drug has been administered is 20 $cmH_2O$ in these two resting profiles. The only artifacts in the tracing are the rhythmic pressure decreases seen in the true detrusor pressure channel, the first three of which are represented by the small arrows. These result from vaginal peristaltic movements as seen in the vaginal pressure channel (curved arrow). The very small regular oscillations in pressure seen in the bladder pressure channel throughout the study are from respiratory activity.

## 35.2 Alpha-Adrenergic Profiles

Five minutes after the administration of the alpha-adrenergic stimulant the closure pressure increases to 35–40 $cmH_2O$. In Fig. 35.2 this pressure increase indicates the denervated nature of this urethra. The only artifact in the tracing is the increased urethral pressure induced by Valsalva during the performance of the first profile (arrow). This causes a mild decrease in closure pressure in the first profile compared to the second. Note the absence of significant pressure variations in the true detrusor pressure tracing.

This is one approach to the diagnosis of urethral denervation. Another more direct approach is in the measurement of specific EMG patterns in the skeletal component of the urethral sphincteric mechanism. The diagnosis can be made directly when fibrillation potentials and other evidence of denervation can be found. It has been recently reported that 80% of patients with stress incontinence may have evidence of urethral denervation. The very important question is then raised as to

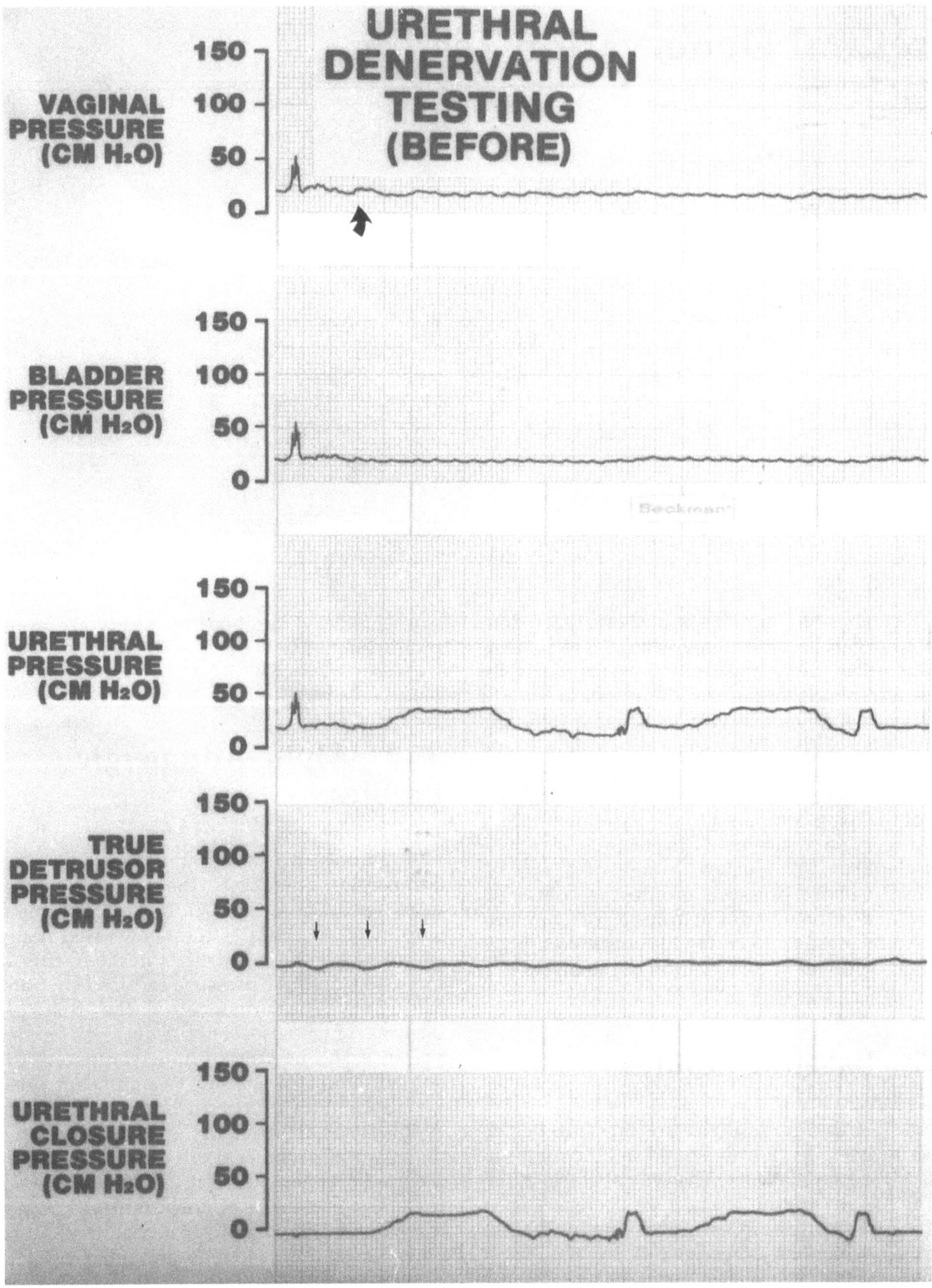


**Fig. 35.1.** Urethral closure pressure profiles in a patient with urethral denervation before ethylphenylephrine testing.

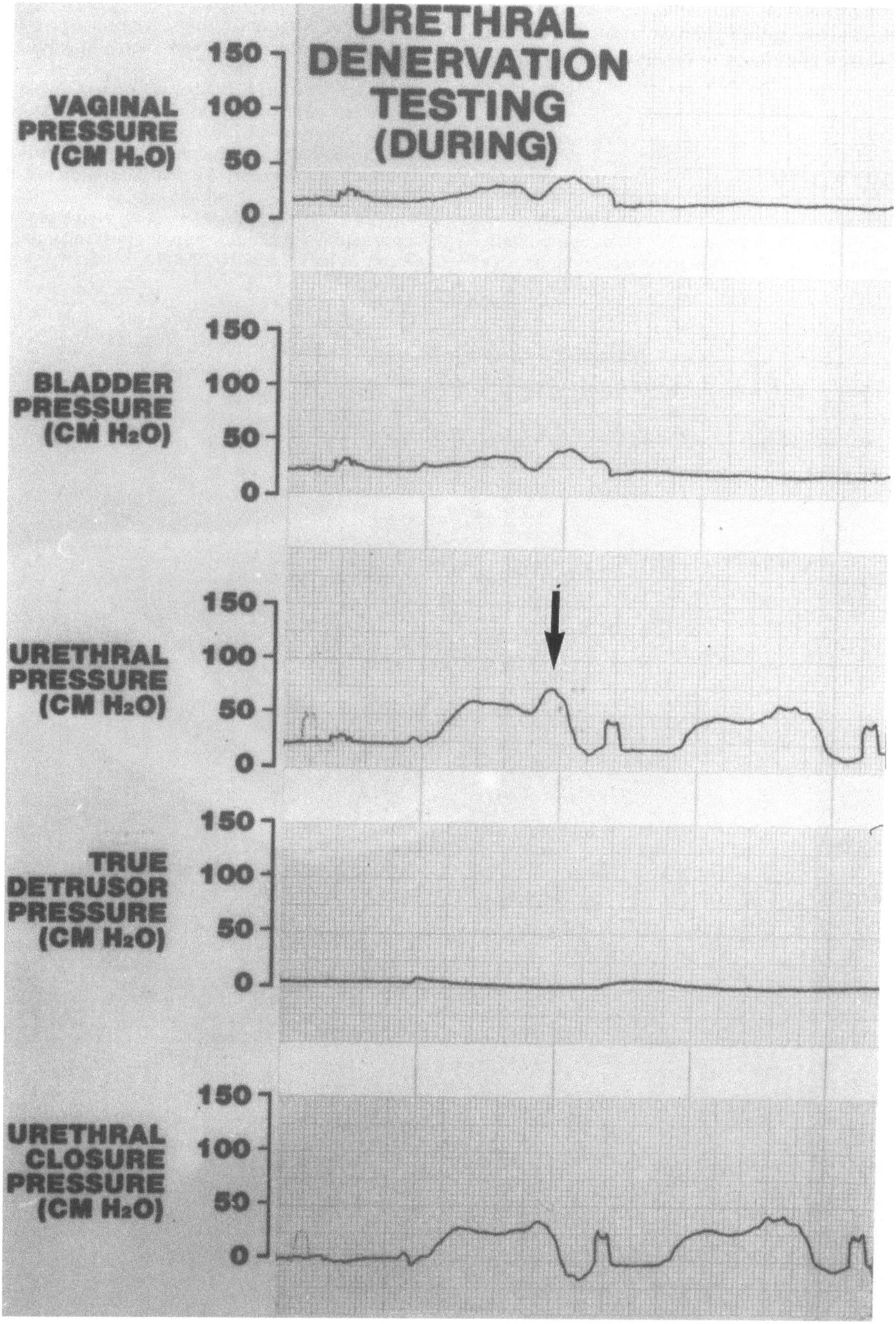


**Fig. 35.2.** Urethral closure pressure profiles in a patient with urethral denervation after ethylphenylephrine administration (same patient as in Fig. 35.1).

whether or not stress incontinence is primarily a neurologic disease rather than an anatomical one. Future research is needed to resolve this issue.

## Bibliography

Awad SA, Downie JW, Lywood DW et al: Sympathetic activity in the proximal urethra in patients with urinary obstruction. J Urol 115:545, 1976.

Cannon WB, Rosenbleauth A: The supersensitivity of denervated structures. New York, Macmillan, 1949, pp. 96–105.

Fanciullacci F, Sandri S, Politi P et al: Sacral evoked potentials in normal women and in women with stress incontinence. Neurourol Urodynam 6:321, 1987.

Snooks SJ, Badenoch DF, Tiptaft RC et al: Perineal nerve damage in genuine stress urinary incontinence. Br J Urol 57:422, 1985.

Varma JS, Fidas A, McInnes A et al: Neurophysiological abnormalities in genuine female stress incontinence. Br J Obstet Gynaecol 95:705, 1988.

# Chapter 36
# Vesical Denervation Testing

This test is similar to urethral denervation testing in that it relies on Cannon's hypothesis that a denervated end organ will give an exaggerated response when re-exposed to its neural transmitter. The test is performed to identify detrusor areflexia in cases of decentralization of the bladder. The test is performed by first obtaining a baseline cystometrogram. This is followed by the administration of 0.03 mg/kg of bethanecol chloride subcutaneously. The usual dose is 2.5 mg. Bethanecol should not be used in patients with asthma, cardiac disease or hyperthyroidism as it may induce bronchospasm, hypotension and atrial fibrillation in these patients. A second postadministration cystometrogram is done 30 min later. Alternatively, the intravesical pressure can be measured continuously after the introduction of a known amount of fluid into the bladder. Recording continues until an increase of 15 $cmH_2O$ occurs or 30 min has passed. A test is considered positive with either method when an increase in detrusor pressure of 15 $cmH_2O$ or more occurs. It is a fairly accurate test for diagnosing detrusor denervation in most series.

In Fig. 36.1 the bladder pressure gradually increases from the arrow and reaches a peak of 15 $cmH_2O$ as seen at the open arrow in the true detrusor pressure channel. Minimal fluctuations of pressure occur in the urethral pressure and urethral closure pressure channels which are of no significance.

Although a pressure rise of 15 $cmH_2O$ is the established criterion for diagnosis of a denervated detrusor, interpretation can be difficult. Rarely is a detrusor so totally denervated that an unequivocally positive test results. The denervation is often partial and may not be detected by the test resulting in a false negative rate as high as 50% in one study.

## Bibliography


Blaivas J, Sabid K, Michalik S et al: Failure of bethanecol denervation supersensitivity test as a diagnostic aid. J Urol 123:199, 1980.

Diokno A, Davis R, Lapides J: Urocholine test for denervated bladders. Invest Urol 13:233, 1975.

Glahn BE: Neurogenic bladder diagnosed pharmacologically on the basis of denervation supersensitivity. Scand J Urol Nephrol 4:13, 1970.

Lidi A, Dykstra D, Peng W: Bethanecol supersensitivity test, rhabdosphincter electromyography, and bulbocavernosus reflex latency in the diagnosis of neuropathic detrusor areflexia. J Urol 140:335, 1988.

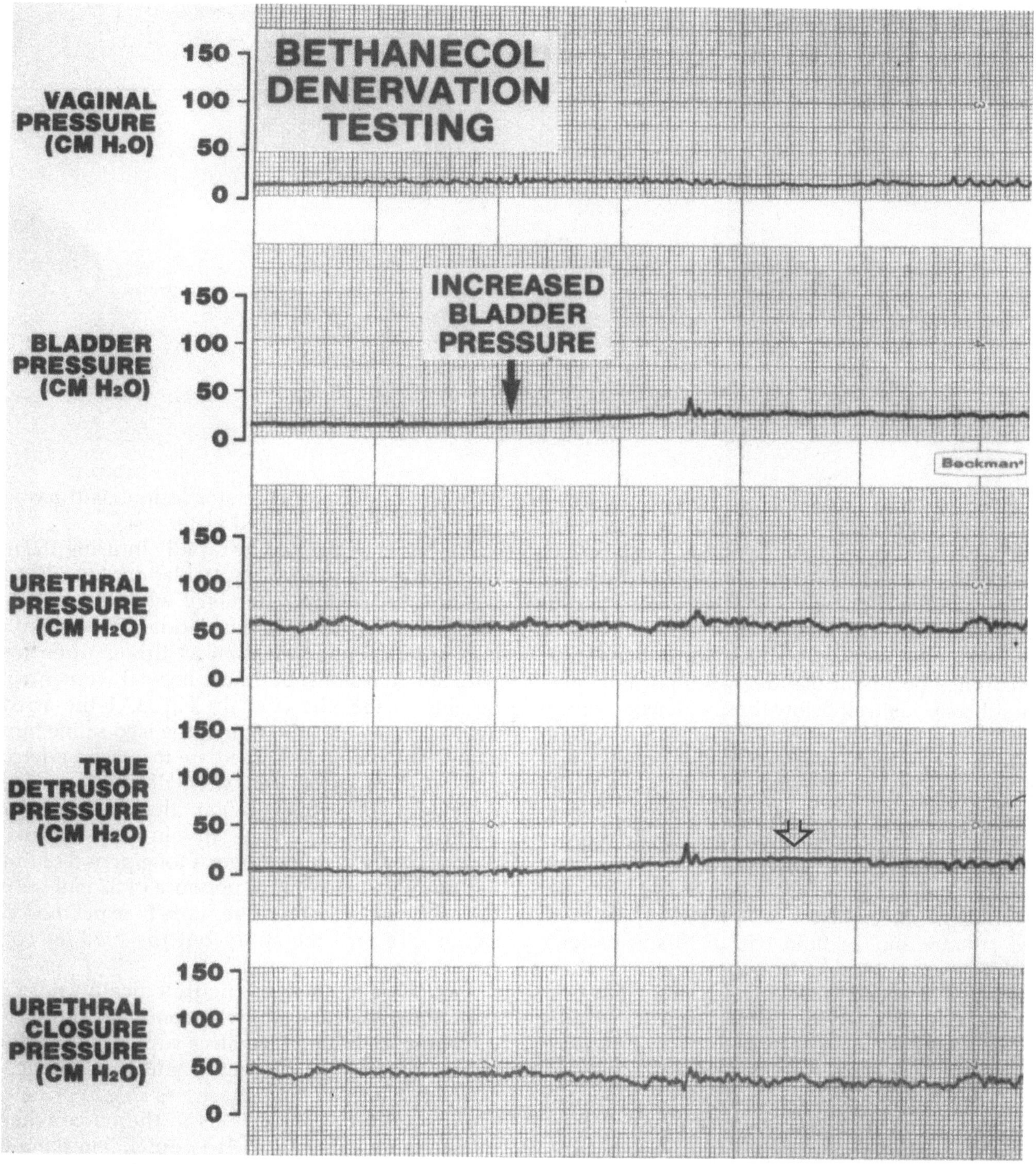


**Fig. 36.1.** Detrusor denervation testing using bethanechol during urethrocystometry.

# Chapter 37
# The Bladder Cooling Test

It is well recognized that people, especially those with detrusor overactivity, will note an increase in urinary urgency and frequency when exposed to cold. Studies in felines have demonstrated specific cold receptors in the bladder which when stimulated with low volumes of an iced solution will trigger an immediate bladder emptying reflex. This reflex occurs at bladder volumes and pressure thresholds well below those of tension receptors in the bladder suggesting an afferent limb different from that associated with the micturition reflex and detrusor overactivity. Bors originally described the classical ice water test in 1956 to distinguish between parasympathetic upper motor neuron lesions and lower motor neuron lesions. Instillation of 100 ml of sterile ice water through an 18F catheter led to rapid expulsion of the catheter and/or fluid within 10 s in patients with suprasacral lesions but was negative in those with sacral or peripheral lesions. The test has been modified to a urodynamic test from its simpler original clinical version over the years to avoid missing low pressure-evoked contractions and false negative tests caused by the presence of detrusor sphincter dyssynergia in many of these patients with detrusor hyperreflexia. It is still a simple test that should be negative in normal individuals but does not appear to distinguish clearly between patients with detrusor instability and detrusor hyperreflexia. In addition, it is not as accurate in distinguishing between upper and lower motor neuron disease largely because not all women with upper motor lesions will have a positive iced saline or iced water test.

The test is performed by rapidly infusing 100 ml of saline at 0°C into an empty bladder over 20 s at the time of urethrocystometry while monitoring the pressure increase in the bladder. The patient is also asked about sensation as this is often lost with spinal lesions, but most normal women will be able to feel the cold. In Fig. 37.1 the arrow demonstrates the initiation of the iced saline infusion with an almost immediate increase in detrusor pressure associated with delayed urethral relaxation (curved arrow) in this woman with detrusor instability. The involuntary detrusor contraction is sustained over a long period of time and reaches a maximum pressure of 37 $cmH_2O$ at the open curved arrow. She starts to expel the iced saline 12 s into the study but the bladder continues to contract throughout.

This woman was a neurologically normal patient on clinical exam who complained of urge incontinence but had negative supine, sitting and standing urethrocystometry studies. The iced saline or bladder cooling test was able to provoke the involuntary contractions in the office where other maneuvers failed. It is quick, simple and easy to perform with or without urodynamic monitoring and may help detect detrusor instability where urethrocystometry cannot. The bladder cooling test may also be used to try to distinguish between upper and lower motor neuron lesions.

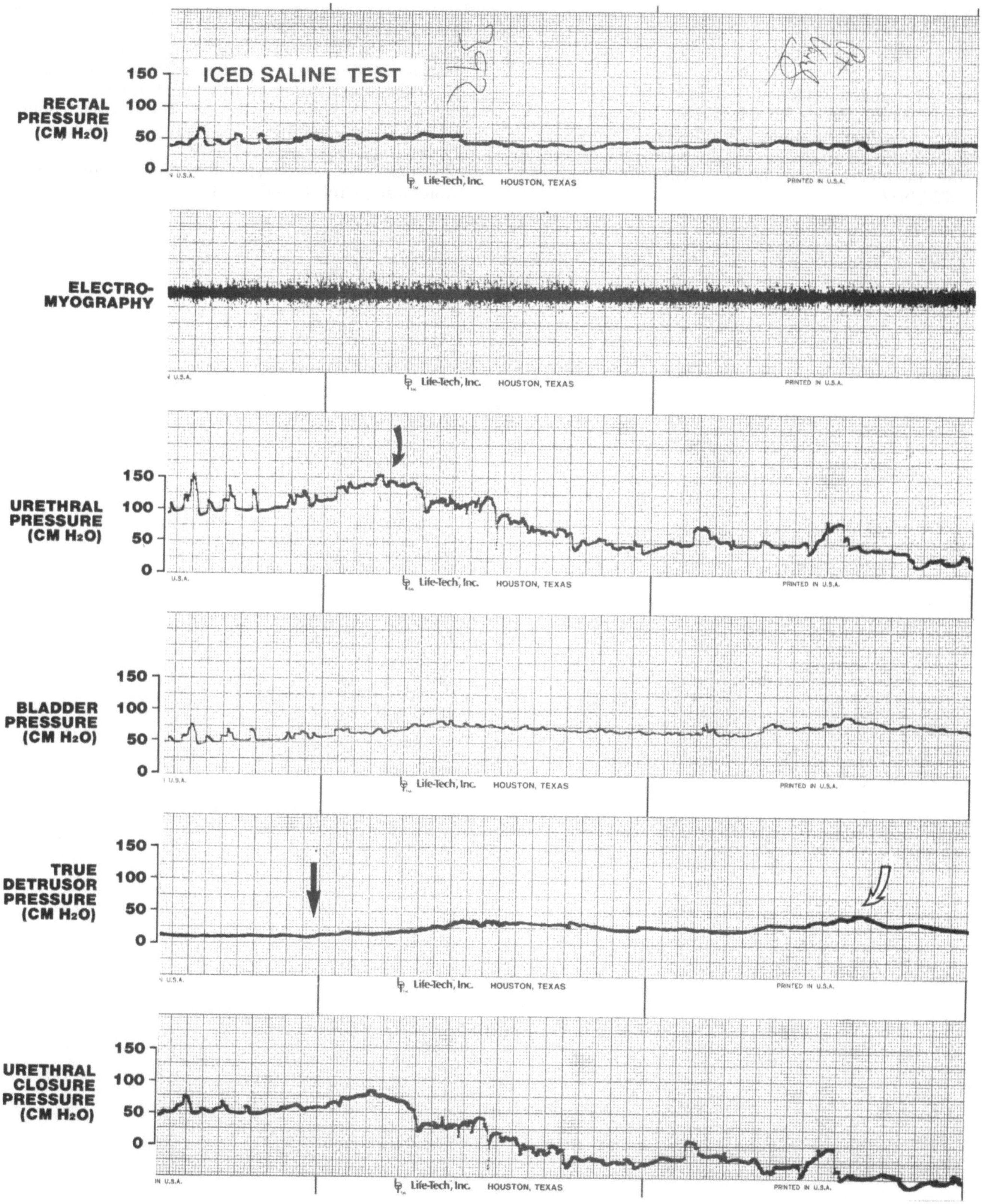


**Fig. 37.1.** The bladder cooling test with iced saline infusion to detect detrusor overactivity.

# Bibliography

Bors E: Neurogenic bladder. Urol Surv 7:177, 1957.

Bors E, Ma KT, Parker RB: Observations on some modalities of bladder sensation. J Urol 76:566, 1956.

Fall M, Lindstrom S, Mazieres L: Experimental aspects on the bladder cooling reflex. Neurourol Urodynam 6:228,1987.

Hellstrom PA, Tammela TLJ: The bladder cooling test. Int Urogynecol J 4:116, 1993.

Hellstrom PA, Tammela TLJ, Kontturi MJ et al: The bladder cooling test for urodynamic assessment: analysis of 400 examinations. Br J Urol 67:275, 1991.

Lindstrom S, Mazieres L, Fall M: The bladder cooling reflex: characterization of afferent mechanisms. Neurourol Urodynam 7:248, 1988.

Raz S: Objective assessment of bladder response in ice water test. J Urol 109:603, 1973.

Chapter 38

# The Stop Test

The stop test demonstrates isometric detrusor contractions in situations where the pressure generated by a detrusor contraction cannot be measured under ordinary circumstances. Pressure recording under such conditions is not possible due to the absence of urethral resistance with unobstructed free flow through the bladder neck. This test allows for the observation of the hidden contraction and the measurement of the intravesical pressure it generates. This test is helpful when it is important to know precisely whether or not the detrusor is actually contracting.

The test is performed during a voiding effort when the patient is asked to stop her urinary stream. The patient responds by increasing urethral closure pressure through a voluntary contraction of her pelvic floor musculature. This increases urethral resistance. Since the detrusor is now contracting against a closed bladder neck a pressure rise is seen in the true detrusor pressure which is due to the recording of the isometric detrusor contraction. Alternatively, urinary flow can be stopped by mechanical digital compression of the urethra.

In Fig. 38.1 the patient's voiding effort begins at the curved arrow with urethral relaxation. Simultaneously the patient begins a Valsalva effort (open curved arrow). Urine flow continues until the distal urethra is mechanically obstructed by digital pressure at the external meatus (open arrow). The isometric bladder contraction becomes immediately evident (arrow) and measures 45 $cmH_2O$. Prior to obstruction of the urethra it appeared that the patient was voiding by Valsalva without a bladder contraction. But the bladder contraction is present throughout the voiding effort even though unregistered until the bladder neck was obstructed.

## Bibliography

Coolsaet BLRA: Cystometry. In Stanton SL (ed) Clinical gynecologic urology. St Louis, CV Mosby, 1984, pp. 59–81.

Frigerio L, Ferrari A, Candiani GB: The significance of the stop test in female urinary incontinence. Diagn Gynecol Obstet 3:301, 1981.

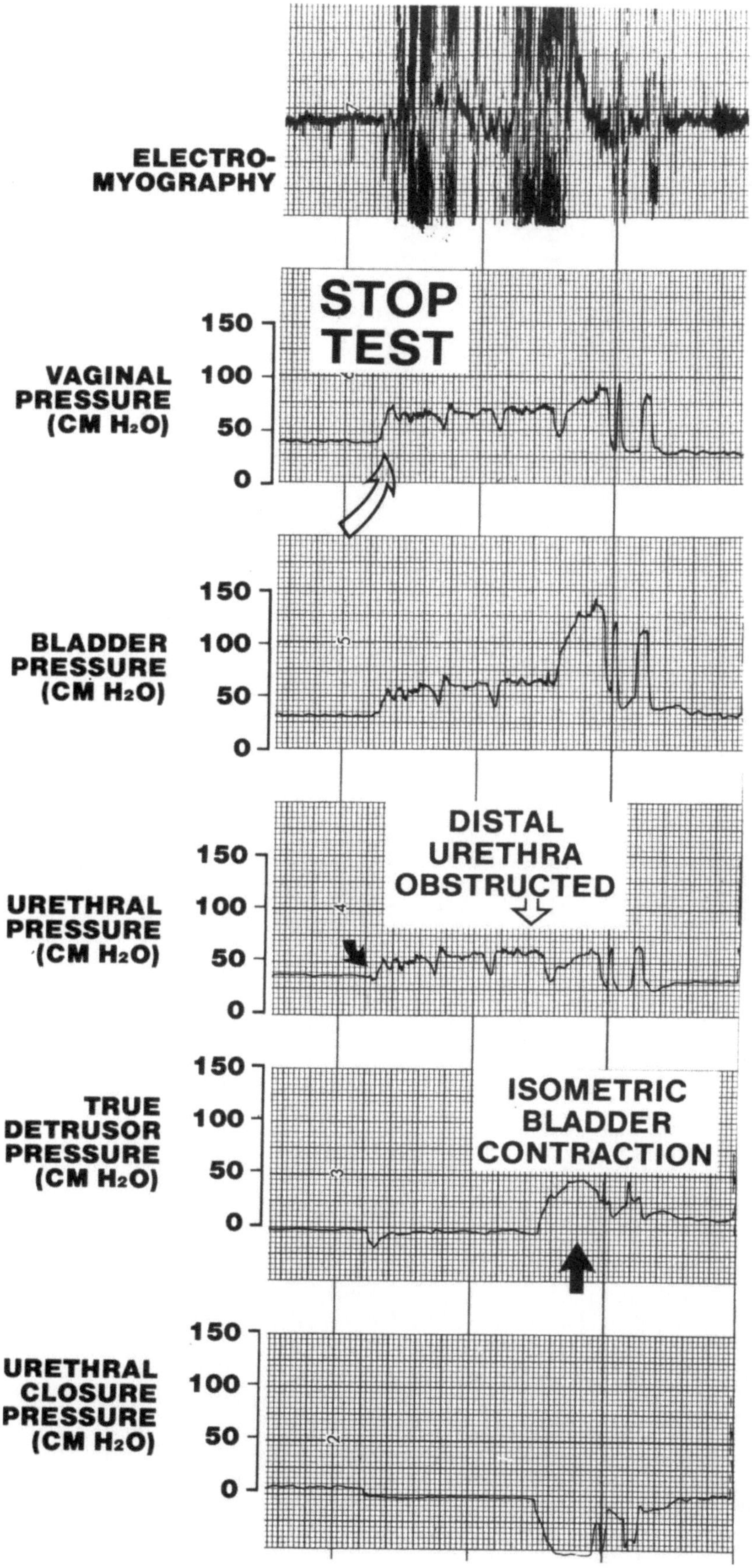


**Fig. 38.1.** The stop test during a voiding pressure study to detect the isometric bladder contraction.

# Chapter 39
# Pelvic Floor Stimulation: Effect on Detrusor Activity

Electrical stimulation of the pelvic muscles has been used for over 25 years to control detrusor overactivity and genuine stress incontinence. From studies in cats, it is believed that the mechanism of detrusor inhibition is through reflex inhibition of the pelvic nerve after stimulating afferently along the pudendal nerve. This mechanism takes advantage of the vesicoinhibitory reflexes which allow one to stop a bladder contraction at the end of micturition by contracting the periurethral skeletal muscle. Transvaginal and transanal electrical stimulation has been reported to be successful in improving or curing detrusor overactivity in up to 90% of patients.

The effects of pelvic floor stimulation on the detrusor may be evaluated with multichannel urethrocystometry studies as described in Chapter 20. The patient in Fig. 39.1 was noted on a prior urethrocystometry study to have involuntary uninhibited detrusor contractions occurring at a bladder volume of around 200 ml. During this study, the urethral pressure transducer has been placed in the mid urethra where it registers a low urethral closure pressure of 12 cm$H_2O$ (Chapter 20). The bladder pressure at the beginning of the study is also about 10 cm$H_2O$ with the true detrusor pressure zeroed at the beginning of the study. During the study water is progressively infused into the bladder, as is routinely done during urethrocystometry, to a maximum capacity of 500 ml at the end of the study. Meanwhile, the patient is being given alternating pulses of electrical energy through a transvaginal electrical stimulator set at a frequency of 10 Hz. With each stimulus the amperage is progressively increased to a maximum of 90 mA (as shown in the top electromyography channel), at which point the patient feels discomfort from the stimulation. One millisecond alternating stimulus pulses are given for 5 s with a 5 s rest period in between. This office technique of acute maximal stimulation may be used for therapy or as a screening study. When it is used for therapy, repetitive sessions are done weekly for 20–30 min with the stimulator for six weeks. This particular study was being done to evaluate whether this patient would be a good candidate for chronic home stimulation with a device and method similar to that described in Appendix A, p. 180. Results during this initial 30 min stimulation period show that the patient had a significant increase in her maximal cystometric capacity and suppression of her involuntary bladder contractions, thus making her a good candidate for pelvic floor stimulation.

Also, of interest is the change in urethral pressure with progressive stimulation. This will be discussed in the next chapter but this urodynamic tracing demonstrates a marked increase in urethral closure pressure which rises during stimulation from 12 cm$H_2O$ up to 90 cm$H_2O$ (arrow).

Small negative changes are seen in the true detrusor pressure throughout the study (small arrows) which are caused by increases in rectal pressure caused by the 5 s pulses of electrical stimulation which cause the rectum to contract. This technique may also be used in patients with fecal incontinence.

Urethrocystometry may be used to monitor the effect of pelvic floor stimulation in the treatment of detrusor instability. Studies may be done

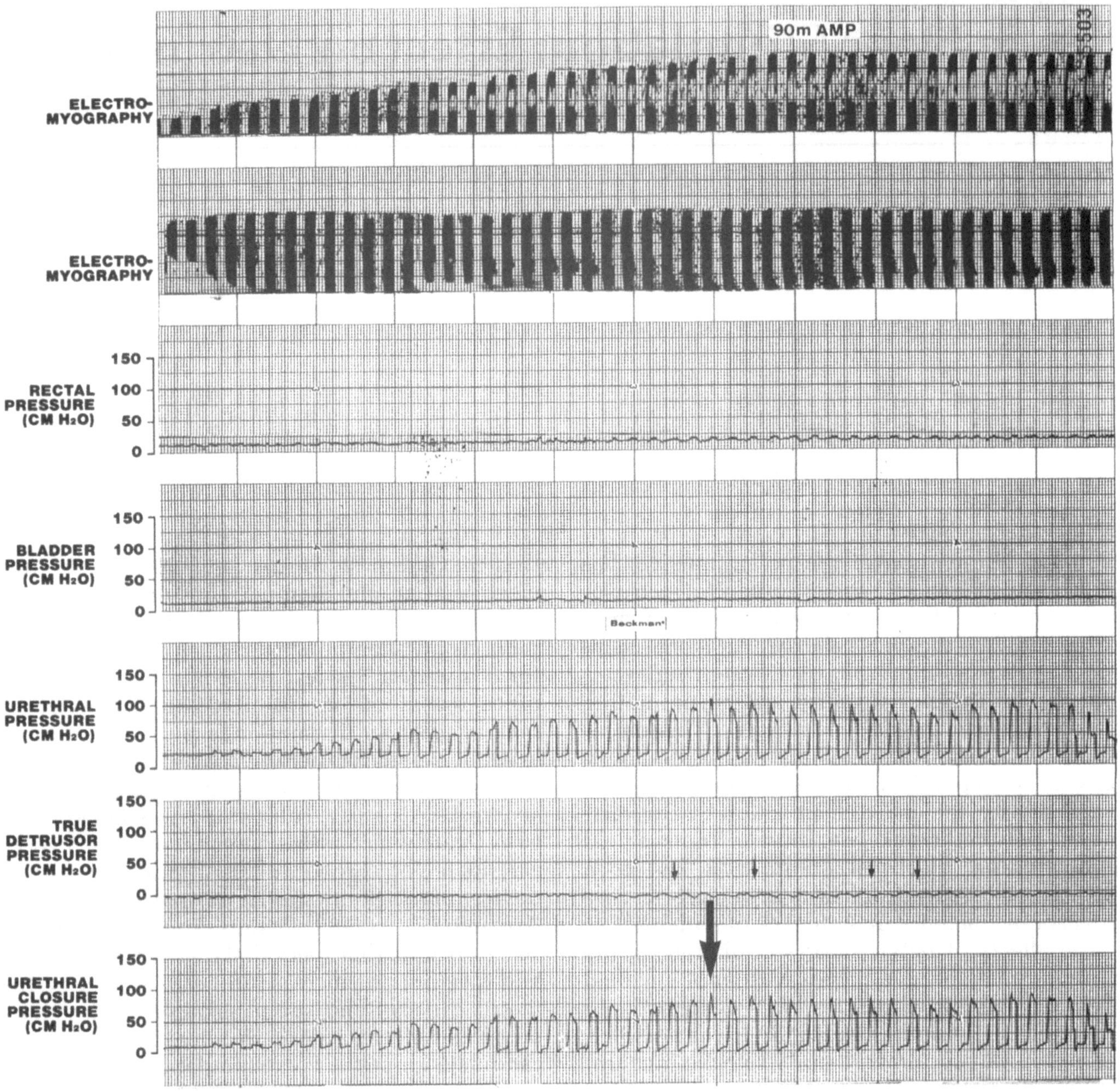


**Fig. 39.1.** Acute maximal functional electrical stimulation during urethrocystometry to treat detrusor overactivity and genuine stress incontinence with a low pressure urethra.

during electrical stimulation such as seen here or they may be done following a 20–30 min session of electrical stimulation to document poststimulation detrusor suppression.

## Bibliography

Eriksen BC, Bergmann S, Eik-Nes SH: Maximal electrostimulation of the pelvic floor in female idiopathic detrusor instability and urge incontinence. Neurourol Urodynam 8:219, 1989.

Jonasson A, Larsson B, Pschera H et al: Short term maximal electrical stimulation – a conservative treatment of urinary incontinence. Gynecol Obstet Invest 30:120, 1990.

Kralj B: Selection of female patients for treatment with functional electrical stimulation (FES). Urogynaecologica 1:41, 1985.

Lindstrom S, Fall M, Carlsson CA et al: The neurophysiological basis of bladder inhibition in response to intravaginal electrical stimulation. J Urol 129:405, 1983.

Nakamura M, Sukarai T, Sugsoh et al: Maximal electrical stimulation for urge incontinence. Urol Int 42:285, 1987.

Vereecken RL, Das J, Grisar P: Electrical sphincter stimulation in the treatment of detrusor hyperreflexia of paraplegics. Neurourol Urodynam 3:145, 1984.

Vodusek DB, Light JK, Libby JM: Detrusor inhibition induced by stimulation of pudendal nerve afferents. Neurourol Urodynam 5:381, 1986.

Chapter 40

# Pelvic Floor Stimulation: Effect on Urethral Closure Pressure Profile

Pelvic floor stimulation (as discussed in Appendix A) can be utilized to treat not only detrusor overactivity but also genuine stress incontinence. It is believed that the primary effect of electrical stimulation for treatment of genuine stress incontinence is to cause activation of the pelvic floor and periurethral musculature via the pudendal nerve. Repetitively contracting the skeletal muscle around the urethra should create muscular hypertrophy with increasing muscle strength. This translates into an increase in intraluminal urethral pressure with intra-abdominal pressure elevations. Similar to physiotherapy with progressive resistance exercises, it allows patients to develop strong guarding reflexes to prevent leakage of urine with anticipated voluntary increases in intra-abdominal pressure.

Fig. 40.1 shows the traces from a patient being studied in the supine position with a relatively empty bladder (150 ml) before and during electrical stimulation with a Contelle® (Crafon Medical AB, Lund, Sweden) inflatable pessary stimulator. This is one of numerous stimulators which have been used successfully to relieve genuine stress incontinence in 30%–60% of patients. Initially, two urethral closure pressure profiles are done at rest as described previously in Chapter 15 and the patient is noted to have a closure pressure of 18 $cmH_2O$ with a functional urethral length of 11 mm. The second two urethral closure pressure profiles are done with a Contelle® device activated in the vagina. In this situation the patient is noted to have an increase in closure pressure to 25 $cmH_2O$ and an increase in functional urethral length to 15 mm.

An acute change such as this suggests that pelvic floor stimulation is able to activate the voluntary skeletal muscle of the pelvic floor leading to an elevation of the intraluminal urethral pressure. One would assume, from this study that this patient might benefit from continued electrical stimulation with an improved response to rises in intra-abdominal pressure with resolution or improvement of her genuine stress incontinence.

Of interest during this study is the rectal peristalsis that is noted during the measurement of all four urethral closure pressure profiles. This variation in the rectal pressure is also reflected in the calculation of the true detrusor pressure where the patient is noted to have pressure variations of up to 25 $cmH_2O$ (arrow). We know that this does not represent involuntary detrusor activity during this study because examination of the bladder pressure channel shows no such pressure increases. The pressure increases in bladder pressure occur only with coughing at the beginning of the pressure profiles (small arrows). This artifact is due to rectal peristalsis as described in Chapter 44.

## Bibliography

Eriksen BC, Eik-Nes SA: Long-term electrostimulation of the pelvic floor: primary therapy in female stress incontinence? Urol Int 44:90, 1989.

Fall M, Ahlstrom K, Carlsson CA et al: Contelle: pelvic floor stimulation for female stress-urge incontinence. Urology 17:282, 1986.

Hahn I, Sonmar S, Fall M: A comparative study of pelvic floor training and electrical stimulation for the treatment of genuine stress urinary incontinence. Neurourol Urodynam 10:545, 1991.

Plevnik S, Janez J, Urtacnik P et al: Short-term electrical stimulation: home treatment for urinary incontinence. World J Urol 4:24, 1986.

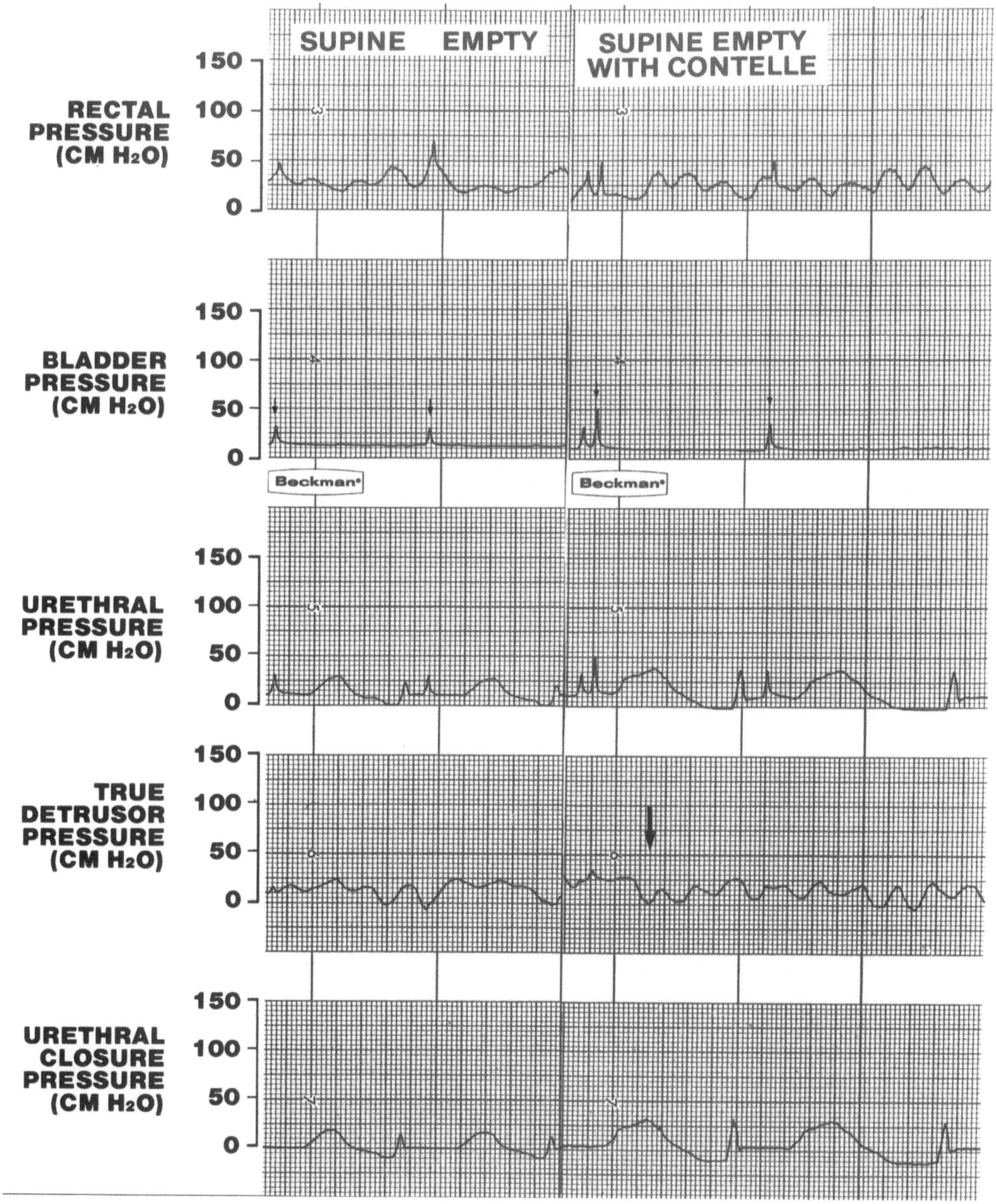


**Fig. 40.1.** Resting urethral closure pressure profiles before and during pelvic floor stimulation.

Chapter 41

# The Effect of Hypogastric Nerve Block on Detrusor Instability

When all medical therapies for detrusor instability have failed partial denervation of the detrusor by surgical hypogastric nerve resection may be indicated for some patients. Although good results may be obtained in up to 90% of selected patients initially, recurrences are frequent in these and other nerve resections or neurologic procedures. If hypogastric nerve resection or phenol injection is to be considered, preliminary evaluation of the patient with unilateral and bilateral hypogastric nerve blocks is indicated to determine the anticipated response of the detrusor muscle to surgical resection or phenol injection of these nerves. Assessment of detrusor function during filling and micturition is accomplished after anesthetic nerve block to look for resolution of detrusor overactivity and to rule out detrusor areflexia.

In Fig. 41.1 the bladder is filled during a sitting urethrocystometry study before hypogastric nerve block. After a cough (arrow) urethral instability becomes evident with wide, prolonged decreases in urethral closure pressure without coincident vesical pressure increases. Uninhibited detrusor contractions begin at a volume of 200 ml during bladder filling (open arrow) with concomitant urethral relaxation (curved arrow). Further filling of the bladder is not possible.

After a bilateral hypogastric nerve block (Fig. 41.2) bladder filling to 500 ml is accomplished without evidence of detrusor contractions or urethral instability. It is anticipated that such a patient would have a good therapeutic response to partial hypogastric nerve resection with resolution of her detrusor overactivity. Periodic coughing, running water and handwashing fail to trigger any involuntary contractions in this study. At the arrow the urethral transducer is moved to record maximal urethral pressure.

The hypogastric nerve block is performed by injection of 5 ml of local anesthetic solution into the bladder pillars. If the cervix is present injections are done at 10 and 2 o'clock relative to the cervix about 1–2 cm deep. If the cervix is absent, the approximate location of the urethrovesical junction is determined and the same solution is injected at 4 and 7 o'clock position about 1 cm posterior to the urethrovesical junction and about 5 mm deep. After giving the block unilaterally, the cystometrogram is repeated. The patient is then asked to void and the residual urine volume is determined by catheterization. This procedure is repeated after bilateral blockade. The residual urine determination is particularly important to detect those patients who may not be able to void after the procedure and who will require intermittent self-catheterization on a permanent basis if a denervation procedure is performed.

## Bibliography

Hogdkinson CP: Intravesical nerve resection for detrusor dyssynergia. The Ingelman–Sundberg operation. Acta Obstet Gynecol Scand 56:401, 1976.

Ingelman-Sundberg A: Partial bladder denervation for detrusor dyssynergia. Clin Obstet Gynecol 21:797, 1978.

Mundy AR: The surgical treatment of detrusor instability. Neurourol Urodynam 4:357, 1985.

Murray K, Mundy AR, Blackford HN et al: Transvesical phenolization of the pelvic plexuses: a simple technique for the treatment of refractory detrusor instability and hyperreflexia. Urol Int 41:202, 1986.

Torrens MJ: The role of denervation in the treatment of detrusor instability. Neurourol Urodynam 4:353, 1985.

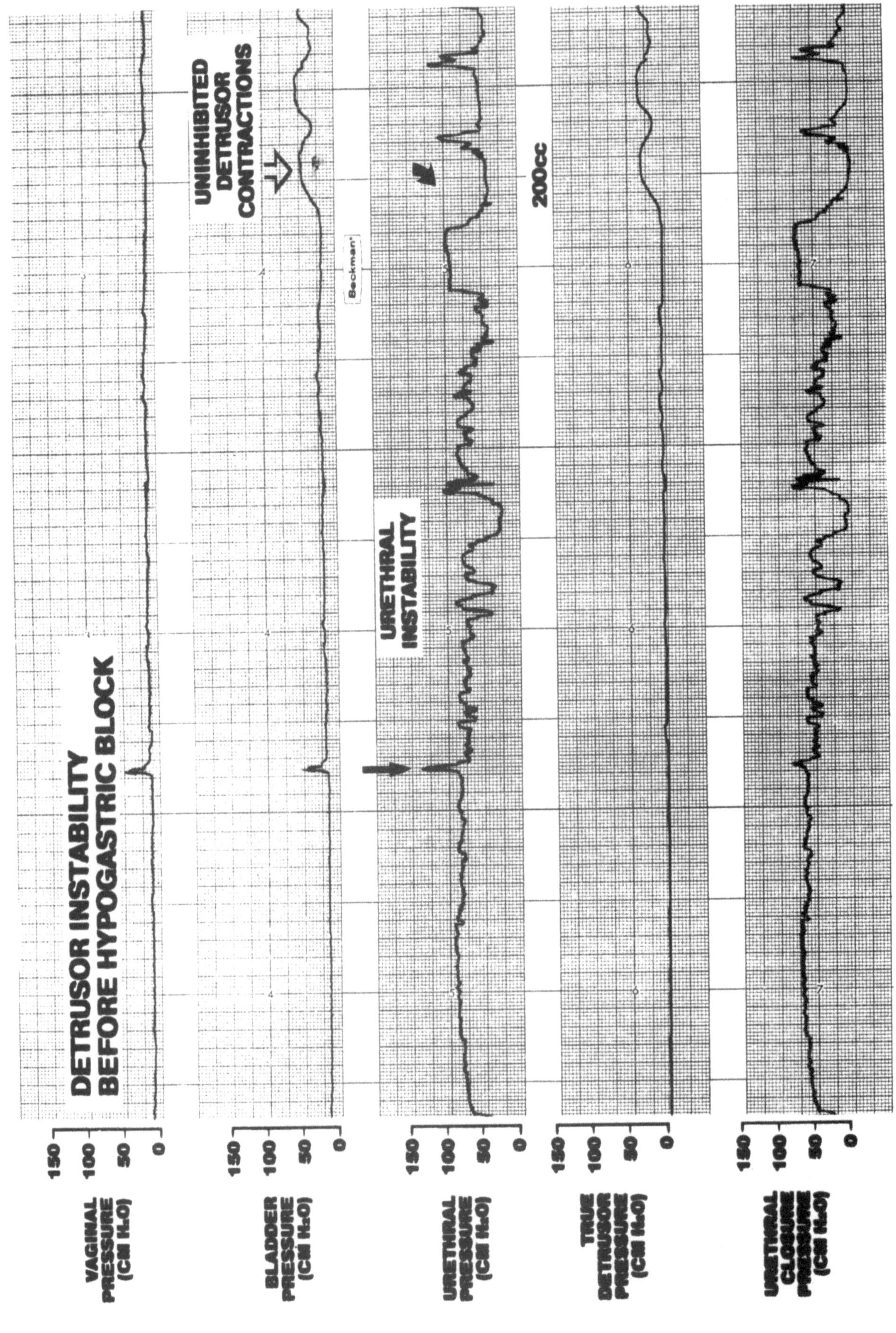


**Fig. 41.1.** Urethrocystometry in a patient with detrusor instability prior to hypogastric anesthetic block.

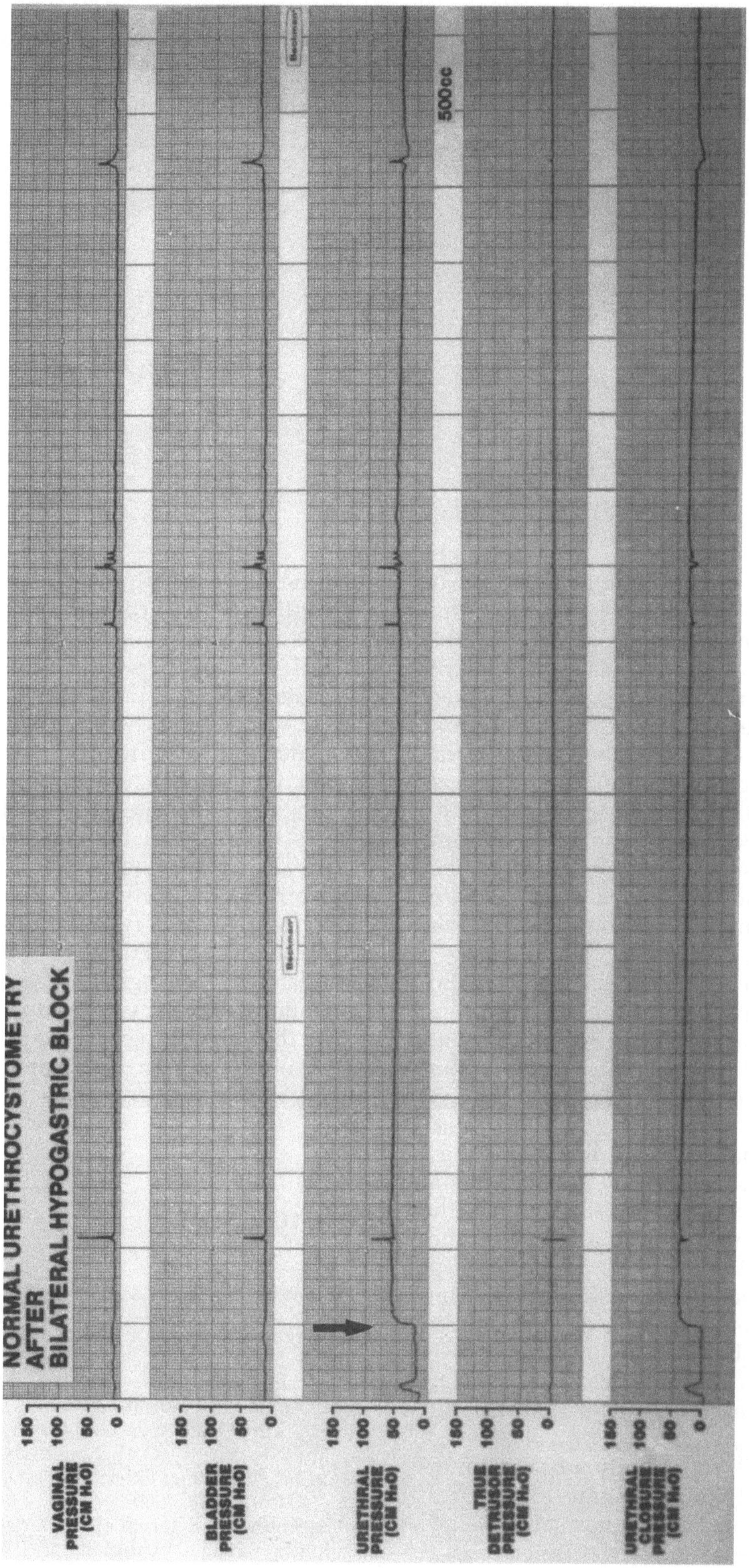


**Fig. 41.2.** Normal urethrocystometry following hypogastric block in the same patient as in Fig. 41.1.

Chapter 42

# The Effect of Pudendal Block on the Urethral Closure Pressure Profile

Certain patients will present with irritative lower urinary tract symptoms that defy conventional therapies. Under these circumstances, urodynamic evaluation may reveal a marked elevation of the urethral closure pressure suggesting overactivity of one of the components of the urethral sphincteric mechanism. Frequently it is the voluntary skeletal muscle component which is responsible. By performing a bilateral pudendal block, the contribution of the skeletal muscle to the urethral sphincteric mechanism can be determined.

Fig. 42.1 demonstrates two urethral closure pressure profiles in the sitting position at maximum cystometric capacity before doing a pudendal block. The closure pressure is 130 $cmH_2O$ (arrow). Vascular pulsations (open arrow) can be seen at peak pressure which are coincident with the cardiac rate. Note the true detrusor pressure channel where the baseline is not properly placed on the chart paper.

Fig. 42.2 shows that the urethral closure pressure has decreased to 35 $cmH_2O$ after pudendal block indicating that the contribution of the voluntary skeletal muscle to the urethral sphincteric mechanism is 95 $cmH_2O$. Note the improperly located baselines in each pressure measuring channel (curved open arrows). Zero pressure in each channel should be keyed to the zero point on the graph recorder or computer screen at the start of each tracing and each channel should be read with this in mind.

Considering the 73% contribution of the voluntary skeletal muscle to total urethral closure pressure (which is far more than its normal 30%–35% contribution) treatment should be directed toward lowering this skeletal muscle spasm. This can be accomplished by central relaxants such as diazepam given in a short two-week dosage schedule. Diazepam should be used with caution due to its hepatic toxicity. Alpha blockers, smooth muscle relaxants and true skeletal muscle relaxants, such as baclofen may be used to relax the urethra. Biofeedback may also be useful in lowering this voluntary skeletal muscle activity. Local sources of irritation and chronic inflammation should also be searched for and treated, such as, urethrotrigonitis, chronic cystitis, urethral diverticula, intravesical foreign bodies, and interstitial cystitis. Elevated urethral pressures may also be secondary to an exaggerated guarding reflex in association with detrusor instability. It is apparent that a thorough urogynecological evaluation is essential to provide for proper diagnosis and therapy in these patients.

## Bibliography

Gerstenberg TC, Lykkegaard Nielsen M, Lindenberg J: Spastic striated external sphincter syndrome imitating recurrent urinary tract infection in females. Eur Urol 9:87, 1983.

Hebert DB, Francis LN, Ostergard DR: Significance of urethral vascular pulsations in genuine urinary incontinence. Am J Obstet Gynecol 144:828, 1982.

Kaplan WE, Firlit CG, Schoenberg HW: The female urethral syndrome: external sphincter spasm as etiology. J Urol 124:48, 1980.

Raz S, Smith RB: External sphincter spasticity syndrome in female patients. J Urol 115:443, 1976.

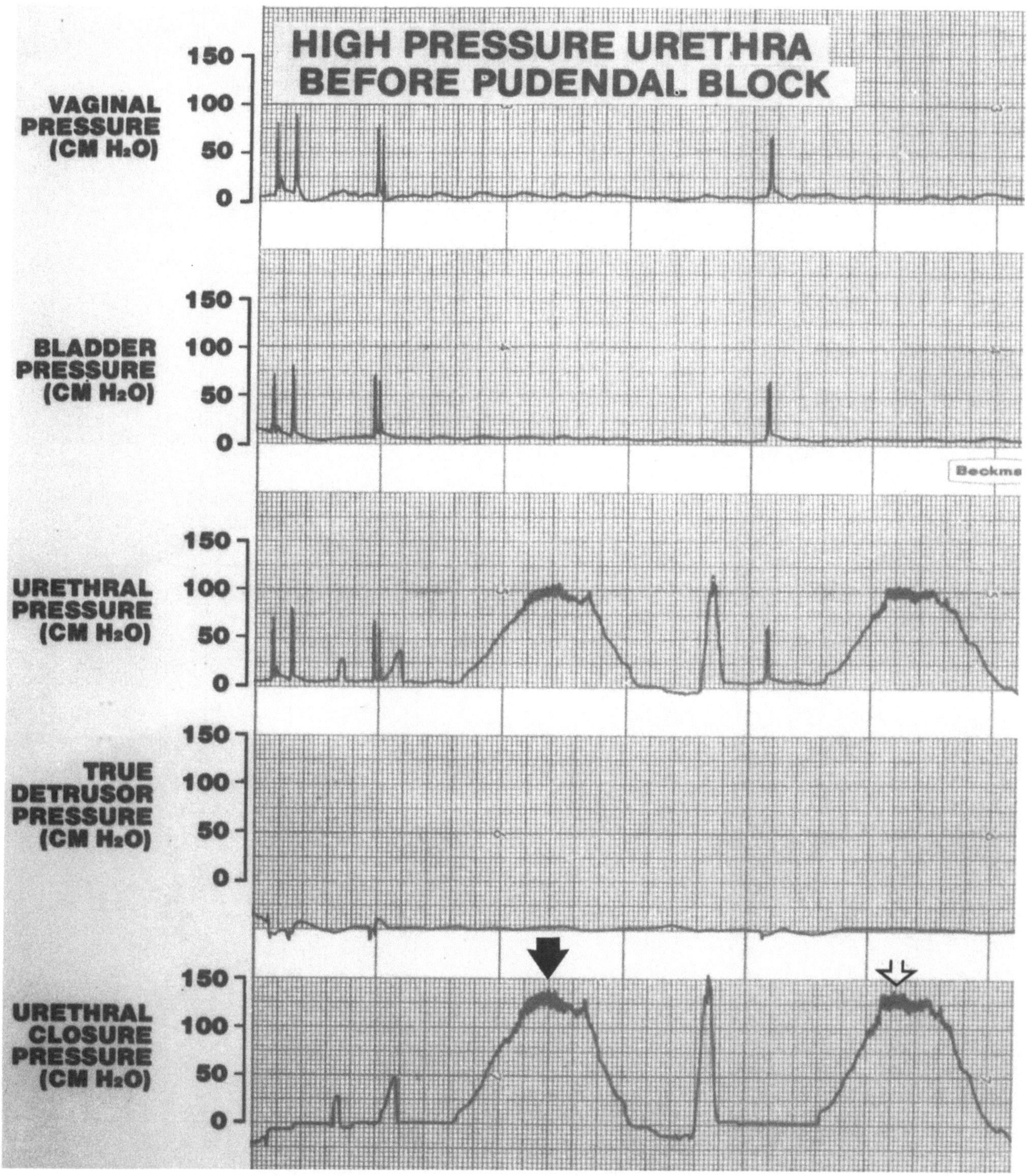


**Fig. 42.1.** Urethral closure pressure profiles before pudendal block.

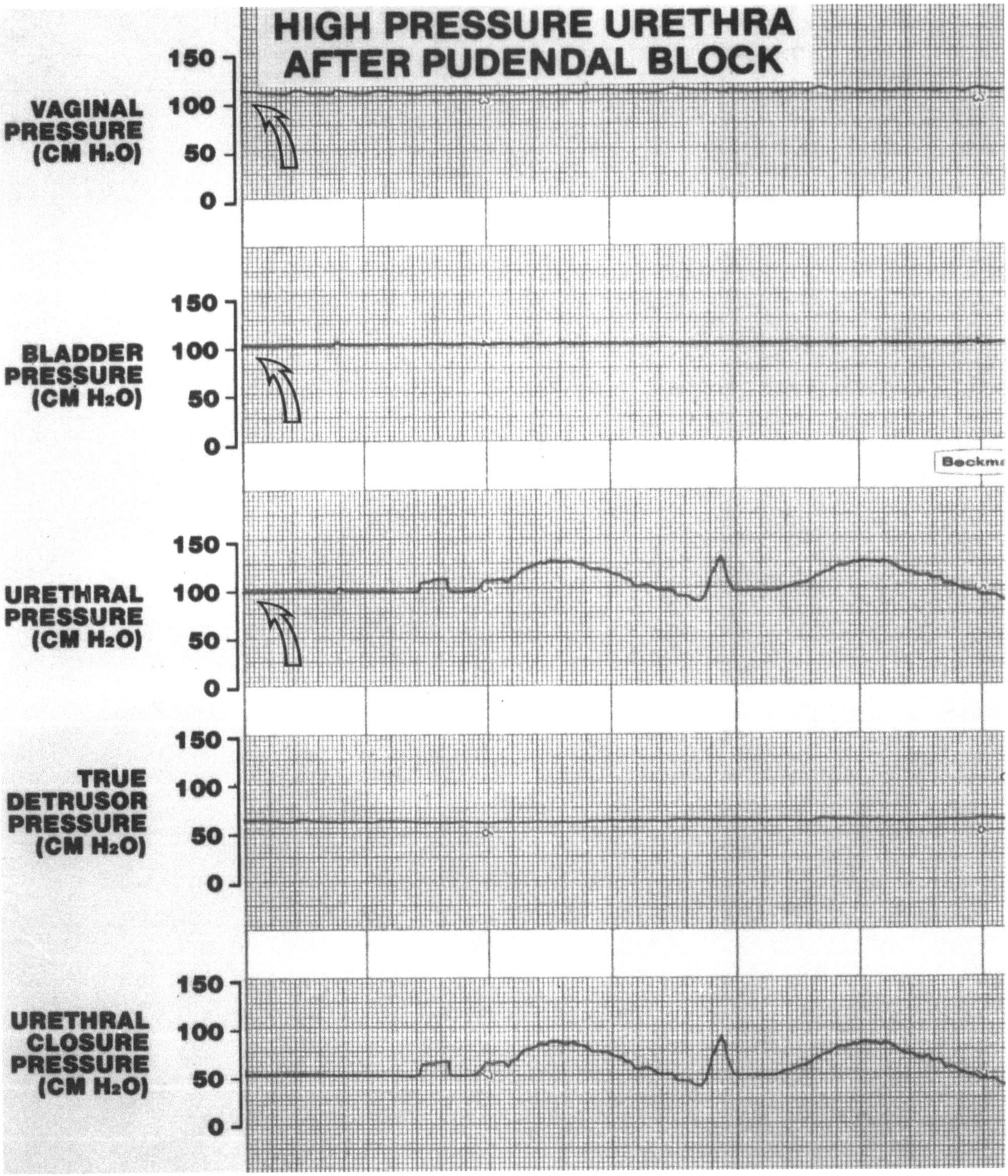


**Fig. 42.2.** Urethral closure pressure profiles after pudendal block in the same patient as in Fig. 42.1.

Chapter 43
# Leak Point Pressure Testing

The leak point pressure is defined as the threshold bladder pressure necessary to cause urinary leakage during increases in intra-abdominal pressure. It acts as a global assessment of the integrity of urinary sphincteric function. Urethral closure pressure is a measurement of the intraurethral force generated by the muscular, elastic and vascular components of the urethra and surrounding pelvic floor musculature; it does not assess factors such as mucosal coaptation which contributes to the continence mechanism. The leak point pressure acts as a measure of urethral opening pressure, the pressure necessary to force urine out of the bladder into the urethra. It is an easy test to perform but its reproduceability may be limited unless the investigator is compulsively consistent in performing this test.

A leak point pressure can easily be performed following a subtracted cystometry study (in any position) by removing the transurethral catheter and measuring intra-abdominal pressure with a rectal or vaginal catheter. Alternatively, a small transurethral pressure catheter may be used to measure bladder pressure directly during leak point pressure calculations. In patients without detrusor instability, both abdominal and bladder pressure should be equally effective in measuring increases in bladder pressure. Although there is no more effective method of approximating bladder pressure than measuring bladder pressure directly, the use of a transurethral pressure catheter may act as a wick to alter mucosal coaptation and the leak point pressure. However, comparative methodology and reproduceability testing has not been done to answer these questions.

Fig. 43.1 is the leak point pressure testing of a 43-year-old woman with pure genuine stress incontinence. Her intra-abdominal pressure was measured continuously with a transvaginal catheter after removal of a dual microtransducer catheter from the urethra. The patient is carefully instructed to gradually strain harder and harder until urinary leakage is first noted. It is a gradient stress test with measurement of intra-abdominal pressure. The slope of the gradient may greatly alter the threshold at which the leak point pressure is measured. As seen in Fig. 43.1, a lower slope increasing Valsalva effort results in urinary leakage at a lower pressure than a more rapid Valsalva effort. Thus, unless the patient consistently strains harder at the same rate and gradient, the leak point pressure may vary significantly. We attempt to repeat the test until the lowest pressure which can produce stress incontinence is noted (curved arrow). The leak point pressure at this point is 128 $cmH_2O$. Alternatively, if maximal straining does not cause urinary incontinence, the test is considered negative and the highest abdominal (or bladder) pressure achieved is recorded.

## Bibliography


Ghoneim GM, Roach MB, Lewis VH et al: The value of leak pressure and bladder compliance in the urodynamic evaluation of meningomyelocele patients. J Urol 144:1140, 1990.

Wan J, McGuire EJ, Bloom DA et al: Stress leak point pressure: a diagnostic tool for incontinent children. J Urol 150:700, 1993.

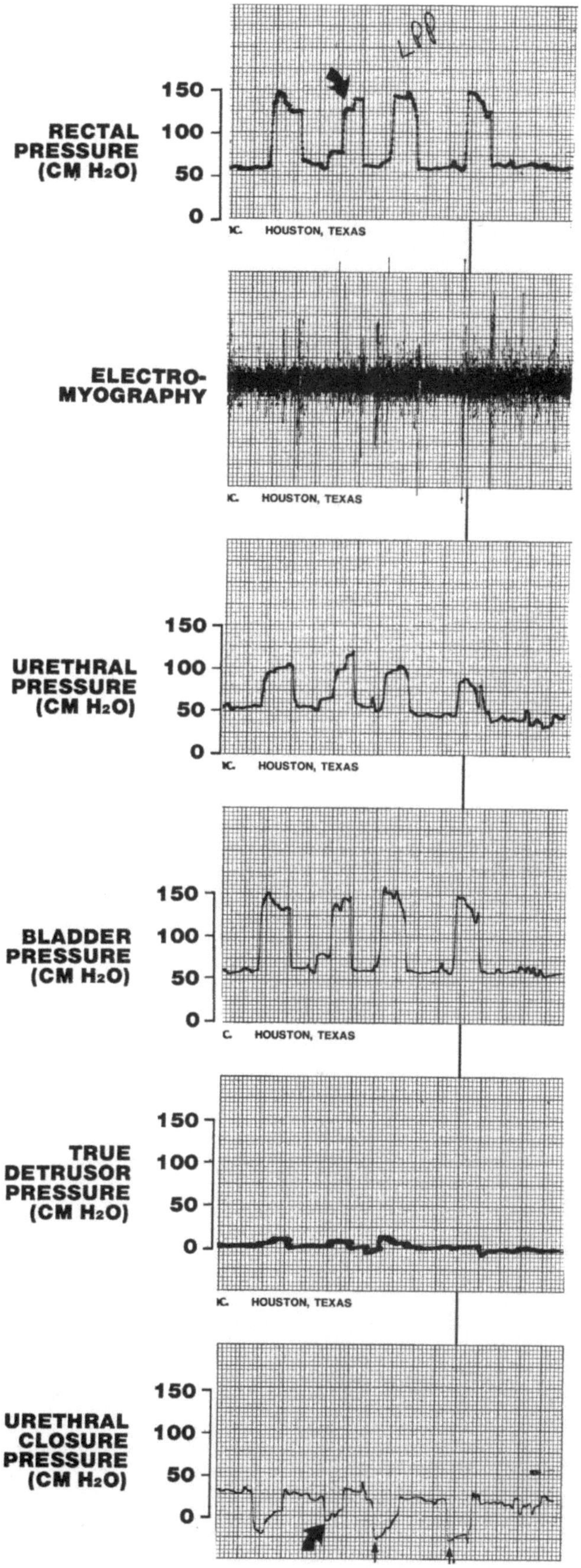


**Fig. 43.1.** Leak point pressure measurements.

# Section VI
# Urodynamic Artifacts

Chapter 44

# Rectal and Vaginal Peristalsis

Rectal and vaginal peristaltic activity frequently obscures urodynamic tracings and complicates interpretation. It is a common source of artifact and its effects must be taken into account whenever it occurs. Due to the fact that the true detrusor pressure is derived by subtraction of rectal or vaginal pressure from bladder pressure, any increase in rectal or vaginal pressure results in a decrease of recorded pressure in the true detrusor channel. A small increase in the bladder pressure channel due to detrusor activity would ordinarily be manifested in the true detrusor channel even when the baseline intra-abdominal pressure increases due to Valsalva or coughing because they are equally recorded by the abdominal (rectal or vaginal) pressure and bladder pressure transducers. In the presence of intrinsic rectal or vaginal peristaltic activity, such an increase in bladder pressure may be obscured by randomly occurring increases in pressure produced by this peristaltic activity. Whenever intrinsic rectal or vaginal peristaltic activity is present, the primary bladder pressure channel must be carefully examined for evidence of intrinsic detrusor activity.

In Fig. 44.1 the marked rectal peristaltic waves are evident in the rectal pressure channel (open arrow). These are accompanied by an inverse pressure response in the true detrusor pressure channel (curved open arrow). Rectal peristaltic pressure waves periodically have cough pressure spikes superimposed (curved solid arrow).

These pressure waves are so intense that detrusor activity cannot be appreciated in the true detrusor pressure channel. However, the bladder pressure channel reveals the presence of detrusor contractions as indicated (arrows). Note the absence of detrusor pressure activity in the true detrusor pressure channel. The urethral closure pressure profiles are essentially uninfluenced by the marked rectal peristaltic activity. Note that the intrinsic bladder overactivity does not coincide with actual urethral closure pressure profile measurement. If it did coincide, it would result in a decrease in measured urethral pressure, thereby artifactually altering closure pressure. Under these circumstances urethral closure pressure would have to be manually determined from the primary urethral pressure channel.

In Fig. 44.2 there are multiple rhythmic vaginal peristaltic waves of pressure increase in the vaginal pressure channel (arrow). These are distinguished from regular Valsalva activity by the fact that there is no pressure change seen in the bladder pressure tracing. These vaginal peristaltic pressure waves are reflected by mirror image decreases in the true detrusor pressure also occurring in wave-like form (open arrow). The urodynamicist must be alert to this type of artifact due to its potential effect on the interpretation of the tracing. Care must be taken to continuously evaluate all pressure channels as the study progresses. When such artifacts are found, the urodynamic tracing must be interpreted carefully accounting for the impact of the artifactual changes.

This accentuates the need to examine fully all pressure channels to completely evaluate the urodynamic tracing especially when there is marked rectal or vaginal peristaltic activity. The physician will have to subtract pressures manually and rely on the primary pressure channels under these circumstances to reveal any coexistent detrusor activity.

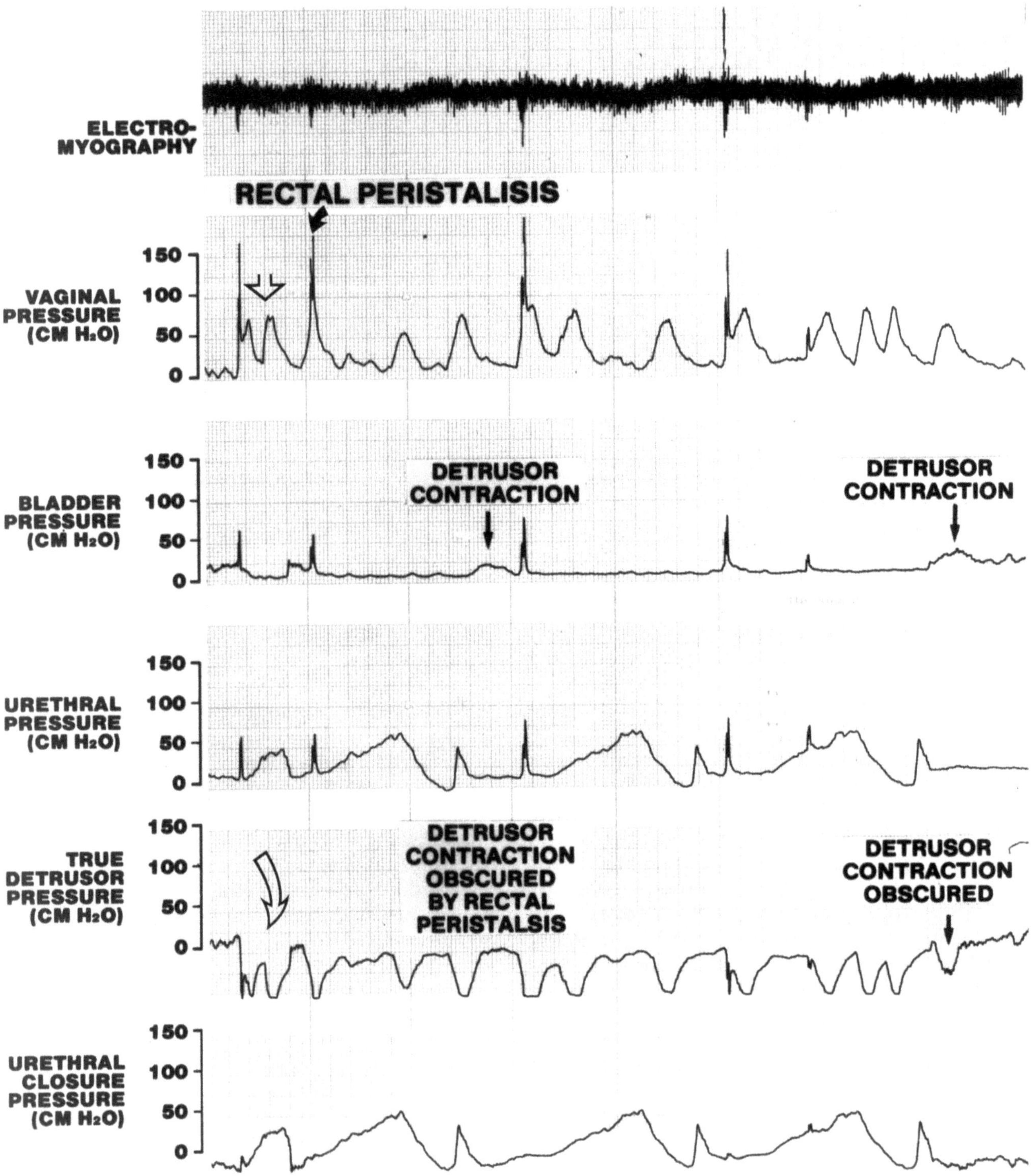


**Fig. 44.1.** Rectal peristalsis obscuring detrusor overactivity during urethral closure pressure profiles.

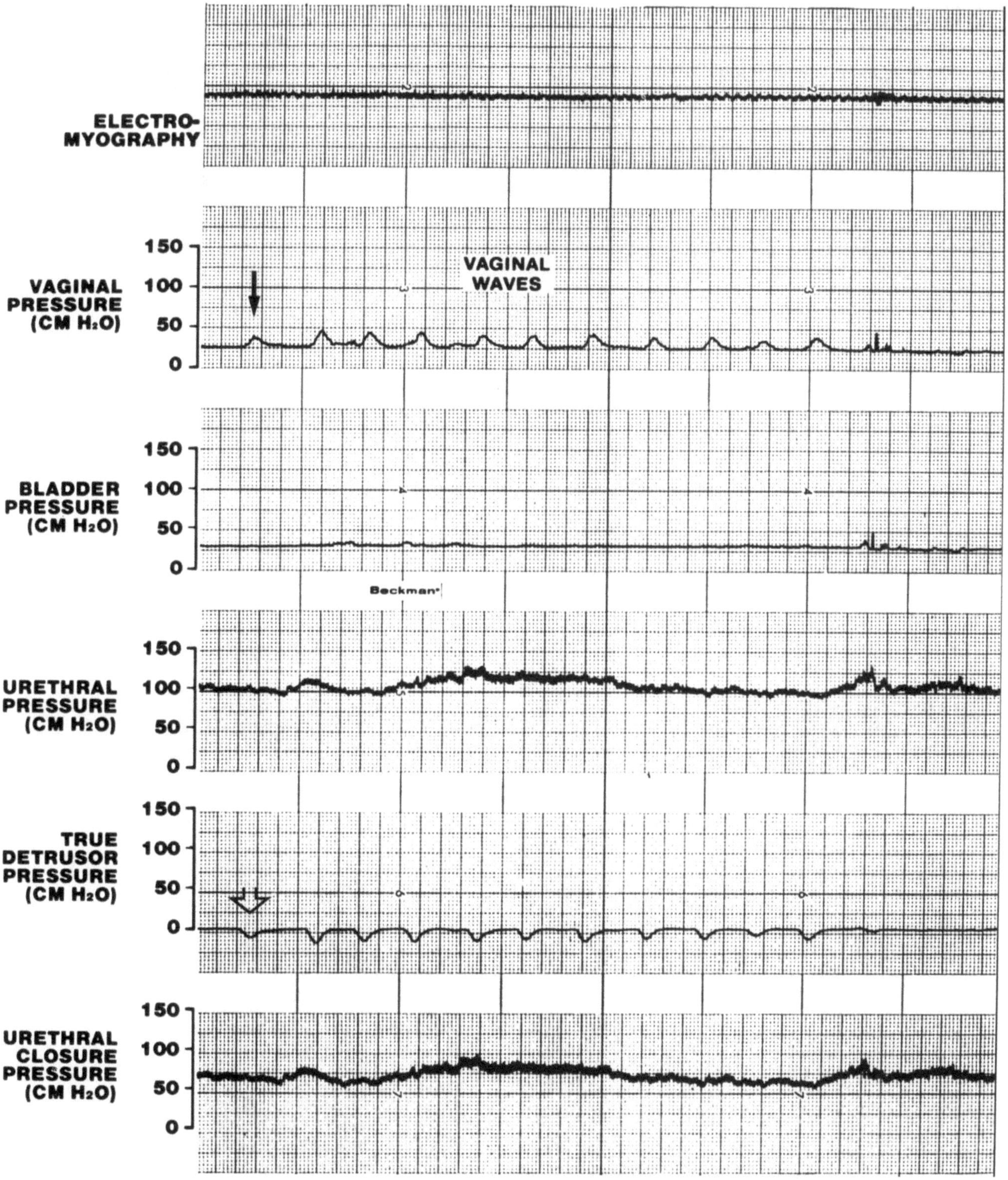


**Fig. 44.2.** Vaginal contractions during urethrocystometry distorting true detrusor pressure measurements.

# Bibliography

Bhatia NN, Bergman A: Urodynamic appraisal of vaginal pressure versus rectal pressure recording as indication of intraabdominal pressure changes. Urology 27:482, 1986.

McCarthy TA: Validity of rectal pressure measurements as indication of intraabdominal pressure changes during urodynamic evaluation. Urology 20:657, 1982.

Chapter 45
# Transducer Placement and Poor Calibration

Transducer placement and measurement artifacts occasionally interfere with the interpretation of urodynamic tracings. The orientation of the microtransducer catheter (lateral, anterior, posterior) may dramatically alter the pressure measured within the urethra, especially during urethral closure pressure profiles. In addition, the placement of the abdominal pressure measuring transducer in a scarred vagina or into stool in the rectum may greatly influence the ability to measure the total intra-abdominal pressure. Routinely, care is taken to avoid these artifacts by constantly checking transducer placement before any type of profile is recorded. A lateral orientation of the urethral microtransducer should be used to ensure consistent results. However, even with these precautions transducer placement may change during the profile, particularly during the dynamic measurements associated with Valsalva and cough profiles. More rapid paper speeds (5 mm/s) used during Valsalva profiles also accentuate this artifact. Placement of the intra-abdominal pressure transducer in the vagina or rectum should be checked for equal pressure transmission when compared to the bladder and the catheter site changed if transmission is not optimal.

As shown in Fig. 45.1, transducer placement and response is first checked by asking the patient to cough (arrow). Essentially the same pressure is measured in each of the primary pressure measuring channels. No significant changes are seen in the subtracted pressure channels (curved arrows) indicating equal pressure being measured by all transducers, and, therefore, good placement and pressure pick-up by the individual transducers. During the Valsalva profile, there is a pressure increase measured in the true detrusor pressure channel which starts at the open arrow. This might be misinterpreted as a detrusor contraction. If this is the only evidence of a contraction in the tracing then further investigation is needed. Further evaluation is best accomplished by a series of brief Valsalva–inspire–Valsalva maneuvers. Differences between pressure transmission through the vagina and through the bladder to reach these respective transducers has caused this subtraction artifact. This is evident in the true detrusor channel where the pressure increases show an exact temporal relationship to the Valsalva effort. The intervening nadir (curved open arrow) represents the decreased pressure associated with the inspiratory effort in between Valsalva efforts. Further inspection of the primary pressure measuring channels reveals that the vaginal transducer is not registering as much pressure as the intravesical transducer. At the end of the first Valsalva effort the intravaginal pressure is 25–30 $cmH_2O$ (long arrow) whereas at the curved arrow the intravesical pressure is 45 $cmH_2O$. This accounts for the 15–20 $cmH_2O$ difference recorded in the subtracted true detrusor pressure channel at this point in the study. Such analysis clarifies these pressure increases and indicates that they are due to the imperfect transmission of intra-abdominal pressure to the vagina and to the intravaginal pressure transducer. The cough profile further substantiates this conclusion since the differential pressure artifacts are recorded (small arrows) in the true detrusor pressure tracing for the very same reason.

Careful analysis of the urodynamic pressure tracing is always indicated with continuous inspection of all pressure and EMG measuring

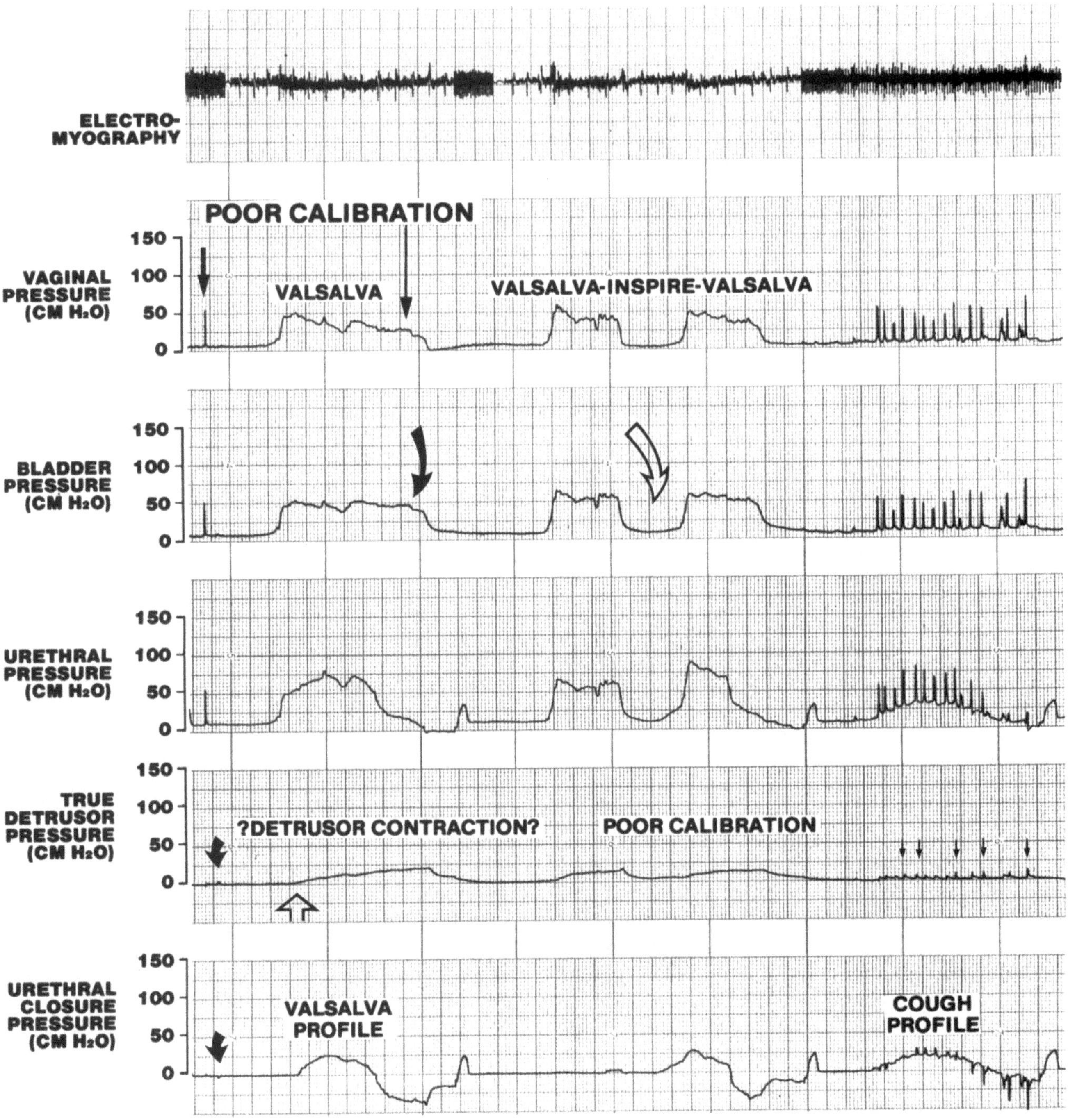


**Fig. 45.1.** Poor pressure pick-up by vaginal pressure transducer during dynamic urethral closure pressure profiles.

channels as the test is being performed. The tracing may reveal many artifactual pressure measurements which may lead to misinterpretation and the establishment of erroneous diagnoses. As seen in this example, one of the most difficult artifacts to interpret is when pressure transmission between organs is equal one minute and unequal the next. This occurs more frequently with the dynamic cough and Valsalva profiles and must be searched for when unusual pressure events are seen to occur on the subtracted tracings. The physician performing the urodynamic study must be alert to these possibilities and constantly alter his study techniques as the need arises to prove or disprove his diagnostic impression.

## Bibliography

Anderson RS, Shepherd AM, Feneley RCL: Microtransducer urethral profile methodology: variations caused by transducer orientation. J Urol 130:727, 1983.

Tanagho EA, Stoller ML: Urodynamics: cystometry and urethral closure pressure profile. In Ostergard DR, Bent AE (eds), Urogynecology and urodynamics, Baltimore, Williams & Wilkins, 1991, pp. 122–142.

# Chapter 46
# Filling Catheter Artifacts

Cystometry and urethrocystometry may be accomplished in a number of different ways. One of the variables that influence the performance of urethrocystometry is the size of the catheter or catheters in the urethra utilized to perform the cystometrogram. Research has shown that the larger the catheter or catheters in the urethra, the larger is the artifact that is introduced into the study. Any movement of the catheter distending the urethra will increase skeletal muscle activity as reflected by periurethral EMG activity. Distention of the urethra will normally increase intraurethral pressure to varying degrees depending on the elasticity of the urethra. Ideally one would like to perform urethrocystometry with an infinitessimally small catheter which is immobile relative to the urethra. Mictrotransducer catheters with central filling apertures are available as shown in Fig. 46.1, but these are more expensive than single lumen water catheters or microtransducer catheters with separate filling catheters. Urethrocystometry can be done with a urodynamic pressure measuring catheter together with a filling catheter, usually either a pediatric feeding tube (5F) or an angiocath (12 or 14 gauge). The addition of secondary filling catheters may produce a considerable amount of artifact in the recording of urethral pressure and may influence detrusor activity. This catheter-induced artifact is demonstrated in Figs. 46.2 and 46.3. Fig. 46.2 shows the most common pattern, where the patient's intraurethral pressure and closure pressure are markedly elevated with the filling catheter in and significantly reduced when the filling catheter is removed. However, the opposite picture can also be seen, as in Fig. 46.3 where the urethral closure pressure actually rises when the filling catheter is removed. Here, it is likely that the filling catheter dampens any increase in intraluminal urethral force as sensed by the microtransducer membrane. The dampening effect is most likely to occur if the filling catheter lies between the pressure-measuring transducer and the urethral wall.

If separate filling catheters are used, one should be careful to remove these catheters before the performance of urethral closure pressure profiles. In addition, one needs to recognize that urethrocystometry done with a second catheter in the urethra may alter quantitative results when compared to studies done with a single small microtransducer catheter. Care should be taken to ensure that the filling catheter is not lying in front of the microtransducer membrane.

## Bibliography


Koraitim M: Catheter as source of error in urodynamic study. Urol 20:223, 1982.

Sand PK, Bowen LW, Ostergard DR: The effect of a filling catheter during urodynamics. Int Urogynecol J 1:124, 1990.

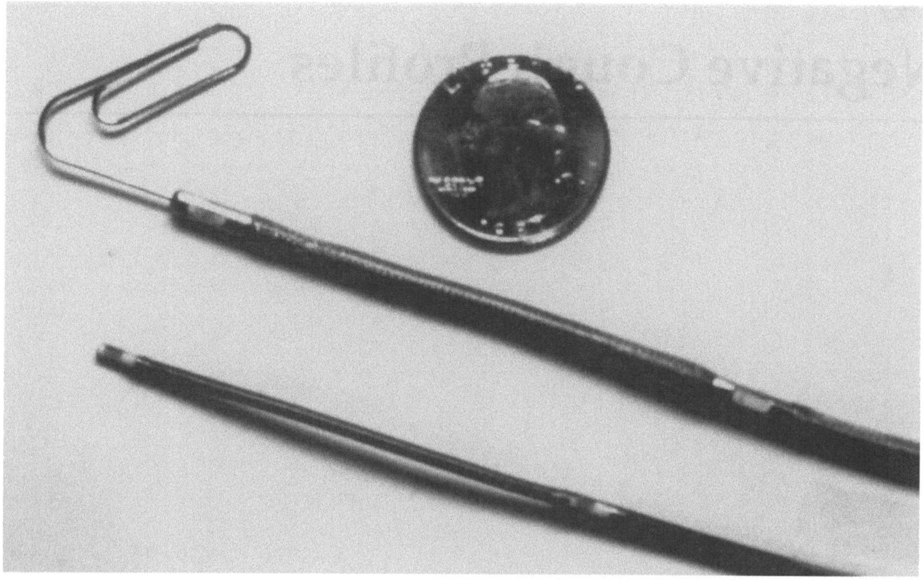

**Fig. 46.1.** Dual channel microtransducer catheters with and without central filling port.

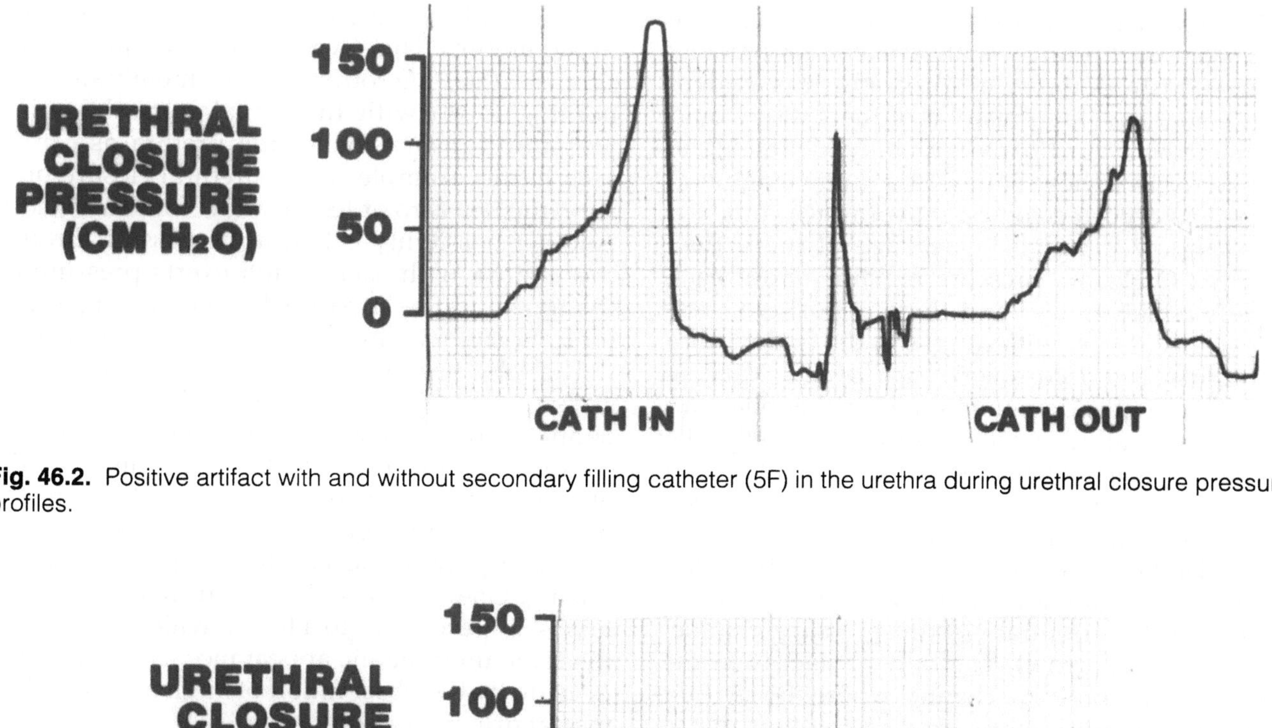


**Fig. 46.2.** Positive artifact with and without secondary filling catheter (5F) in the urethra during urethral closure pressure profiles.

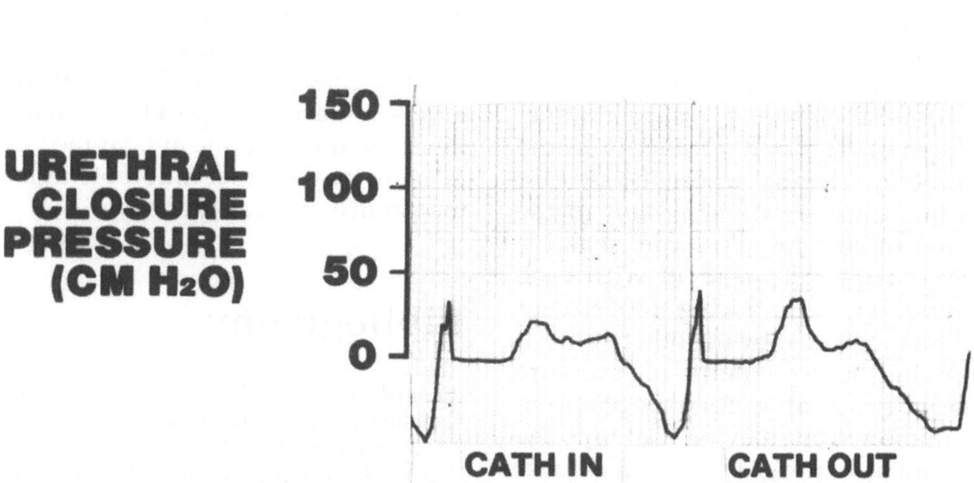


**Fig. 46.3.** Negative artifact with and without secondary filling catheter (5F) in urethra during urethral closure pressure profiles.

# Chapter 47
# False Negative Cough Profiles

Occasionally cough profiles will demonstrate a positive margin to leakage under the curve and yet each cough will be associated with coincident urine loss. This emphasizes the need to correlate urodynamic findings with clinical parameters continuously as the study proceeds. It is evident that erroneous interpretation of the study would be made by a third party with only the tracing of the study to review without the knowledge that urine loss occurred coincident with each cough.

In Fig. 47.1 margin to leakage of more than 15 $cmH_2O$ closure pressure remains under each profile (small arrow) and there is positive pressure transmission with coughs in the mid urethra yet urine loss occurs with each cough. Varying cough strengths do not account for this phenomenon since all coughs produce essentially the same pressure increases in the vaginal and bladder pressure recordings. The transducer localization cough of the second cough profile (solid curved arrow) does not demonstrate a subtraction error since no alteration of pressure measurement results in the urethral closure pressure channel (open curved arrow). The only artifact is in the true detrusor pressure channel where the slightly greater abdominal pressure transmission to the vagina compared to bladder results in negative deflections (large arrows) coincident with each cough. Throughout the entire tracing the detrusor remains inactive as indicated by the otherwise flat pressure curve in the true detrusor pressure tracing. The exact explanation for this phenomenon remains unknown, but may be related to the use of unidirectional semirigid microtransducer catheters. These catheters measure force in a non-fluid-filled space like the urethra and may measure elevated "pressures" in the urethra secondary to impact of the microtransducer against the urethral wall with coughing. This is especially likely if there is some flexion or kinking in the urethra. This measurement of impact force against the microtransducer membrane has nothing to do with the actual intra-abdominal pressure transmission to the urethra as can be seen in this example where urethral closure pressure must be zero or less to allow for urinary loss. Another possibility is that urine passing through the urethra with each cough exerts pressure on the transducer as it passes by, thus giving a false indication of remaining positive closure pressure.

The false negative cough profile again emphasizes the importance of recognizing that urodynamic studies must be interpreted in view of coexisting clinical observations. In this case, the observation that urine was lost through the urethra during coughing in the absence of detrusor activity was critical to the interpretation of the tracing. One must also be careful that such urine loss is not secondary to a fistula which would give the same urodynamic appearance. Differentiation is made by the observation of vaginal rather than meatal urinary leakage.

## Bibliography


Richardson DA: Value of cough pressure profile in the evaluation of patients with stress incontinence. Am J Obstet Gynecol 155:808, 1986.

Versi E, Cardozo L, Studd J et al: Evaluation of urethral pressure profilometry for the diagnosis of genuine stress incontinence. World J Urol 4:6, 1986.

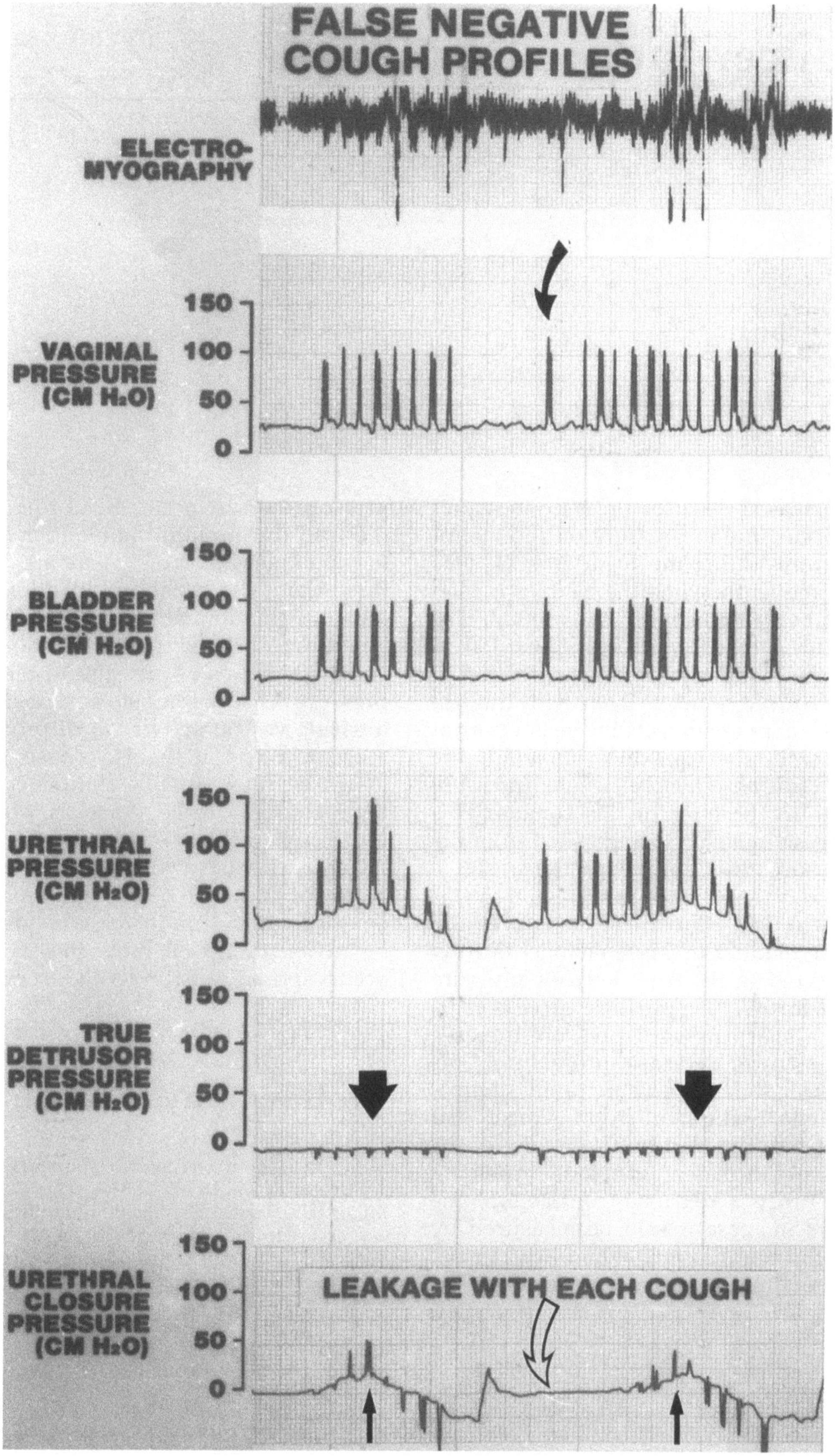


**Fig. 47.1.** False negative cough urethral closure pressure profiles in a patient with genuine stress incontinence.

# Chapter 48
# Transducer-Induced Artifacts

Artificially increased detrusor pressure measurements may occur due to pressure on the microtransducers from hitting the bladder wall. This occurs more frequently when the bladder is relatively empty and the transducer is in motion. This artifact is usually avoided by placing at least 150 ml of fluid into the bladder prior to introduction of the microtransducer catheter. Even with fluid in the bladder, if there are defects in the support of the bladder wall, the transducer may hit the bladder wall creating a falsely elevated pressure recording due to the force of this contact. This pressure increase must be distinguished from the elevated pressure associated with the unstable bladder.

As shown in Fig. 48.1 there is a pressure increase in the bladder pressure channel (arrow) which is reflected in the true detrusor pressure channel (large arrow). The pressure curve is characterized by a sharp upward pressure increase followed by a slower decrease in pressure. This occurred between the two pressure profiles immediately after the urethral microtransducer had been replaced into the bladder. Therefore, if this recorded pressure increase in the bladder pressure tracing were truly a detrusor contraction, the same pressure increase would be measured by the urethral microtransducer which was in the bladder at the time (open curved arrow). The pressure increase occurring during replacement of the transducers into the bladder is indicated by the solid curved arrow. There are mild variations throughout the rectal and bladder pressure tracings due to minimal increases in intra-abdominal pressure associated with respiration.

Any increases of pressure in the true detrusor pressure channel must be considered due to intrinsic vesical activity until proven otherwise. Since artifacts may also cause such pressure increases, they must be eliminated as a cause of the pressure increase. When the pressure increase is directly associated with movement of the transducer, particularly when the bladder is relatively empty or known to be poorly supported, the etiology of the pressure increase is quickly known to be artifactual. Generally this type of artifact occurs sporadically under these circumstances.

## Bibliography


Bump RC: The urodynamics laboratory. Obstet Gynecol Clin North Am 16:795, 1989.

Miller HD, Baker LE: A stable ultraminiature catheter-tip pressure transducer. Med Biol Eng 11:86, 1973.

Teague CT, Merrill DC: Laboratory comparison of urethral profilometry techniques. Urology 13:221, 1979.

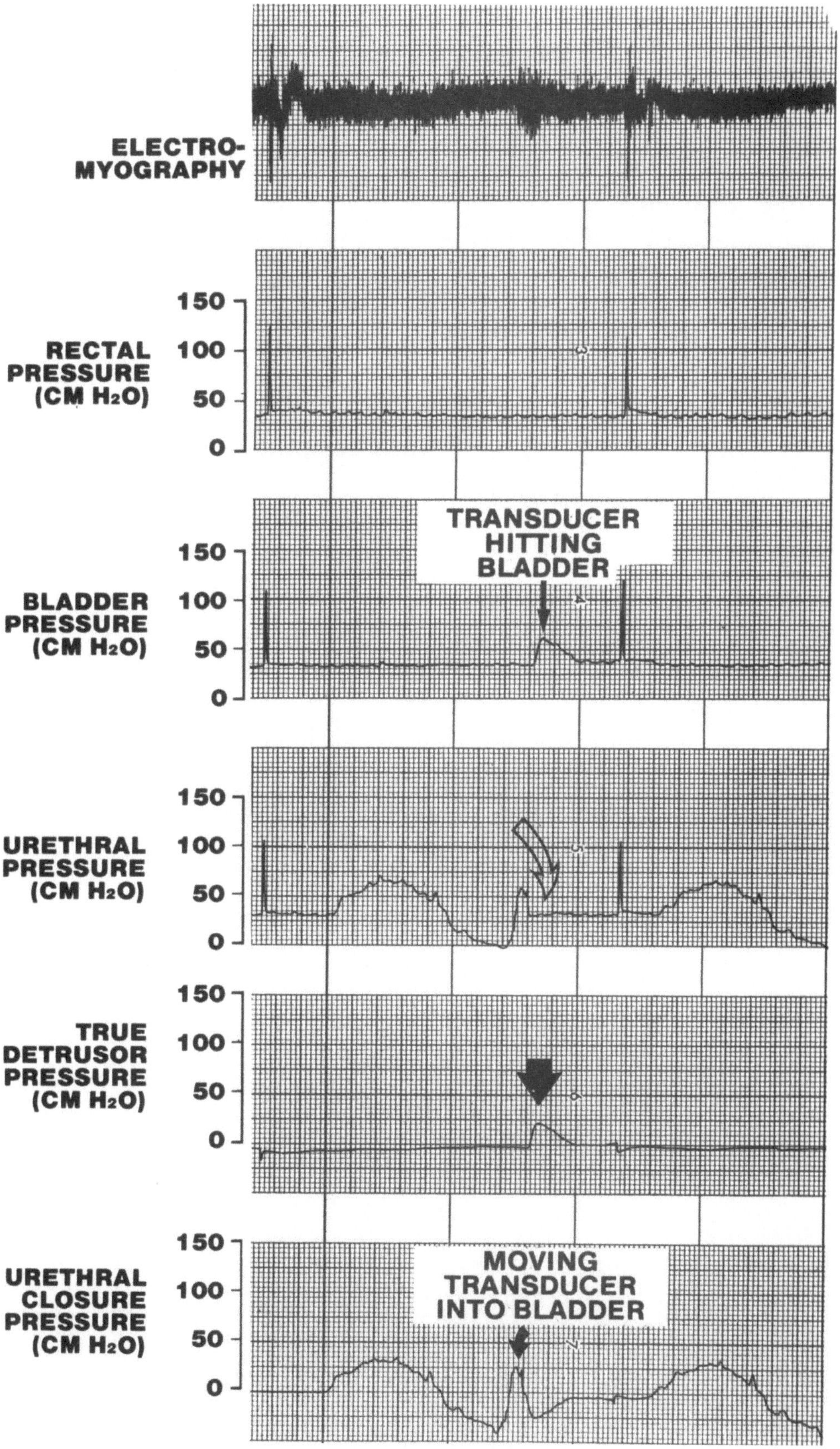


**Fig. 48.1.** Artifact during urethral closure pressure profiles secondary to transducer contact with the bladder wall.

# Section VII

# Postoperative Urodynamics

Chapter 49

# The Effect of Retropubic Urethropexy on the Resting Urethral Closure Pressure Profile

The effect of the Burch retropubic urethropexy on the urethral closure pressure profile is variable from patient to patient. Only occasionally is an increase in closure pressure observed when postoperative urodynamic studies are performed. More commonly functional length increases, although this is also a variable finding. Most of the studies in the literature have not divided patients according to various presurgical events. Especially important is the patient who has had previous surgery for incontinence. Since these procedures may alter the normal function of the urethra through the production of fibrosis, denervation and devascularization, they are especially important and may affect the response of the urethral sphincteric mechanism to the present surgical procedure. The recent realization that a high proportion of patients with genuine stress incontinence may have a primary neurological disease, as evidenced by denervation potentials in the skeletal musculature of the pelvic floor and altered nerve conduction velocities is especially important and must be considered.

In Fig. 49.1 the preoperative resting urethral closure pressure in the first two profiles is 35 $cmH_2O$ and the functional length is 3.2 cm. After performance of a Burch retropubic urethropexy, the closure pressure increased to 65 $cmH_2O$ and the functional length increased to 3.5 cm as seen in the second two profiles. It is unusual to find an increase in both closure pressure and functional length postoperatively in nonobstructing procedures like the Burch procedure.

An artifact is present in the preoperative tracing from unequal pressure registration of abdominal pressure between the bladder and vagina resulting in a negative deflection in the true detrusor pressure tracing (arrow) during the transducer localization cough. Note the artifact in the postoperative tracings produced by the erratic vaginal pressure recording from peristalsis (solid curved arrow) which produces a mirror image in the true detrusor channel (open curved arrow). Since this may obscure intrinsic detrusor activity due to the unstable bladder, the primary bladder pressure tracing must be reviewed for evidence of possible detrusor overactivity (Chapter 44). In this example none is found.

Postoperative urodynamic studies are now considered essential for the proper analysis of the results of a surgical procedure performed to correct urinary incontinence. Any other statements of cure must be considered subjective and subject to change when the appropriate studies are done.

## Bibliography

Faysal MH, Constantinou CE, Rather LF et al: The impact of bladder neck suspension on the resting and stress urethral pressure profile: a prospective study comparing controls with incontinent patients preoperatively and postoperatively. J Urol 125:55, 1987.

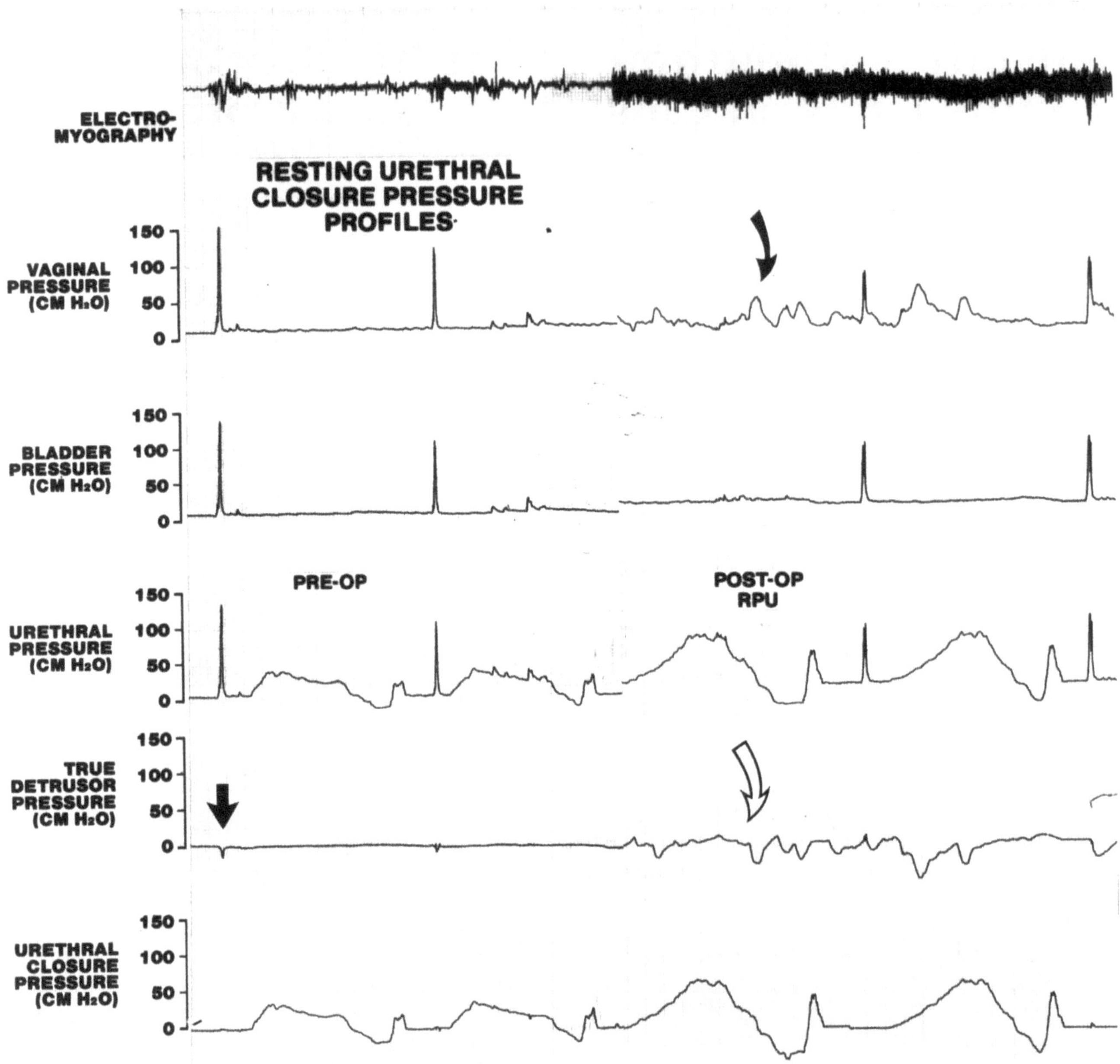


**Fig. 49.1.** Resting and dynamic urethral closure pressure profiles before and after retropubic urethropexy.

Hilton P: A clinical and urodynamic assessment of the Burch colposuspension for genuine stress incontinence. Br J Obstet Gynaecol 90:934, 1983.

van Geelen JM, Theeuwes AGM, Eskes TKAAB et al: The clinical and urodynamic effects of anterior vaginal repair and Burch colposuspension. Am J Obstet Gynecol 159:137, 1988.

Weil A, Reyes H, Bischoff P et al: Modifications of the urethral rest and stress profiles after different types of surgery for urinary stress incontinence. Br J Obstet Gynaecol 91:46, 1984.

Chapter 50

# The Effect of Retropubic Urethropexy on the Dynamic Urethral Closure Pressure Profile

The most consistent finding in the postoperative period in successfully treated patients is the presence of positive pressure transmission during increases in intra-abdominal pressure. The usual profile preoperatively is characterized by pressure equalization with each cough and no margin to leakage. Various dynamic profiles are done routinely in the urodynamic evaluation of the incontinence patient. These may include rectal and urethral sphincter tightening, Valsalva and cough profiles (Chapters 15–17). The sphincter tightening profiles are compared to the resting profile in order to determine whether or not the patient has the voluntary ability to tighten the skeletal muscles of the pelvic floor and urethra. When this ability exists an increase of pressure in the respective profile will be measured. The Valsalva and cough profiles are dynamic recordings done during constant or intermittent increases in intra-abdominal pressure as discussed in Chapter 17. These profiles are done primarily to stress the urethral sphincteric mechanism and to determine the presence or absence of pressure equalization causing incontinence.

In this patient (Figs. 50.1 and 50.2) the reestablishment of positive pressure transmission as demonstrated in both the Valsalva and cough profiles accounts for restoration of continence. The proximal urethra has been appropriately repositioned in an intra-abdominal location where it can now properly receive transmitted intra-abdominal pressure. This improved transmission of abdominal pressure to the urethral lumen is the mechanism by which continence is restored. This urethral stabilization is helped by the increased urethral closure pressure and the increased functional ability to augment closure pressure voluntarily. The patient may also regain the ability reflexively to increase closure pressure during stress by more efficient voluntary contraction of the pelvic floor.

The preoperative tracing in Fig. 50.1 begins with the resting urethral closure pressure profile which demonstrates a maximal closure pressure of 20 $cmH_2O$. The patient retained the ability to contract the urethral sphincter voluntarily as demonstrated in the rectal and urethral sphincter tightening profiles which have maximal closure pressures of 35 $cmH_2O$ (small curved arrows). This pressure increase is seen primarily in the proximal urethra. There is an accompanying increase in EMG activity with each profile (arrows). As is the case with many women there is a coincident Valsalva effort (large arrow) with each profile. The Valsalva activity interferes with the proper measurement of the augmenting profile and the patient must be coaxed to minimize it and encouraged to relax her abdominal wall while contracting her urethra or rectum.

During the Valsalva profile a short distance of positive closure pressure is observed which rapidly gives way to pressure equalization and urine loss (curved arrow). Similarly the cough profile demonstrates pressure equalization with each cough (small arrows). Although there is a pressure differential artifact between the bladder and rectum which is demonstrated in the true detrusor pressure channel (open arrow), there is no intrinsic detrusor activity present during any of the profiles.

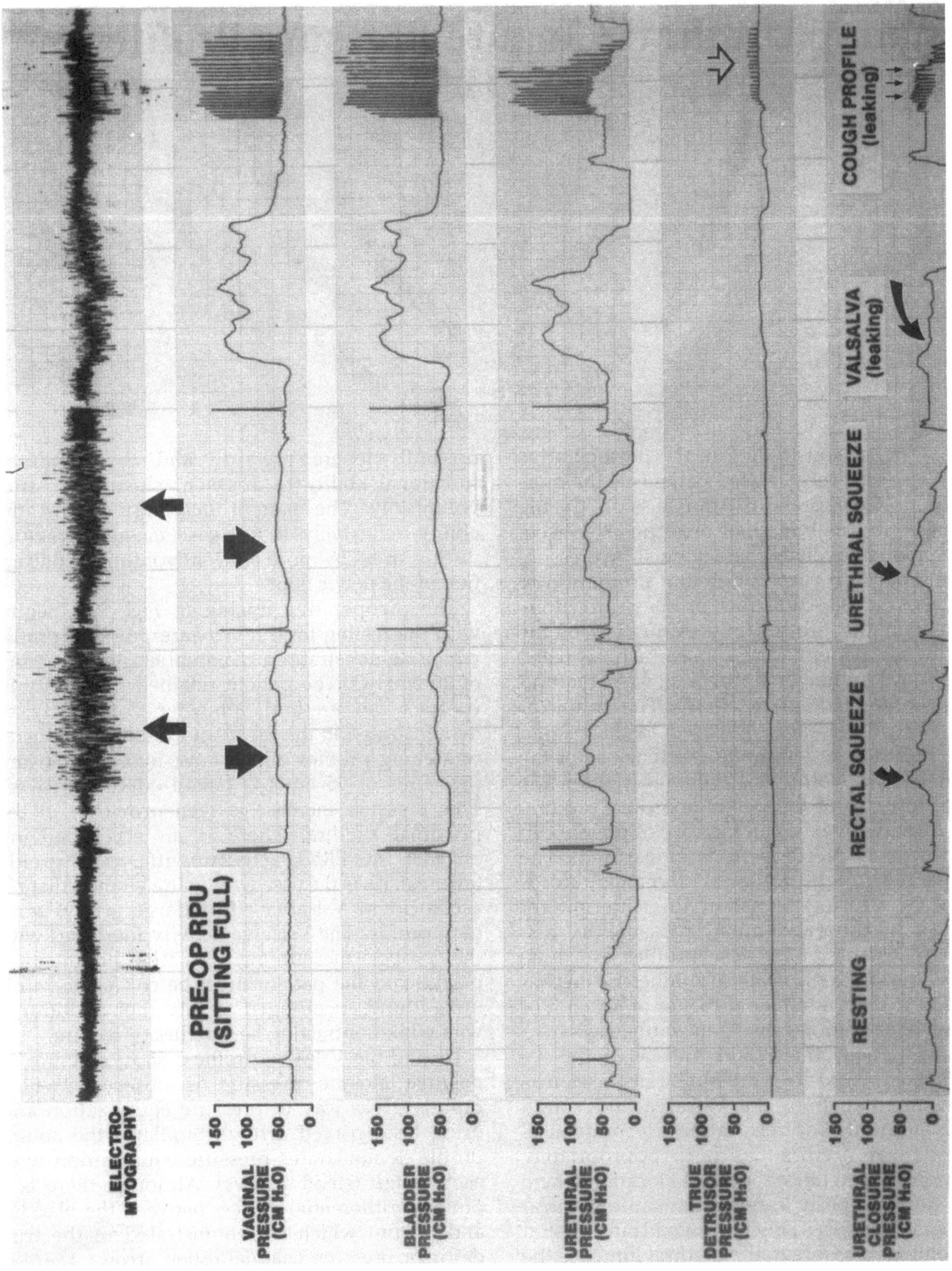


**Fig. 50.1.** Resting and dynamic urethral closure pressure profiles before retropubic urethropexy in a woman with genuine stress incontinence.

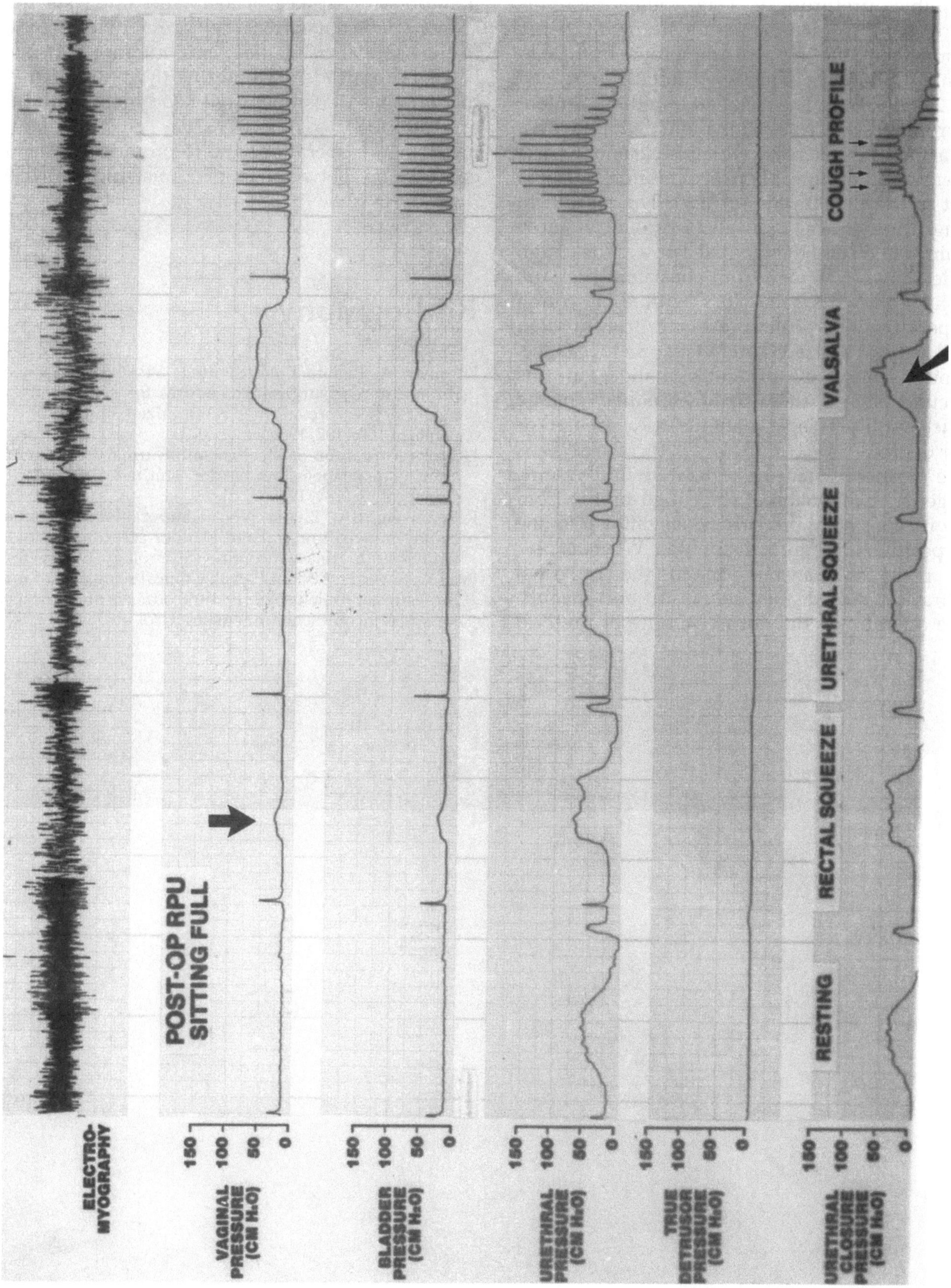


**Fig. 50.2.** Resting and dynamic urethral closure pressure profiles after successful retropubic urethropexy in the same patient as in Fig. 50.1.

In the postoperative urodynamic tracing after retropubic urethropexy (Fig. 50.2) there is improvement in each parameter studied. Closure pressure increased in the resting profile from 20 to 35 $cmH_2O$ and the functional length increased from 2.8 to 3.0 cm. The rectal and urethral tightening profile responses became more definite with a similar pressure increase which is sustained for a longer period of time. There is a minimal Valsalva effort in the first profile (arrow). The margin to leakage under the Valsalva profile is now sustained at 55 $cmH_2O$ (angled arrow). The cough profile shows a change from consistent pressure equalization with urine loss with each cough preoperatively to positive pressure transmission (small arrows) and a 35 $cmH_2O$ margin to leakage. Although these are dramatic changes in this particular patient, these parameters may change in successfully treated patients to a greater or lesser degree.

The most consistent postoperative urodynamic change is a conversion of the cough profile from one with consistent pressure equalization into one with positive pressure transmission. Whereas positive pressure transmission to the proximal urethra is restored after successful anti-incontinence operations, the normal timing of urethral pressure increases preceding bladder and abdominal pressure spikes is lost. This suggests that surgery does not correct the normal reflex activity of the skeletal pelvic floor musculature that may be compromised in women with genuine stress incontinence. Postoperative urodynamic studies are essential to objectify the results of anti-incontinence operations and to provide a basis for comparison between institutions and between procedures.

## Bibliography

Bergman A, Ballard CA, Koonings PP: Comparison of three different surgical procedures for genuine stress incontinence: prospective randomized study. Obstet Gynecol 160:1102, 1989.

Hertogs K, Stanton S: Mechanism of urinary continence after colposuspension: barrier studies. Br J Obstet Gynaecol 92:1184, 1985.

Rosenzweig BA, Bhatia NN: Temporal separation of cough-induced urethral and bladder pressure spikes in women with urinary incontinence. Urology 39:165, 1992.

Weil A, Reyes H, Bischof P et al: Clinical relevance of urethral stress profile using microtransducers after surgery for stress incontinence in females. Urol Int 38:363, 1983.

# Chapter 51
# The Effect of Suburethral Sling Procedure on the Dynamic Urethral Pressure Profile

The low pressure urethra is defined as a urethra with a closure pressure of equal to or less than 20 $cmH_2O$ in the sitting position at maximum cystometric capacity. Its importance lies in the fact that it is associated with an increased rate of surgical failure when standard surgical approaches are used. Urodynamic evidence of cure is present in <50% of patients when a Burch retropubic urethropexy procedure is performed in patients with genuine stress incontinence with low urethral pressure. This high risk of failure has also been found with other routine anti-incontinence operations which do not attempt to obstruct the urethra. These patients respond more predictably to a suburethral sling procedure or artificial sphincter which may directly increase urethral resistance by intermittent or continuous urethral obstruction.

In this example (Fig. 51.1) the urodynamics of a patient with low urethral closure pressure is shown pre- and postoperatively. In the preoperative tracing the Valsalva and cough profiles are shown which demonstrate continuous incontinence. The slight increase of pressure in the true detrusor pressure channel (curved arrow) is related to unequal pressure transmission between the bladder and the vagina. The small pressure increase at the end of this Valsalva urethral closure pressure profile on the urethral pressure tracing is the pressure curve recorded as the urethral microtransducer is returned to the bladder in preparation for the next cough profile. The resting urethral closure pressure profile is not shown. The maximal closure pressure for this patient was 5 $cmH_2O$ preoperatively. The cough profile demonstrates pressure equalization with each cough and negative pressure transmission (arrow).

In the postoperative tracing, done 6 months after a suburethral sling procedure, the Valsalva profile demonstrates a positive closure pressure of 10 $cmH_2O$ (open curved arrow) which is enough to maintain continence. Similarly the cough profile demonstrates a solitary positive pressure spike (small arrow) and a margin to leakage of <10 $cmH_2O$. This is also sufficient to maintain continence and no urine loss is seen during this profile.

A significant advance in our knowledge of urinary incontinence has been the recognition that patients with low urethral closure pressure do not respond as well to standard anti-incontinence procedures as those with "normal" closure pressure. Suburethral sling procedures produce much better results when used as surgical therapy for these patients with cure rates of 80%–90%. Only minimal areas of positive pressure transmission and minimal pressure increases are necessary to restore continence as seen in this example.

## Bibliography

Beck RP, Grove D,Annusch D et al: Recurrent urinary stress incontinence treated by the fascia lata sling procedure. Am J Obstet Gynecol 120:613, 1974.

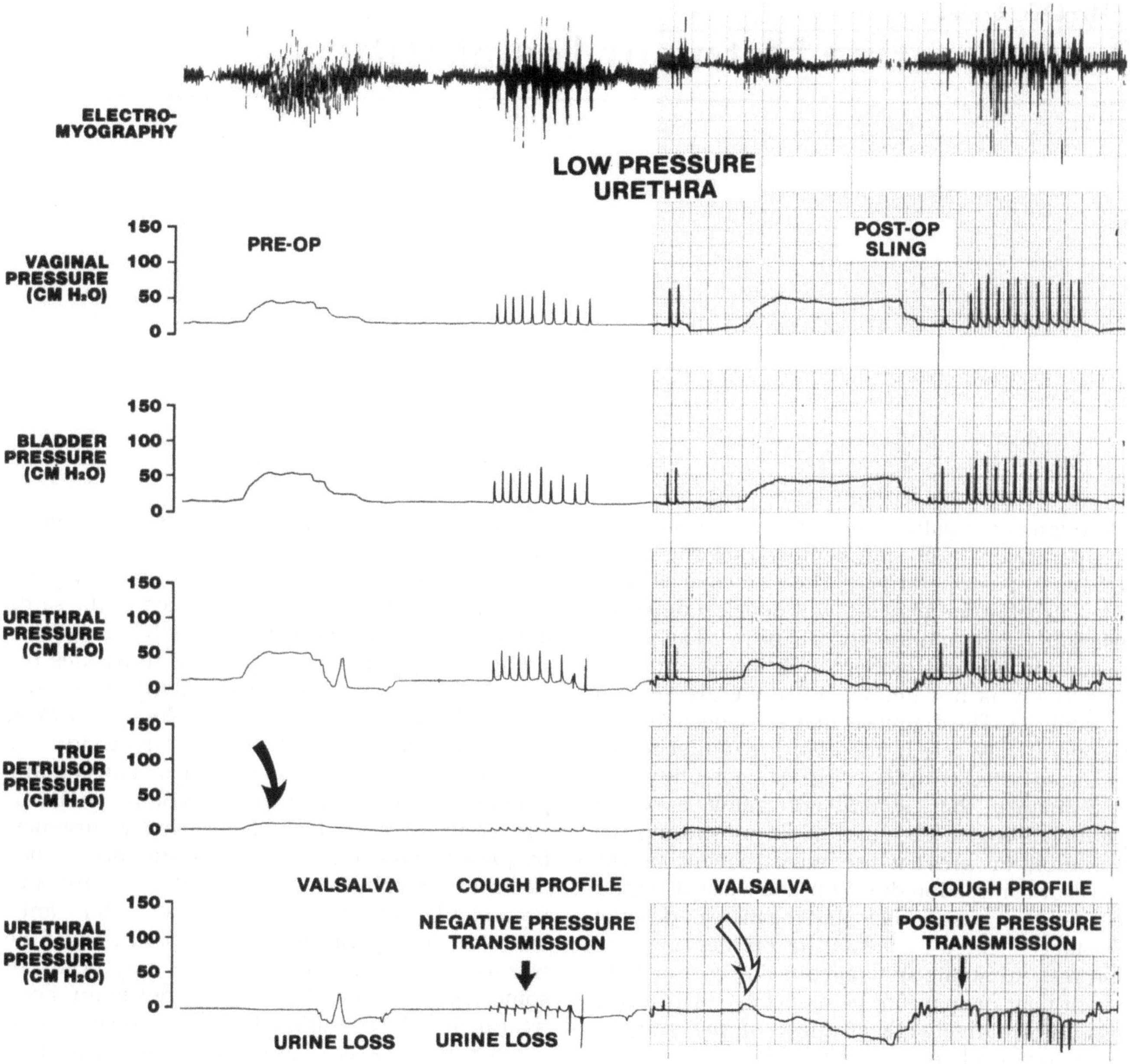


**Fig. 51.1.** Dynamic urethral closure pressure profiles in a patient with a low pressure urethra before and after a suburethral sling procedure.

Henriksson C, Ulmsten U: A urodynamic evaluation of the effects of abdominal urethrocystopexy and vaginal sling urethroplasty in women with stress incontinence. Am J Obstet Gynecol 131:77, 1978.

Hilton P: A clinical and urodynamic study comparing the Stamey bladder neck suspension and suburethral sling procedures in the treatment of genuine stress incontinence. Br J Obstet Gynaecol 96:213, 1989.

Horbach NS, Blanco JS, Ostergard DR: A suburethral sling procedure with polytetrafloroethylene for the treatment of genuine stress incontinence in patients with low urethral closure pressure. Obstet Gynecol 71:648, 1988.

Summitt RL, Bent AE, Ostergard DR et al: Suburethral sling procedure for genuine stress incontinence and low urethral closure pressure. A continued experience. Int Urogynecol J 3:18, 1992.

# Chapter 52
# Postoperative Detrusor Instability

Although some patients with detrusor instability preoperatively will still demonstrate the same condition postoperatively, the converse is also true in that some patients will develop detrusor instability postoperatively de novo. The exact reason for the development of this problem postoperatively is not known but there are several possibilities. The diagnosis may have been missed preoperatively due to the very low outlet resistance associated with the coexisting genuine stress incontinence that would not allow maximal bladder filling to the point of demonstrating the condition or prevent the measurement of the detrusor contraction during urinary loss (Chapter 38). Another possibility is that the increased outlet resistance created by the anti-incontinence operation may stimulate spontaneous detrusor activity which may or may not be associated with urine loss. Alternatively, the trauma of the surgical procedure itself may be sufficient to cause this uninhibited detrusor activity from partial denervation.

The patient in Fig. 52.1 had complaints of urinary urgency and frequency with rare episodes of urge incontinence following a modified Pereyra procedure. As seen in this example, a cough has stimulated detrusor activity (arrow) in this patient who preoperatively had a stable detrusor. There is concomitant urethral relaxation (open arrow) which persists intermittently for the duration of the contraction. At the curved arrow there is an attempt by the patient to contract the urethra to try to inhibit the bladder contraction and severe sense of urgency which is accompanied by a momentary decrease in detrusor activity (curved arrow). Incontinence did not result from this contraction since urethral resistance never dropped enough to allow for pressure equalization (zero closure pressure).

Patients who develop detrusor instability postoperatively are evaluated and treated in the same manner as those who evidence this condition preoperatively. This example also illustrates the principle that detrusor overactivity need not always be associated with urine loss. However, the diagnosis of detrusor overactivity by definition cannot be made in asymptomatic patients. In this woman these involuntary detrusor contractions cause her urinary urgency, frequency and rare urge incontinence. Since detrusor instability occurs with a low but predictable frequency (5%–20%) after anti-incontinence operations each patient should be warned of the possibility that this may occur. In some cases this may be transient but many need treatment if the condition does not resolve spontaneously. Recurrence of incontinence in the postoperative period when urethrovesical anatomy seems normal should lead the clinician to suspect the de novo development of a new cause of incontinence which should become apparent through thorough urodynamic testing.

## Bibliography


McGuire EJ, Savastano JA: Stress incontinence and detrusor instability/urge incontinence. Neurourol Urodynam 4:313, 1985.

Mundy AR: A trial comparing the Stamey bladder neck suspension procedure with colposuspension for the treatment of stress incontinence. Br J Urol 55:687, 1983.

Sand PK, Bowen LW, Ostergard DR et al: The effect of retropubic urethropexy on detrusor stability. Obstet Gynecol 71:818, 1988.

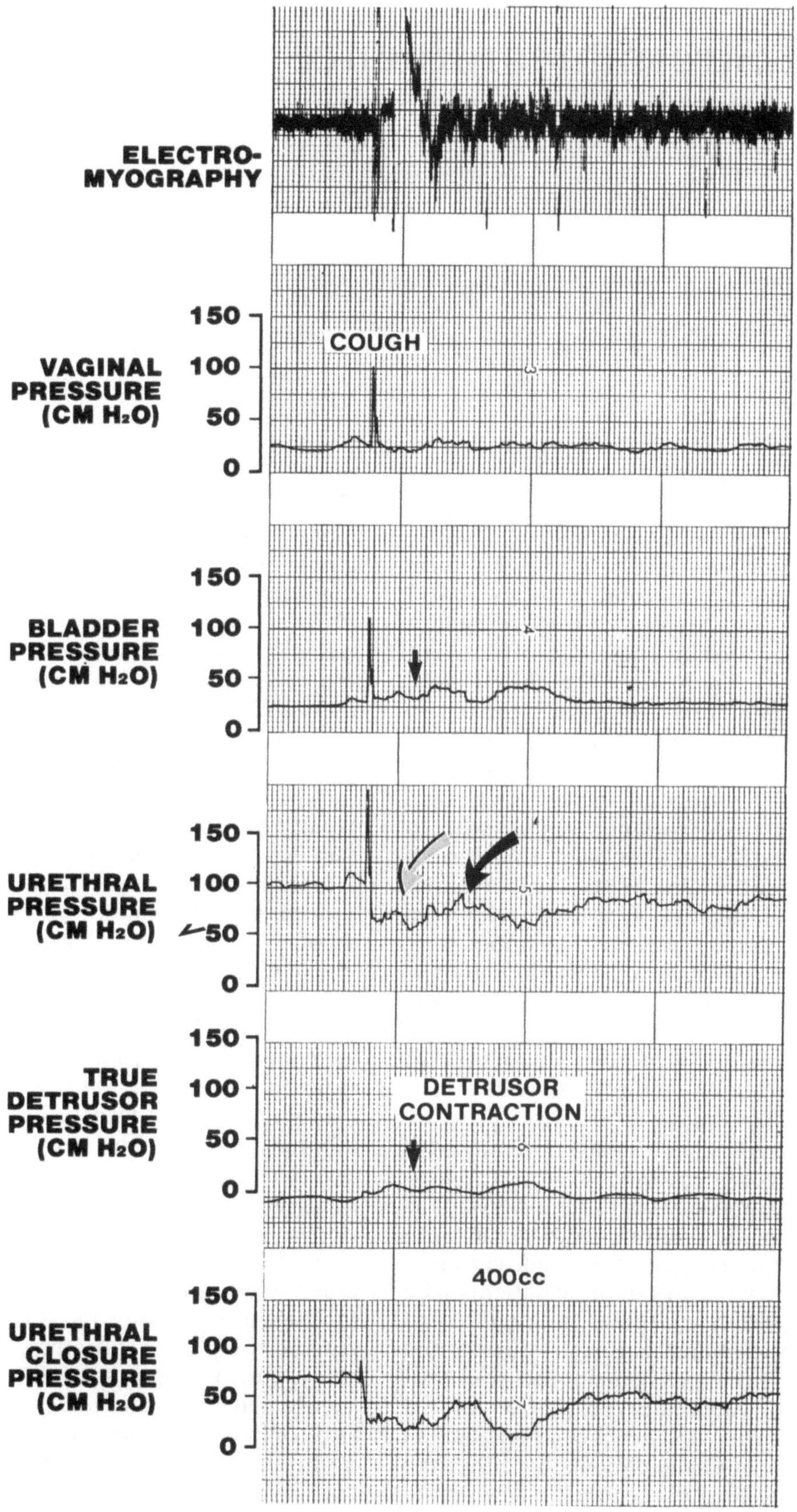


**Fig. 52.1.** Cough induced detrusor instability on postoperative urethrocystometry following a modified Pereyra procedure.

Chapter 53

# Type III Stress Incontinence

As described in Chapter 29, the loss of intrinsic sphincteric function may result in a urethra with remarkably decreased urethral resistance and closure pressure. Such loss of urethral resistance may cause stress incontinence even in a well-supported urethra. The patient who has a well-supported proximal urethra, with little or no urethral mobility, associated with urinary leakage during increases in intra-abdominal pressure is said to have Type III stress incontinence. On radiographic studies these patients will be seen to have an open bladder neck, at rest, at maximum cystometric capacity. On urodynamic testing, these patients look identical to patients who have a low pressure urethra. These two conditions are distinguished by the absence of urethral hypermobility in patients who have Type III stress incontinence. Some examiners distinguish between Type III stress incontinence and Type III stress incontinence with mobility. We believe that the latter is more accurately called a low pressure urethra which avoids confusion. Patients with Type III stress incontinence should not be treated with routine anti-incontinence operations. It is inappropriate to do routine retropubic urethropexies, needle suspensions, and certainly primary vaginal procedures in these patients who have well-supported urethras to begin with because these operations work by resupporting the urethra. These patients benefit only from relative urethral obstruction or coaptation of the urethral mucosa. This can best be accomplished in Type III stress incontinent patients by either the use of obstructive sling procedures, placement of artificial urinary sphincters or the use of periurethral injections of heterologous and autologous materials. Recent advances in the use of heterologous and autologous periurethral injections should soon make obstructive anti-incontinence operations, such as suburethral slings and artificial sphincters almost obsolete in these patients. These operations, although effective in treating Type III stress incontinence, are associated with increased morbidity in comparison and the frequent need for self-catheterization. Periurethral injections can be done in the outpatient setting, are far less costly, morbid, and usually allow for normal voiding after treatment.

In Fig. 53.1, we see the urethral closure pressure profiles of a 74-year-old multiparous female who had previously undergone an anterior colporrhaphy with Kelly–Kennedy plication and Marshall–Marchetti–Krantz procedure on two separate occasions to try to control urinary incontinence. Despite these two different operations, the patient's urinary incontinence increased rather than decreased. Currently, she wears five adult diapers a day and loses urine involuntarily with minimal activity. The severity of this problem severely limits her activities and social interactions, leading to secondary depression. Urethral closure pressure profiles in these patients may be very difficult to perform without fluoroscopic guidance, because it is often difficult to tell when the urethral pressure measuring transducer has entered the proximal urethra. This is noted at the arrow during the first urethral closure pressure profile, when the urethral closure pressure subtly rises only to fall, soon after, to below zero at the midurethra. During the first urethral closure pressure profile registered here, the patient has a closure pressure of approximately 3 $cmH_2O$. During the second urethral closure pressure profile, she is noted to have a closure pressure of

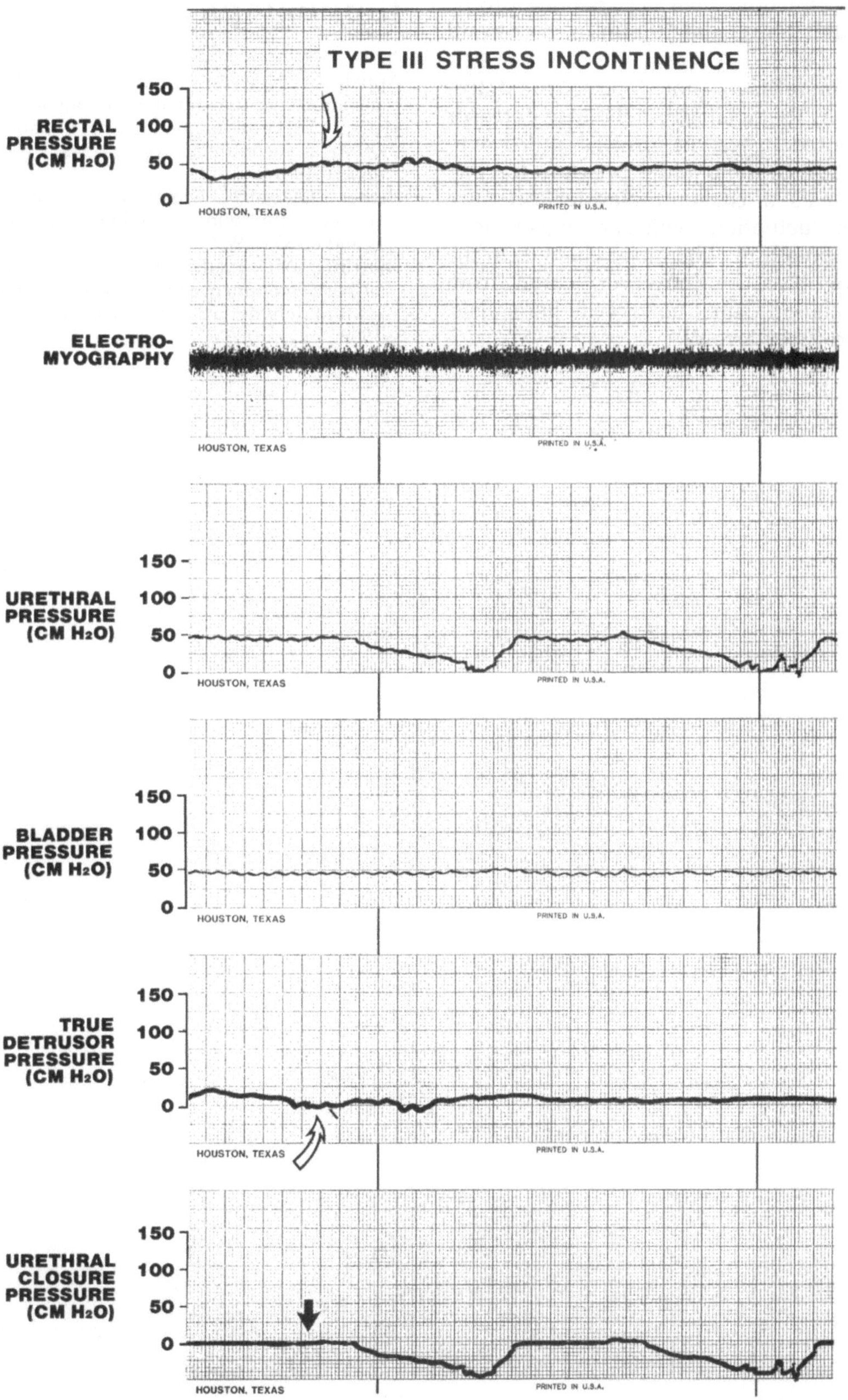


**Fig. 53.1.** Resting urethral closure pressure profiles in a patient with Type III incontinence following two failed operations.

4 $cmH_2O$. The functional length of the first profile is approximately 8 mm and 10 mm in the second profile.

A subtraction artifact is noted in the true detrusor pressure. At the open arrow the true detrusor pressure is noted to waiver upward and downward. Inspection of the bladder pressure tracing, however, reveals a constant bladder pressure despite minor fluctuations which are registrations of the patient breathing. The major changes in the true detrusor pressure, however, come from changes in rectal pressure due to rectal peristalsis, as is indicated (open arrow).

# Bibliography

Appell RA: New developments: injectables for urethral incompetence in women. Int Urogynecol J 1:117, 1990.

McGuire EJ: Urodynamic findings in patients after failure of stress incontinence operations. Prog Clin Biol Res 78:351, 1981.

Osther PJ, Rohl H: Female urinary stress incontinence treated with teflon injections. Acta Obstet Gynecol Scand 66:333, 1987.

Shortliffe LMD, Freiha FS, Kessler R et al: Treatment of urinary incontinence by the periurethral implantation of glutaraldehyde cross-linked collagen. J Urol 141:538, 1989.

# Appendices

# Appendix A
# Office Treatment of Urinary Incontinence

This part of the text is intended to present the reader with some commonly used methods to treat the abnormalities described in the text. It is not meant to be a definitive treatise on these treatments nor the research surrounding their use. For such information, the reader is directed to the references listed in the appropriate areas of this text for a more involved discussion of these treatment modalities.

## A.1 Bladder Drill

One of the most common forms of behavior modification utilized to treat incontinent women was described by Frewen as bladder drill. Bladder drill is used primarily for detrusor instability but may also be used for sensory urgency quite effectively. Like all forms of behavior modification, successful bladder drill requires a motivated and compliant patient. This is best achieved by the physician adequately explaining the basis for behavior modification and giving the patient the confidence that bladder drill will work.

We start by informing the patient that control of micturition is initially gained in early childhood when children first realize that they can identify an impending bladder contraction and inform their parents of this event. Children later learn that they are able not only to recognize an impending bladder contraction but sometimes inhibit it. Beyond this, at around the fourth year of life, the child learns not only to inhibit unwanted bladder contractions but also is able to initiate and inhibit bladder contractions at will. This adult pattern of micturition is lost in patients who have detrusor instability. They need to understand that they have lost this voluntary control and they are voiding when their bladder tells them to and not when their frontal cortex dictates.

The first step to restore bladder control using bladder drill is to assess the patient's normal intervoiding interval and then to have them void at a shorter interval, based on a cortical signal rather than a bladder signal. If the patient normally voids every 2–3 hours during the day then she is instructed instead to void on an hourly basis by the clock. She is told to void only at the designated times and not at other times. In this way we begin to have the patient assert cortical control not only over the initiation of micturition but also to begin to negate afferent bladder signals of "urgency" and restore cortical control over these episodes. Should the patient feel the urge to urinate at a non-assigned time, she is instructed to sit down and to try to contract her periurethral musculature to indirectly inhibit the bladder contraction. The patients are given bladder drill cards such as seen in Fig. A.1, and they record when they urinate as well as when they have accidents during their wakeful hours. They do not continue bladder drill during the night but instead merely record when they voided during the night and if they had urge incontinence during the night. As with bladder control in children, night time control seems to follow the establishment of daytime control in adults. By using this technique and having patients come back every 2–4 weeks to assess their progress and gradually lengthen their intervoiding interval, success has been reported in 60%–92% of patients.

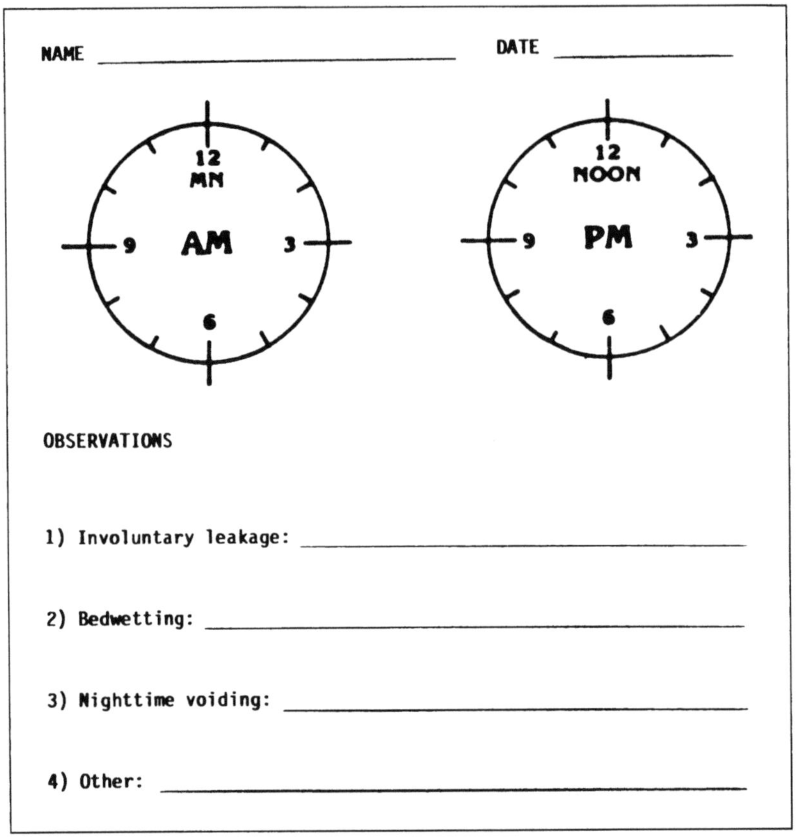


**Fig. A.1.** Both sides of a bladder drill card used for behavior modification in the treatment of detrusor instability.

## Bibliography

Fantl JA, Wyman JF, McClish DK et al: Efficacy of bladder training in older women with urinary incontinence. JAMA 256:609, 1991.

Frewen WK: Role of bladder training in the treatment of the unstable bladder in the female. Urol Clin North Am 6:273, 1979.

Frewen WK: The significance of the psychosomatic factor in urge incontinence. Br J Urol 56:330, 1984.

# A.2 Biofeedback

Using auditory and visual biofeedback several groups have been able to show significant improvement in patients with detrusor instability. Like other forms of behavioral therapy it is used for people with non-neurologic conditions (detrusor instability). Cures rates as high as 50% with improvement in up to 90% of patients have been reported. Patients undergo bladder filling either retrograde or orthograde and are presented with information regarding their pelvic floor electromyographic activity, their urethral pressure and/or detrusor pressure. They are trained to recognize what happens prior to their episodes of urge incontinence. By recognizing urethral relaxation before an involuntary leakage episode, by identifying decreased EMG activity or a drop in urethral pressure, the patient can be taught to contract the periurethral striated muscle in an attempt to inhibit the bladder contraction. Repetitive filling studies are done to educate the patient to inhibit the detrusor reflexively by contracting the periurethral skeletal musculature. Sessions of 1–2 h are repeated weekly for up to three months. Although this is a very successful therapy, it is labor intensive and expensive in comparison to other behavioral therapies. In addition, long-term follow-up data are lacking.

## Bibliography

Burgio KL, Whitehead WE, Engel BT: Urinary incontinence in the elderly: bladder–sphincter biofeedback and

toileting skills training. Ann Intern Med 104:507, 1985.
Cardozo LD, Abrams PD, Stanton SL et al: Idiopathic bladder instability treated by biofeedback. Br J Urol 50:521, 1978.
O'Donnell PD, Doyle R: Biofeedback therapy technique for treatment of urinary incontinence. Urology 37:432, 1991.

## A.3 Prompted Voiding

Another form of behavior modification, prompted voiding has been used successfully, mostly in institutions, to reduce the number of involuntary voiding episodes and to help control costs for diapers and laundry. In patients who are not cognatively appropriate candidates for bladder drill, their caretakers may prompt them to void on a regular basis (i.e., every 2 hours) to avoid urge incontinence from detrusor instability or detrusor hyperreflexia. Although detrusor hyperreflexia will not respond to behavior modification such as bladder drill with resolution of involuntary bladder contractions, prompted voiding may help these patients avoid being wet. Once an appropriate interval is discerned, if fluid intake is constant, excellent control may be achieved even in large populations of patients (i.e., nursing homes).

### Bibliography

Hadley EC: Bladder training and related therapies for incontinence in older people. JAMA 256:372, 1986.
Hu T, Igou JF, Kaltreider L et al: A clinical trial of a behavioral therapy to reduce urinary incontinence in nursing homes. JAMA 261:2656, 1989.
Ouslander JG, Blaustein J, Connor A, et al: Habit training and oxybutynin for incontinence in nursing home patients. J Am Geriatr Soc 36:40, 1988.

## A.4 Pharmacologic Therapy for Detrusor Overactivity

The most common therapy for urge incontinence due to detrusor instability and detrusor hyperreflexia is currently pharmacotherapy. However, this is not necessarily the most successful form of therapy and it is often complicated by side effects. One must be especially careful with the use of such pharmacologic agents in elderly persons where their half-life may be dramatically extended because of relative hepatic and renal insufficiency.

Medications may be grouped into five different categories for the treatment of urge incontinence as shown in Table A.1. The beta-sympathomimetics, although theoretically bladder relaxants, have not been shown to be effective in vivo for controlling detrusor instability. In the future, it is likely that we will see more and more combination medications with anticholinergic and calcium channel blocking effects. In Table A.1, different medications commonly used to treat urge incontinence are listed along with dosage ranges. Table A.2 lists the common side effects of these medications. Most of these side effects are due to the anticholinergic properties of these medications.

### Bibliography

Castleden CM, Duffin HM, Gulati RS: Double-blind study of imipramine and placebo for incontinence due to bladder instability. Age Ageing 15:299, 1986.
Gerstenberg TC, Klarskov P, Ramirez D et al: Terodiline in the treatment of women with urgency and motor urge incontinence. Br J Urol 58:129, 1986.
Lose G, Jorgensen L, Thinedborg P: Doxepin in the treatment of female detrusor overactivity: a randomized double-blind crossover study. J Urol 142:1024, 1989.
Lukkarinen O, Grohn P, Wilen-Rosenquist G et al: A controlled, double-blind crossover study of terodiline in motor urge incontinence. Ann Chir Gynaecol 76:128, 1987.
Rud T, Anderson KE, Ulmsten U: Effects of nifedipine in women with unstable bladders. Urol Int 34:421, 1979.
Sand PK, Brubaker L: Non-surgical treatment of detrusor overactivity in postmenopausal women. J Reprod Med 35:758, 1990.
Tapp AJS, Cardozo LD, Versi E et al: The treatment of detrusor instability in post-menopausal women with oxybutynin chloride: a double blind placebo controlled study. Br J Obstet Gynaecol 97:521, 1990.
Tapp A, Fall M, Norgaard J et al: Terodiline: a dose titrated, multicenter study of the treatment of idiopathic detrusor instability in women. J Urol 142:1027, 1989.
Zeagers AGM, Kiesswetter H, Kramer AEJL et al: Conservative therapy of frequency, urgency and urge incontinence: a double-blind clinical trial of flavoxate hydrochloride, oxybutynin chloride, emepronium bromide and placebo. World J Urol 5:57, 1987.

## A.5 Pharmacologic Therapy for Genuine Stress Incontinence

Medications used for the treatment of genuine stress incontinence fall primarily into two categories. These are the sympathomimetics and the tricyclic antidepressants which also appear to have some alpha-adrenergic activity. The primary sympathomimetic in this group utilized for the

**Table A.1** Drugs utilized for the treatment of detrusor overactivity

| | | Dose | Frequency |
|---|---|---|---|
| *Anticholinergics* | | | |
| Propantheline bromide | P.O. | 13–30 mg | q 4°–6° |
| Methantheline bromide | P.O. | 50 mg | q 12°–24° |
| Emepronium bromide | I.M. | 25–50 mg | |
| *Antispasmodics* | | | |
| Dicyclomine HCl | P.O. | 10–30 mg | q 6°–24° |
| Oxybutynin chloride | P.O. | 2.5–10 mg | q 6°–24° |
| Flavoxate HCl | P.O. | 100–200 mg | q 6°–12° |
| Hyoscyamine sulfate | P.O. | 0.125–0.375 mg | q 6°–12° |
| *Tricyclic antidepressants* | | | |
| Imipramine HCl | P.O. | 25–75 mg | q 8°–24° |
| Doxepin HCl | P.O. | 25–75 mg | q8°–24° |
| *Sympathomimetics* | | | |
| Phenylpropanolamine HCl | P.O. | 25–75 mg | q 8°–12° |
| Midodrine | P.O. | 25–75 mg | q 8°–12° |
| Terbutaline | P.O. | 2.5–5.0 mg | q 4° |
| *Calcium channel blockers* | | | |
| Nifedipine | P.O. | 10–20 mg | q 12°–24° |
| Terodiline | P.O. | 25–75 mg | q 24° |

**Table A.2** Side effects of the drugs used for the treatment of detrusor overactivity

| |
|---|
| Dry mouth |
| Urinary retention |
| Constipation |
| Blurred vision |
| Drowsiness |
| Hallucinations |
| Decreased sweating |
| Tachycardia |
| Headache |
| Dizziness |

treatment of stress incontinence is phenylpropanolamine. This is available by prescription or may be obtained as the primary ingredient in many over-the-counter diet pills and cold remedies such as Dexatrim®, Entex LA®, Ornade®, Contact®, Allerest®, Dimetapp®, Triaminic®, Tavist® and Drixoral®. Phenlypropanolamine is usually given in doses of 25–75 mg bid or tid and has been shown to be more effective than placebo in relieving symptoms of stress incontinence. It appears to cure 10%–20% of patients and to improve symptomatically up to 60% of patients. Its use is largely limited by its effect on their peripheral vascular system. There are numerous reports in the medical literature of normotensive women having cerebrovascular accidents and myocardial infarctions following abuse of these medications. Therefore, baseline blood pressures should be obtained prior to starting alpha-adrenergic medications and blood pressure should be checked with some frequency during the first two weeks of therapy (1-2h after taking medication for 3 days). This side effect of significant hypertension may be less common with midodrine, another alpha-adrenergic agent which has been shown to be effective for the treatment of stress incontinence in European trials and is currently being tested in the United States for the treatment of genuine stress incontinence.

The tricyclic antidepressant imipramine has alpha-adrenergic type effects on the smooth muscle of the urethra. In addition, it is also effective in the treatment of detrusor overactivity. It does not appear to cause hypertension as seen with the alpha-adrenergic drugs but does cause a number of side effects as listed in Table A.2. Therapy is usually initiated with doses of 25–75 mg at bedtime and may be increased slowly to doses as high as 300 mg per day.

## Bibliography

Lose G, Rix P, Diermore E et al: Norfenefrine in the treatment of female stress incontinence. Urol Int 43:11, 1988.

Sand PK, Brubaker L: Nonsurgical treatment of detrusor overactivity in postmenopausal women. J Reprod Med 35:758, 1990.
Schtonen T, Rannicko S. Lindell O et al: The effect of phenylpropanolamine on female stress urinary incontinence. Ann Chir Gynaecol 75:236, 1986.

## A.6 Physiotherapy for Genuine Stress Incontinence

In 1949, Kegel introduced the concept of progressive resistance exercises to treat genuine stress incontinence. He reported cure rates in excess of 70%. Kegel advocated the use of a balloon perineometer which was able to measure increases in vaginal pressure from contraction of the puborectalis muscle. Since that time no one has been able to achieve quite this level of success with physiotherapy. And whereas physiotherapy does not correct the underlying urethral hypermobility in patients with genuine stress incontinence it does aid in the treatment of incontinence by strengthening the striated periurethral muscle and improve its response to increases in intra-abdominal pressure. For many years physicians have suggested that patients try to interrupt the flow of urine during normal micturition to identify which muscles need to be trained. Once they have an idea of how to selectively contract the pubococcygeal musculature while not straining nor increasing gluteal muscle activity, they are instructed to do ten 3 s contractions in a row and then repeat these sets five to ten times a day. Over the last 40 years, many patients have either received these instructions verbally or received tear sheets describing these exercises. Most of these patients either do not comply with the suggested therapy or become rapidly frustrated with their inability to identify the proper muscle groups to exercise. Some may actually strain, instead of contracting the periurethral musculature, which may actually be detrimental. Therefore, only the most motivated and diligent patients will have any chance for success with this therapy in the absence of extensive training or biofeedback. Over the last decade, physiotherapy aided by biofeedback has undergone a resurgence. Several investigators have reported symptomatic improvement in 50%–75% of patients using either vaginal cones, perineometers or EMG directed biofeedback. Success has been roughly the same with all of these groups. Probably the simplest way to initiate physiotherapy with biofeedback is with the use of vaginal cones.

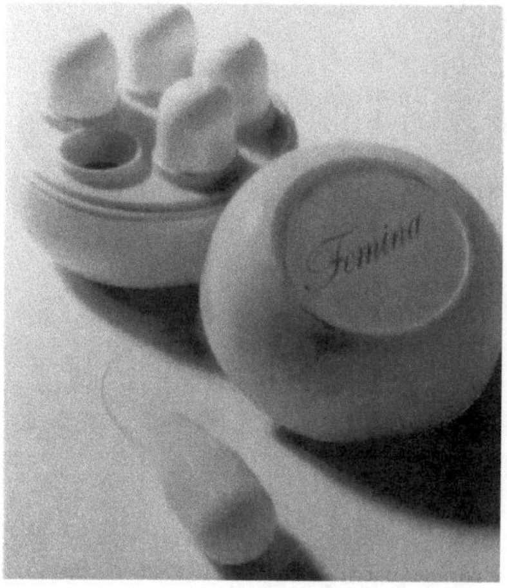


**Fig. A.2.** Set of five weighted vaginal cones (Femina®, Dacomed Inc., Minneapolis, MN) used for biofeedback with physiotherapy.

These are available in sets of five conically shaped weights (Fig. A.2).

When a cone is placed in the vagina with the tapered end down the weight on the levator muscles aids the patient in identifying which muscles to contract. These cones are then worn for 15 min in the morning and 15 min in the evening during light household activities in the sitting and standing positions. If the patient is able to retain the lightest weight cone for both sessions she then moves to the second lightest cone on the following day. The cones are very easy to work with. If the cone slips out, the patient places it back in the vagina and continues with the 15 min session. After initial success with the cones, it is suggested to patients that rapid contraction exercises be initiated at the end of each session for 3–5 min to strengthen fast twitch muscle fibers. Patients are instructed to rapidly contact their levator muscles as strongly as possible while keeping their rectus muscles relaxed. Intermittent 3 s periods of contracting and relaxing exercises are done. Although EMG-directed devices and the perineometer are also excellent for biofeedback they are far more expensive than vaginal cones.

## Bibliography

Bump RC, Hurt WG, Fantl JA et al: Assessment of Kegel pelvic muscle exercise performance after brief verbal instruction. Am J Obstet Gynecol 165:322, 1991.
Kegel AH: The physiologic treatment of poor tone and function of the genital muscles and of urinary stress incontinence. World J Surg Obstet Gynecol Nov: 527, 1949.

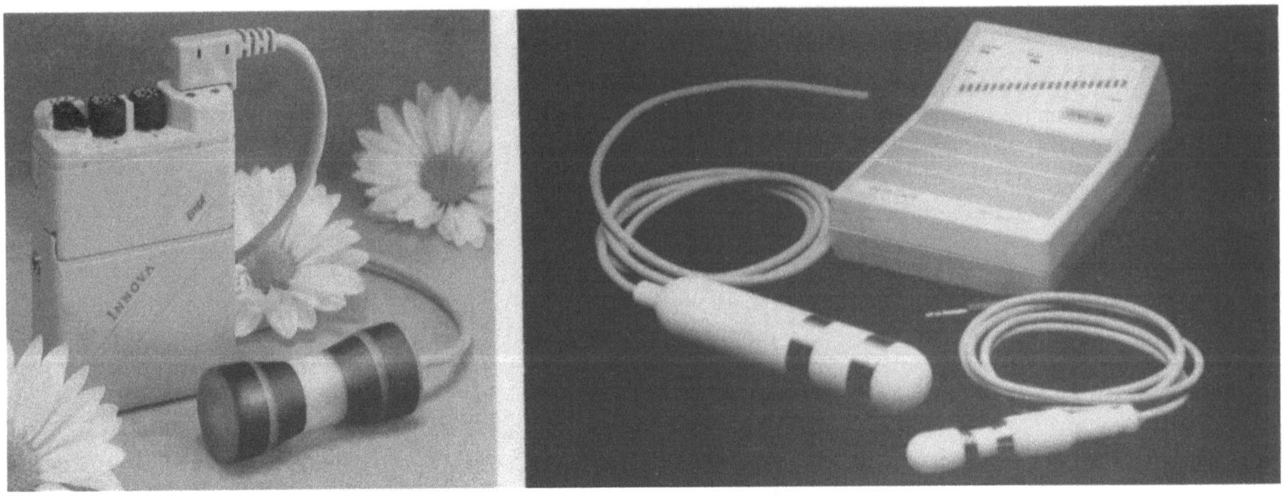


**Fig. A.3.** Two home pelvic floor stimulation units marketed in the United States for the treatment of genuine stress incontinence and detrusor overactivity.

Klarskov P, Nielsen KK, Kromann-Andersen B et al: Long-term results of pelvic floor training and surgery for female genuine stress incontinence. Int Urogynecol J 2:132, 1991.
Peattie AB, Plevnick S, Stanton SL: Vaginal cones: a conservative method of treating genuine stress incontinence. Br J Obstet Gynaecol 95:1049, 1988.
Sandri SD, Biggiogero L, Fanciullacci F et al: Long-term follow-up results of pelvic floor rehabilitation in female stress urinary incontinence. Int Urogynecol J 1:188, 1990.
Susset JG, Galea G, Read L: Biofeedback therapy for female incontinence due to low urethral resistance. J Urol 143:1205, 1990.
Tchou CH, Adams C, Varner RE et al: Pelvic floor musculature exercises in treatment of anatomical urinary stress incontinence. Phys Ther 68:652, 1988.

## A.7 Pelvic Floor Stimulation for Treatment of Urinary Incontinence

Pelvic floor stimulation has been utilized for over 25 years to treat both genuine stress incontinence as well as urge incontinence due to detrusor instability and detrusor hyperreflexia. Although the mechanism by which electrical stimulation treats detrusor instability and genuine stress incontinence is not perfectly clear, it is believed that afferent stimulation along the pudendal nerve directly inhibits pelvic nerve activation of the detrusor and stimulation of hypogastric nerve activity may also inhibit bladder contractions. In the treatment of genuine stress incontinence, it is believed that pelvic floor stimulation acts to electronically maximally contract the periurethral striated musculature in an intermittent fashion. Successful treatment of stress incontinence with various devices has been reported in 30%–60% of patients whereas treatment of detrusor overactivity has been reported to be successful in 50%–90% of cases. Although quite popular in some areas of Europe, pelvic floor stimulation has only been minimally utilized in the United States.

Electrical stimulation can be delivered either by vaginal, rectal or implanted electrodes. All three methods seem to offer good success in women but most patients prefer a vaginal approach. Numerous devices are available throughout the world but very few devices are readily available in the United States. Fig. A.3 shows two devices which are commonly used in the United States. The vaginal devices are tampon like in their shape and are placed in the vagina and activated usually for 15–30 min either two or three times per day. The amperage is controlled by the patient so that stimulation should not be painful. Different frequencies have been shown to be optimal for differing conditions. Most authors agree that low frequencies (5–10 Hz) are optimal for detrusor instability whereas higher frequencies (50–100 Hz) appear to be optimal for the treatment of genuine stress incontinence. Treatment with electrical stimulation should yield results in 4–6 weeks. Once success is achieved it may be maintained with less frequent administration of electrical stimulation. Most patients are able to decrease their therapy to three or four days a week, rather than twice daily therapy. Approximately 20% of patients with detrusor instability may achieve long-lasting resolution of their urge incontinence after 8–12 weeks of pelvic floor stimulation.

Acute maximal electrical stimulation for the treatment of detrusor overactivity has been reported to create permanent re-education with relief of symptoms in up to 60% of patients. With acute maximal stimulation, electrical stimulation is delivered with a much stronger current than found in most home units and stimulation is painful yet tolerable. Sessions are done on a weekly basis for 20–30 min and usually repeated for 4–6 weeks.

## Bibliography


Bent AE, Sand PK, Ostergard DR et al: Transvaginal electrical stimulation in the treatment of genuine stress incontinence and detrusor instability. Int Urogynecol J 4:9, 1993.

Eriksen BC, Bergmann S, Eik-Nes SH: Maximal electrostimulation of the pelvic floor in female idiopathic detrusor instability and urge incontinence. Neurourol Urodynam 8:219, 1989.

Eriksen BC, Eik-Nes SH: Long-term electro-stimulation of the pelvic floor: primary therapy in female stress incontinence? Urol Int 44:90, 1989.

Hahn I, Sommer S, Fall M: A comparative study of pelvic floor training and electrical stimulation for the treatment of genuine female stress urinary incontinence. Neurourol Urodynam 10:545, 1991.

Nakamura M, Sakurai T, Sugo H et al: Maximal electrical stimulation for urge incontinence. Urol Int 42: 285, 1987.

Plevnik S, Janez J, Urtacnik P et al: Short-term electrical stimulation: home treatment for urinary incontinence World J Urol 4:24, 1986.

Tanagho EA, Schmidt RA: Electrical stimulation in the clinical management of the neurogenic bladder. J Urol 140:1331, 1988.

# Appendix B
# Terminology of Lower Urinary Tract Function

This section is modified from work produced by the International Continence Society Committee on Standardization of Terminology

In 1973 the International Continence Society established a committee for the standardization of terminology of lower urinary tract function. Their work is summarized here. These standards are recommended to facilitate comparison of results by investigators who use urodynamic methods. These terms and standards are recommended not only for urodynamic investigations carried out on human patients but also during animal studies. When performing urodynamic studies in animals, the type of any anesthesia used should be stated. It is suggested that acknowledgement of these standards in written publications be indicated by a footnote to the Methods and Materials section or its equivalent, to read as follows: "Methods, definitions, and units conform to the standards recommended by the International Continence Society, except where specifically noted."

Urodynamic studies are tests involving the assessment of the function and dysfunction of the urinary tract by any appropriate method. Aspects of urinary tract morphology, physiology, biochemistry, and hydrodynamics affect urine transport and storage. Other methods of investigation such as the radiographic visualization of the lower urinary tract may be useful adjuncts to conventional urodynamics.

This Appendix reviews the urodynamics of the lower urinary tract.

## B.1 Classification of Urinary Tract Dysfunction

The lower urinary tract is composed of the bladder and urethra which together form a functional unit. Each has two functions; the bladder to store and void, and the urethra to control and convey. When a reference is made to the hydrodynamic function or to the whole anatomical unit as a storage organ (the vesica urinaria) the correct term is the bladder. When the smooth muscle structure known as the m. detrusor urinae is being discussed, the correct term is detrusor. For simplicity, the bladder/detrusor and the urethra will be considered separately so that a classification based on a combination of functional anomalies can be reached. Sensation cannot be precisely evaluated but should be assessed. This classification depends on the results of various objective urodynamic investigations which will be discussed in this appendix. A complete urodynamic assessment is not necessary in all patients. However, studies of the filling and voiding phases are essential for each patient. The bladder and urethra may behave differently during the storage and micturition phases. Therefore, it is helpful to examine bladder and urethral activity separately during each phase.

Terms used should be objective, definable, and, ideally, should be widely applicable. When authors use terms that have not been defined here, their meaning should be made clear.

Assuming the absence of inflammation, infection, and neoplasm, lower urinary tract dysfunction may be caused by disturbance of the pertinent nervous or psychological control systems, disorders of muscle function or structural abnormalities.

It is most important that urodynamic diagnoses based on this classification should correlate with the patient's symptoms and signs. For example, the presence of an unstable detrusor contraction in an asymptomatic, continent patient does not warrant a diagnosis of detrusor overactivity during storage.

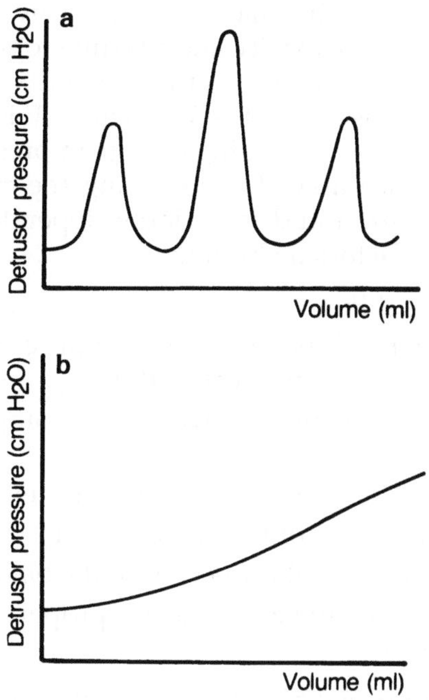


**Fig. B.1.** Diagrams of retrograde cystometry to illustrate (**a**) the typical phasic contractions in patients with detrusor instability and (**b**) the gradual rise in detrusor presence seen in patients with decreased bladder compliance during bladder filling.

# B.2 The Storage Phase

## Detrusor Activity

In this context, detrusor activity is interpreted from the measurement of detrusor pressure (Pdet) and may be described as normal or overactive.

### *Normal Detrusor Function*

During the filling phase, the bladder volume increases without a significant rise in pressure (accommodation). No involuntary contractions occur despite provocation.

A normal detrusor may be described as "stable".

### *Overactive Detrusor Function*

Overactive detrusor function is characterized by involuntary detrusor contractions during the filling phase, which may be spontaneous or provoked and which the patient cannot completely suppress. Involuntary detrusor contractions may be provoked by rapid filling, alterations of posture, coughing, walking, jumping, and other triggering manuevers. Various terms have been used to describe these features, and they are defined as follows:

The unstable detrusor is one that is shown objectively to contract, spontaneously or on provocation, during the filling phase while the patient is attempting to inhibit micturition. Unstable detrusor contractions may be asymptomatic or may be interpreted by the patient as urgency. The presence of these contractions does not necessarily imply a neurological disorder. Unstable contractions are usually phasic in type (Fig. B.1a). A gradual increase in detrusor pressure without subsequent decrease is best regarded as a change of compliance (Fig. B.1b).

Detrusor hyperreflexia is defined as overactivity due to a disturbance of neurologic control. The term detrusor hyperreflexia should only be used when there is objective evidence of a relevant neurological disorder temporally related to the onset of detrusor overactivity. The use of conceptual and undefined terms such as hypertonic, systolic, uninhibited, spastic, neurogenic and automatic should avoided.

## Bladder Sensation

Bladder sensation during filling can be classified in qualitative terms (first desire to void, etc.) and by objective measurement (sensory evoked potentials and reflex latencies). Sensation can be classified broadly as follows:

1. Normal
2. Increased (hypersensitive)
3. Reduced (hyposensitive)
4. Absent

Bladder capacity may be defined by its functional maximal capacity and maximal cystometric capacity described later in this appendix.

*Compliance* is defined as $V/P$ where $V$ is volume and $P$ is the corresponding change in pressure.

Compliance may change during the cystometric examination and is variably dependent on a number of factors including:

1. Rate of filling
2. The part of the cystometrogram curve used for the compliance calculation
3. The volume interval over which compliance is calculated
4. The geometry (shape) of the bladder
5. The thickness of the bladder wall
6. The mechanical properties of the bladder wall
7. The contractile and relaxant properties of the detrusor

During normal bladder filling, little or no pressure change occurs and this is termed "normal compliance". However, at the present time, there are insufficient data to define normal, high, or low compliance.

When reporting compliance one should specify the rate of bladder filling and the bladder volumes at which compliance is calculated.

## Urethral Function During Storage

The urethral closure mechanism during storage may be described as normal or incompetent.

The normal urethral closure mechanism maintains a positive urethral closure pressure during filling even in the presence of increased abdominal pressure. Immediately prior to micturition, the normal closure pressure decreases to allow flow.

An *incompetent urethral closure mechanism* is defined as one that allows leakage of urine in the absence of a detrusor contraction. Leakage may occur whenever intravesical pressure exceeds intraurethral pressure (genuine stress incontinence) or when there is an involuntary fall in urethral pressure. Terms such as "the unstable urethra" await further data and precise definition.

## Urinary Incontinence

*Urinary incontinence* is defined as involuntary loss of urine that is objectively demonstrable and a social or hygienic problem. Loss of urine through channels other than the urethra is extraurethral incontinence.

Urinary incontinence denotes a symptom indicating the patient's statement of involuntary urine loss, a sign represents the objective demonstration of urine loss and a condition which is the urodynamic demonstration of urine loss.

### *Symptoms*

*Urge incontinence* is the involuntary loss of urine associated with a strong desire to void (urgency). Urgency may be associated with two types of dysfunction:

1. Overactive detrusor function (motor urgency)
2. Hypersensitivity (sensory urgency)

*Stress incontinence* is the symptom indicated by the patient's statement of involuntary loss of urine during physical exertion.

*"Unconscious" incontinence* is urinary leakage that may occur in the absence of urgency and without conscious recognition of the urinary loss.

*Enuresis* represents any involuntary loss of urine. If it is used to denote incontinence during sleep, it should be qualified as "nocturnal" enuresis.

*Postmicturition dribble* and *continuous leakage* denote other symptomatic forms of incontinence.

### *Signs*

The sign of stress incontinence denotes the observation of urine loss through the urethra during physical exertion (e.g., coughing). Incontinence may also be observed without physical exercise. Postmicturition dribble and continuous leakage denote other signs of incontinence. Symptoms and signs do not indicate the cause of urinary incontinence. Accurate diagnosis often requires urodynamic investigation in addition to careful history and physical examination.

### *Conditions*

*Genuine stress incontinence* is the involuntary loss of urine occurring when the intravesical pressure exceeds the maximum urethral pressure in the absence of a detrusor contraction.

*Reflex incontinence* is loss of urine due to detrusor hyperreflexia and/or involuntary urethral relaxation in the absence of the sensation usually associated with the desire to micturate. This condition is usually only seen in patients with neuropathic bladder and urethral disorders.

*Overflow incontinence* represents any involuntary loss of urine associated with overdistension of the bladder.

# B.3 The Voiding Phase

## Detrusor Function During Voiding

During micturition, the detrusor may be acontractile, underactive or normal.

The *acontractile detrusor* is one that cannot be demonstrated to contract during urodynamic studies. *Detrusor areflexia* is defined as acontractility due to a neurologic problem and denotes the complete absence of a centrally coordinated contraction. In detrusor areflexia due to a lesion of the conus medullaris or sacral nerve outflow, the detrusor should be described as decentralized and not denervated, because the peripheral neurons remain. In such bladders, pressure fluctuations of low amplitude, sometimes known as "autonomous" waves, may occasionally occur. The use of terms such as atonic, hypotonic, autonomic, and flaccid should be avoided.

*Detrusor underactivity* is defined as a detrusor contraction of inadequate magnitude and/or duration to bring about complete bladder emptying within a normal time span. Patients may have underactivity during micturition and detrusor overactivity during filling.

*Normal detrusor contractility* is represented by the ability voluntarily to initiate a detrusor contraction that is sustained and can be suppressed voluntarily. A normal detrusor contraction will result in complete bladder emptying in the absence of obstruction. For a given detrusor contraction, the magnitude of the recorded pressure rise will depend on the degree of outlet resistance.

## Urethral Function During Voiding

During voiding, urethral function may be normal or obstructive due to muscular overactivity or mechanical obstruction.

The normal urethra opens to allow the bladder to be emptied completely.

Obstruction due to urethral overactivity occurs when the urethral closure mechanism contracts against a detrusor contraction or fails to open when the detrusor contracts. Synchronous detrusor and urethral contraction is called detrusor/urethral dyssynergia. This diagnosis should be qualified by stating the location and type of urethral muscles (striated or smooth) that are involved. Despite the confusion surrounding "sphincter" terminology, the use of certain terms is so widespread that they are retained and defined here. The term detrusor/external sphincter dyssynergia or detrusor–sphincter–dyssynergia (DSD) describes a detrusor contraction concurrent with involuntary contraction of the urethral and/or periurethral striated muscle. In the adult, detrusor sphincter dyssynergia is a feature of neurological voiding disorders. In the absence of neurologic disease, the validity of this diagnosis should be questioned. The term detrusor/bladder neck dyssynergia is used to denote a detrusor contraction concurrent with an objectively demonstrated failure of bladder neck opening. No parallel term has been elaborated for possible detrusor/distal urethral (smooth muscle) dyssynergia.

Overactivity of the urethral sphincter may occur during voiding in the absence of neurological disease and is termed dysfunctional voiding. The use of terms such as "non-neurogenic" or "occult neuropathic" should be avoided.

Mechanical obstruction is most commonly anatomical, e.g. urethral stricture.

Using these characteristics of detrusor and urethral function during storage and micturition an accurate definition of lower urinary tract behavior in each patient becomes possible.

# B.4 Office Assessment

The basic clinical assessment of patients with lower urinary tract dysfunction should consist of a detailed history, a frequency/volume chart, and a physical examination. In urinary incontinence, leakage should be demonstrated objectively by some type of stress test.

## History

The general history should include questions relevant to neurological and congenital abnormalities as well as information on previous urinary tract infections, obstetric history and relevant surgery. A list of medications should be obtained focusing on medications with known or possible effects on the lower urinary tract. The general history should also include assessment of menstrual, sexual, and bowel function.

The urinary history must consist of questions about symptoms related to both the storage and the evacuation functions of the lower urinary tract.

### Frequency/Volume Chart

The frequency/volume chart is a specific urodynamic investigation that records fluid intake and urine output per 24-hour period (Fig. B.2). The chart gives objective information on the number of voids, the distribution of voidings between daytime and nighttime, and each voided volume. The chart can also be used to record episodes of urgency and leakage and the number of incontinence pads used. The frequency/volume chart is very useful in the initial qualitative assessment of voiding disorders and in the follow-up of treatment.

### Physical Examination

Besides a general urological and gynecological examination, the physical examination should include a basic lumbosacral neurologic assessment including evaluation of perineal sensation, the perineal reflexes supplied by the sacral segments $S_2$ to $S_4$, and anal sphincter tone and control.

## B.5 Evaluation of the Storage Phase

### Cystometry

Cystometry is the method by which the pressure/volume relationship of the bladder is measured. All systems are zeroed at atmospheric pressure. For external transducers, the reference point is the level of the superior edge of the symphysis pubis. For catheter-mounted transducers, the reference point is the transducer itself.

Cystometry is used to assess detrusor activity, sensation, capacity, and compliance.

Before starting to fill the bladder, the residual urine may be measured. However, the removal of a large volume of residual urine may alter detrusor function, especially in neuropathic disorders. Certain cystometric parameters may be significantly altered by the speed of bladder filling.

During cystometry, it is assumed that the patient is awake, unanesthetized, and neither sedated nor taking drugs that affect bladder function. Any variations should be specified. In addition the following factors should be defined for cystometry:

1. Access (transurethral or percutaneous)
2. Fluid medium (saline, $H_2O$ or $CO_2$ gas)
3. Temperature of fluid (state in degrees Celsius)
4. Position of patient (e.g. supine, sitting, or standing)
5. Filling mode (orthograde by diuresis or retrograde by catheter).

Filling by catheter may be continuous or incremental and the precise filling rate should be stated. When the incremental method is used, the volume increment should be stated. For general discussion, the following terms for the range of filling rate may be used:

Slow-fill up to 10 ml/min
Medium-fill 10–100 ml/min
Rapid fill over 100 ml/min

#### *Technique*

The technique of pressure measurement should be defined, by listing the equipment used.

1. Fluid-filled catheter: specify number of catheters, single or multiple lumens, type of (manufacturer) and size of catheter
2. Catheter tip transducer: list specifications and number of transducers
3. Other catheters: list specifications
4. Measuring equipment

#### *Definitions*

*Intravesical pressure* is the pressure within the bladder which is created by abdominal and detrusor pressure.

*Abdominal pressure* is taken to be the pressure surrounding the bladder. In current practice, it is

## VOIDING DIARY

| TIME | AMOUNT VOIDED | ACTIVITY | LEAK VOLUME | URGE PRESENT | AMOUNT/TYPE OF INTAKE |
|---|---|---|---|---|---|
| | | | | | |
| | | | | | |
| | | | | | |
| | | | | | |
| | | | | | |
| | | | | | |
| | | | | | |
| | | | | | |
| | | | | | |
| | | | | | |
| | | | | | |
| | | | | | |
| | | | | | |
| | | | | | |
| | | | | | |
| | | | | | |
| | | | | | |
| | | | | | |
| | | | | | |
| | | | | | |
| | | | | | |
| | | | | | |
| | | | | | |
| | | | | | |
| | | | | | |
| | | | | | |
| | | | | | |
| | | | | | |

**Fig. B.2.** An example of a voiding diary or frequency volume chart.

estimated from vaginal, rectal, or less commonly, extraperitoneal pressure.

*Detrusor pressure* is that component of intravesical pressure that is created by forces in the bladder wall (passive and active). It is estimated by subtracting abdominal pressure from intravesical pressure. The simultaneous measurement of abdominal pressure, therefore, is essential for the interpretation of the detrusor pressure. However, artifacts on the detrusor pressure tracing may be produced by intrinsic rectal or vaginal contractions.

*Bladder sensation* is difficult to evaluate because of its subjective nature. It is usually assessed by questioning the patient in relation to the fullness of the bladder during cystometry.

Commonly used descriptive terms of bladder sensation include the following.

*First desire to void* is defined as the lowest volume that the patient can identify as being able to void at.

*Normal desire to void* is defined as the feeling that leads the patient to pass urine at the next convenient moment, but voiding can be delayed if necessary.

*Strong desire to void* is defined as a persistent desire to void without the fear of leakage.

*Urgency* is defined as a strong desire to void accompanied by fear of leakage or fear of pain.

*Pain* (the site and character of which should be specified). Pain during bladder filling or micturition is abnormal.

*Maximum cystometric capacity*, in patients with normal sensation, is the volume at which the patient feels she can no longer delay micturition. In the absence of sensation, the maximum cystometric capacity cannot be defined in the same terms and is the volume at which the clinician decides to terminate filling. In the presence of sphincter incompetence, the maximum cystometric capacity may be significantly increased by occlusion of the urethra with a balloon catheter.

The *functional bladder capacity*, or largest voided volume, is more relevant and is assessed from a frequency/volume chart (urinary diary).

The *maximum (anesthetic) bladder capacity* is the volume measured after filling during a deep general or spinal/epidural anesthetic, specifying fluid temperature, filling pressure, and filling time.

*Compliance* indicates the change in pressure during a change in volume. Compliance is calculated by dividing the volume change ($V$) by the change in detrusor pressure ($P_{det}$) during that change in bladder volume ($V/P_{det}$). Compliance is expressed as ml/cm$H_2O$.

## Urethral Pressure Measurement

It should be noted that the urethral pressure and the urethral closure pressure are idealized concepts that represent the ability of the urethra to prevent leakage. In current urodynamic practice, the urethral pressure is measured by a number of different techniques that may be subject to considerable artifact.

*Intraluminal urethral pressure* may be measured while the patient is at rest, coughing, straining or during voiding. Measurements may be made at one point in the urethra over a period of time, or at several points along the urethra consecutively forming a urethral pressure profile (UPP).

Two types of UPP may be measured during the storage phase.

1. The *resting urethral pressure profile* which is measured with the bladder and subject at rest.
2. The *stress urethral pressure profile* which is measured during a defined applied stress (e.g. cough, Valsalva).

In the storage phase, the urethral pressure profile defines the intraluminal pressure along the length of the urethra. All systems are zeroed at atmospheric pressure. For external transducers, the reference point is the superior edge of the symphysis pubis. For catheter mounted transducers, the reference point is the transducer itself. Intravesical pressure should be measured to exclude simultaneous detrusor contractions. The subtraction of intravesical pressure produces the urethral closure pressure profile.

The simultaneous recording of both intravesical and intraurethral pressure are essential during stress urethral profilometry.

The following variables and techniques should be specified when describing urethral pressure profiles:

1. Infusion medium (liquid or gas)
2. Rate of infusion
3. Stationary, continuous, or intermittent withdrawal
4. Rate of withdrawal
5. Bladder volume
6. Position of patient (supine, sitting, or standing)
7. Type of catheter:
   a) Open catheter: specify type (manufacturer), size, number, position, and orientation of side or end hole.
   b) Catheter mounted transducers: specify manufacturer, number of transducers, spacing of transducers along the catheter,

orientation with respect to one another, transducer design (e.g. transducer face depressed or flush with catheter surface), catheter diameter, and material. The orientation of the transducer(s) in the urethra should be stated.

c) Other catheters (e.g. membrane, fiberoptic): specify type (manufacturer), size and number of channels as for microtransducer catheter.

8. Measurement technique: for stress profiles, the particular stress employed should be stated (e.g. cough or Valsalva).
9. Recording apparatus: describe type of recording apparatus. The frequency response of the total system should be stated. The frequency response of the catheter in the perfusion method can be assessed by blocking the eyeholes and recording the consequent rate of change of pressure.

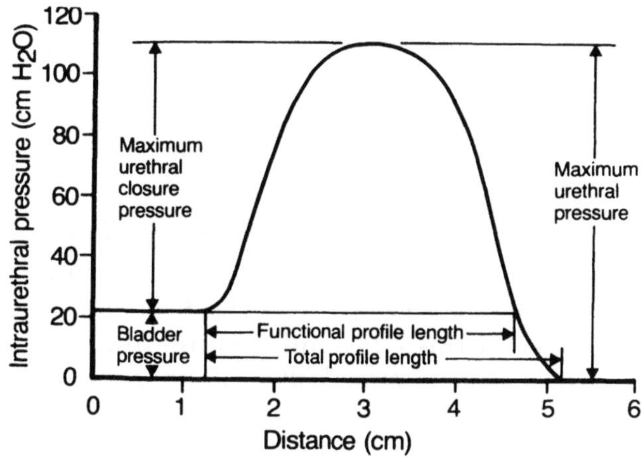


**Fig. B.3.** Diagram of an idealized urethral closure pressure profile with ICS nomenclature.

*Total profile length* is not generally regarded as a useful parameter but is an estimation of the anatomic length of the urethra.

## *Definitions* (Referring to profiles measured in storage phase) (Fig. B.3)

*Maximum urethral pressure* is the maximum urethral pressure of the measured profile.

*Maximum urethral closure pressure* is the maximum difference between the urethral pressure and the intravesical pressure.

*Functional profile length* is the length of the urethra along which the urethral pressure exceeds intravesical pressure.

*Functional profile length (on stress)* is the length over which the urethral pressure exceeds the intravesical pressure on stress.

*Pressure "transmission" ratio* is the increment in urethral pressure on stress as a percentage of the simultaneously recorded increment in intravesical pressure. For stress profiles obtained during coughing, pressure transmission ratios can be obtained at any point along the urethra. If single values are given, the position in the urethra should be stated. If several pressure transmission ratios are defined at different points along the urethra, a pressure "transmission" profile is obtained. During "coughing profiles", the amplitude of the cough should be stated, if possible. Note that the term "transmission" is in common usage and cannot be changed. However, transmission implies a completely passive process. Such an assumption is not yet justified by scientific evidence. A role for muscular activity is likely.

## Quantification of Urine Loss

Subjective grading of incontinence may not always indicate the degree of urinary leakage. In addition, office urodynamic evaluations may not always demonstrate urinary leakage and an objective test which quantifies urinary leakage may be useful.

A simple standard test can be used to measure urine loss objectively in any subject. It may be used to assess and compare the results of the treatment of different types of incontinence in different centers. In order to obtain a representative result, especially in subjects with variable or intermittent urinary incontinence, the test should occupy as long a period as possible; yet, it must practical. It should mimic everyday life as closely as possible yet be similar for all subjects to allow for meaningful comparison.

The ICS has recommended a test occupying a one-hour period during which a set series of standard activities is carried out. This test can be extended by further one-hour periods if the result of the first one-hour test were not considered representative by either the patient or the investigator. Alternatively, the test can be repeated after having filled the bladder to a defined volume.

The total amount of urine lost during the test period is determined by weighing a collecting device such as a nappy, absorbent pad, or condom appliance. A nappy or pad should be worn inside waterproof underpants or should have a waterproof backing. Care should be taken to use a collecting device of adequate capacity.

Immediately before the test begins, the collecting device is weighed on a gram scale.

A typical test schedule is as follows.

1. Test is started without the patient voiding.
2. Preweighed collecting device is put on and first one-hour test period begins.
3. Subject drinks 500 ml sodium-free liquid within a short period (max. 15 min), and then sits or rests.
4. Half-hour period: subject walks, including stair climbing equivalent to one flight up and down.
5. During the remaining period, the subject performs the following activities:
   a) standing up from sitting, 10 times
   b) coughing vigorously, 10 times
   c) running on the spot for 1 minute
   d) bending to pick up small objects from floor, 5 times
   e) washing hands in running water for 1 minute
6. At the end of the one-hour test, the collecting device is removed and weighed.
7. If the test is regarded as representative, the subject voids, and the volume is recorded.
8. Otherwise, the test is repeated, preferably without voiding.

If the collecting device becomes saturated or filled during the test, it should be removed, weighed and replaced by a fresh device. The total weight of urine lost during the test period is taken to be equal to the gain in weight of the collecting device(s). In interpreting the results of the test, it should be borne in mind that a weight gain of up to 2 g may be due to weighing errors, sweating, or vaginal discharge.

The activity program may be modified according to the subject's physical ability. If substantial variations from the usual test schedule occur, this should be recorded so that the same schedule can be used on subsequent occasions.

The subject should not void during the test period. If the patient experiences urgency, she should be persuaded to postpone voiding and to perform as many of the activities in section (5) as possible in order to detect leakage. Before voiding, the collection device is removed for weighing. If inevitable voiding cannot be postponed, the test is terminated. The voided volume and the duration of the test should be recorded. For subjects not completing the full test, the results may require separate analysis, or the test may be repeated.

The test result is given as grams of urine lost in the one-hour test period in which the greatest urine loss is recorded. A loss of one gram or less of urine is within experimental error and should be viewed as normal.

Additional procedures intended to give information of diagnostic value are permissible provided they do not interfere with the basic test. For example, additional changes and weighing of the collecting device can give information about the timing of urine loss: the absorbent nappy may be an electronic recording nappy so that the timing is recorded directly.

When results are presented they should be qualified by specifying the type of collecting device used, the physical condition of the subject (ambulant, chairbound, bedridden), any relevant medical condition or relevant drug treatments as well as the test schedule used.

In some situations, the timing of the test (e.g. in relation to the menstrual cycle) may be relevant.

### Statistical Analysis

When performing statistical analysis of urine loss in a group of subjects, non-parametric statistics should be employed because the values are not normally distributed.

## B.6 Procedures Related to the Evaluation of Micturition

### Measurement of Urinary Flow

Urinary flow may be described in terms of rate and pattern and may be continuous or intermittent. The flow rate is defined as the volume of fluid voided per unit time. It is expressed in ml/s. When reporting uroflowmetry the following data should be specified:

1. Voided volume
2. Patient environment and position (supine, sitting, or standing)
3. How the bladder was initially filled either by diuresis (spontaneous or forced: specify regimen) or by catheter (transurethral or suprapubic)
4. Type of fluid voided

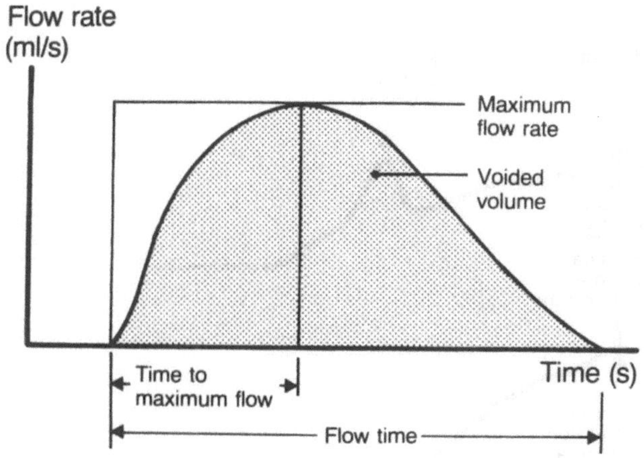


**Fig. B.4.** Uroflowmetry study with ICS recommended descriptive terminology.

A note should also be made of the measuring equipment used and whether the uroflow study was a solitary procedure or combined with other measurements.

## Definitions

### *Continuous Flow Studies* (Fig. B.4)

*Voided volume* is the total volume expelled via the urethra.

*Maximum flow rate* is the maximum measured value of the flow rate.

*Average flow rate* is voided volume divided by the time it takes to void. The calculation of average flow rate is only meaningful if the flow is continuous and without terminal dribbling.

*Flow time* is the time over which measurable flow actually occurs.

*Time to maximum flow* is the elapsed time from onset of flow to maximum flow.

The flow pattern should be described when the flow time and average flow rate are measured.

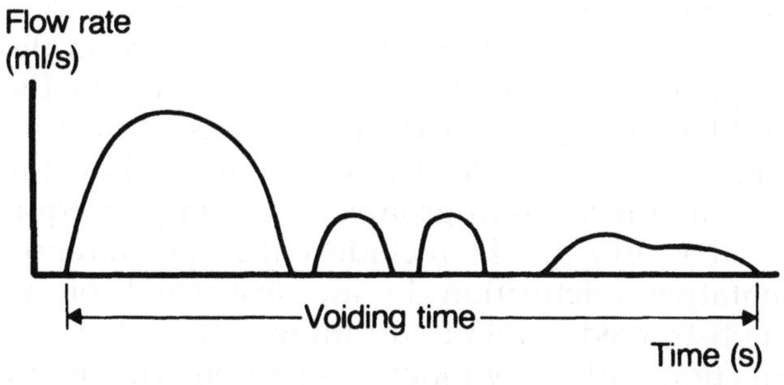


**Fig. B.5.** Interrupted flow pattern during a spontaneous uroflowmetry study.

### *Intermittent Flow Studies* (Fig. B.5)

The same parameters used to characterize continuous flow may be applicable if care is exercised in patients with intermittent flow. In measuring flow time, the time intervals between flow episodes are not counted in the measurement.

*Voiding time* is total duration of micturition including interruptions. When voiding is completed without interruption, the voiding time is equal to flow time.

## Bladder Pressure Measurements During Micturition (Pressure-Flow Studies)

The specifications of patient position, access for pressure measurement, catheter type, and measuring equipment should be defined as is done for cystometry.

The *opening time* is defined as the elapsed time from the initial rise in detrusor pressure to onset of flow (Fig. B.6). This is the initial isovolumetric contraction period of micturition. Time lags should be taken into account because in most urodynamic systems, a time lag occurs equal to the time taken for the urine to pass from the point of pressure measurement to the uroflow transducer.

The following parameters are applicable to measurements of each of the pressure curves: intravesical, abdominal and detrusor pressure.

*Premicturition pressure* is the baseline pressure recorded immediately before the initial isovolumetric contraction.

The *opening pressure* is the pressure recorded at the onset of measured flow.

*Maximum pressure* is the maximum value of the measured pressure.

The *pressure at maximum flow* is the pressure recorded at the point of the maximum measured flow rate. The contraction pressure at maximum flow is the difference between pressure at maximum flow and the premicturition baseline pressure.

## Pressure Flow Relationships

The flow rate and voiding pressure may be used to calculate the urethral resistance but this is reliable only if the urethra behaves as a rigid tube. However, it is an irregular and distensible conduit whose walls and surroundings have active and

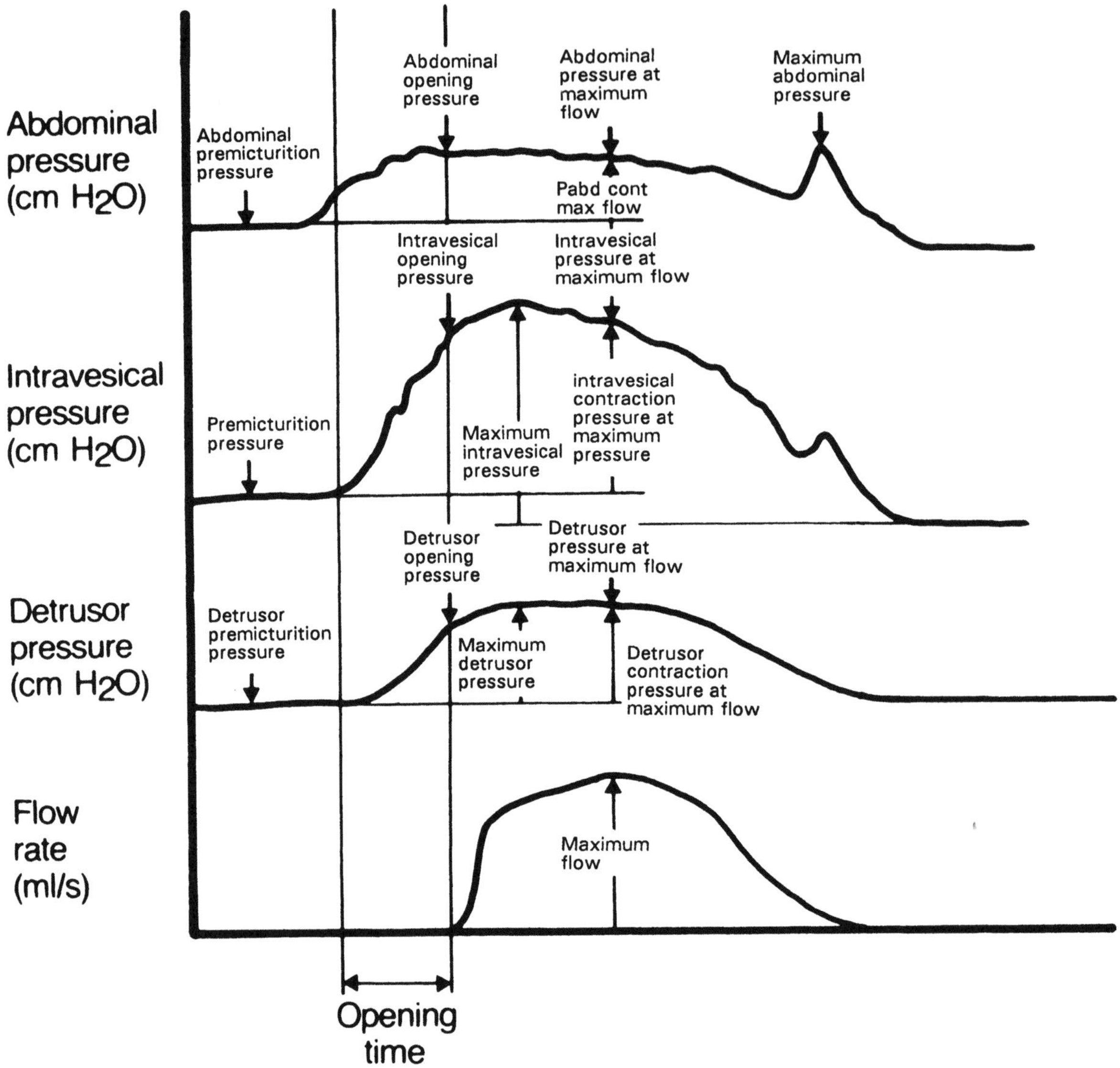


**Fig. B.6.** A pressure/flow voiding study with ICS recommended descriptive terminology.

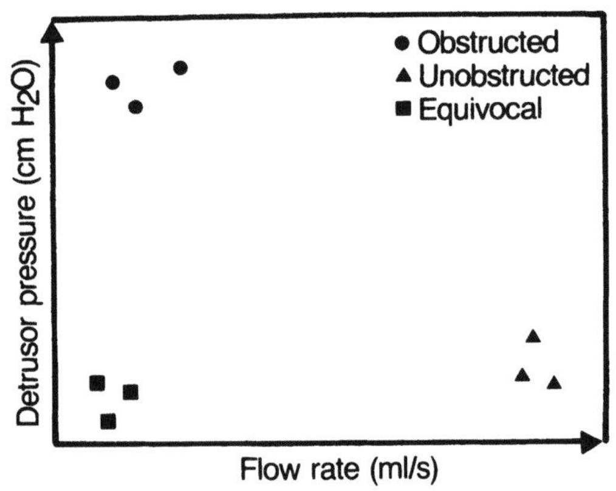


**Fig. B.7.** Diagram illustrating a pressure/flow chart on individual patients in three groups of three patients; obstructed, equivocal and unobstructed.

passive elements and hence influence the flow through it. Therefore, a resistance factor cannot provide a valid comparison between patients.

The relationships between flow and pressure during micturition can be graphically represented as shown Fig. B.7. This form of presentation allows lines of demarcation to be drawn on the graph to separate the results according to the problem being studied. The points shown in Fig. B.7 are purely illustrative to indicate how the data might fall into groups. The group of equivocal results might include either an unrepresentative micturition in an obstructed or an unobstructed patient, or underactive detrusor function with or without obstruction. This is the group that invalidates the calculation of urethral resistance.

## Urethral Pressure Measurements During Voiding (VUPP)

The VUPP is used to determine the urethral pressure as well as any potential site of urethral obstruction. Pressure is recorded in the urethra during voiding. The technique is similar to that used in the UPP measured during storage as described previously during resting urethral pressure profiles.

Accurate interpretation of the VUPP depends on the simultaneous measurement of intravesical pressure and the measurement of pressure at a precisely localized point in the urethra. Localization may be achieved by placing a radiopaque marker on the catheter, which allows the pressure measurements to be related to a visualized point in the urethra.

This technique is not fully developed, and a number of technical as well as clinical problems need to be solved before the VUPP is widely used.

## Residual Urine

*Residual urine* is defined as the volume of fluid remaining in the bladder immediately following the completion of micturition. Its measurement is the most important variable studied during voiding. However, voiding in unfamiliar surroundings may lead to unrepresentative results, as may voiding on command with a partially filled or overfilled bladder. The residual urine is commonly estimated by the following methods.

1. Catheter or cystoscope (transurethral, suprapubic)
2. Radiography (excretion urography, micturition cystography)
3. Ultrasound
4. Radioisotopes (clearance, gamma camera)

When estimating residual urine, the measurement of voided volume and the time interval between voiding and residual urine estimation should be recorded. This is particularly important if the patient diureses rapidly. When vesicoureteric reflux is present urine may re-enter the bladder after micturition and may be falsely interpreted as residual urine. The presence of a bladder diverticulum may also confuse the measurement of residual urine.

The various methods of measurement each have limitations as to their applicability and accuracy in the various conditions associated with residual urine. The absence of residual urine is usually an observation of clinical value, but it does not exclude infravesical obstruction or bladder dysfunction. An isolated elevated residual urine requires confirmation before being considered significant.

# B.7 Electromyography

Electromyography (EMG) is the study of electrical potentials generated by the depolarization of muscle. The functional unit in EMG is the motor unit which comprises a single motor neuron and the muscle fibers it innervates. A motor unit action potential is the recorded depolarization of muscle fibers that results from activation of a single anterior horn cell. Muscle action potentials may be detected either by needle electrodes or by surface electrodes.

Needle electrodes are placed directly into the muscle mass and permit visualization of the individual motor unit action potentials.

Surface electrodes are applied to an epithelial surface as close to the muscle under study as possible. Surface electrodes detect the action potentials from groups of adjacent motor units underlying the recording surface.

EMG potentials may be displayed on an oscilloscope screen or played through audio amplifiers. An accurate permanent record of EMG potentials can only be made using a chart recorder with a high frequency response (in the range of 10 kHz).

When performing EMG the following data should be controlled and specified:

1. Whether EMG was a solitary procedure, or a part of urodynamic or other electrophysiological investigations.
2. Patient position (supine, standing, sitting, or other).
3. Electrode placement:
   a) Sampling site (intrinsic striated muscle of the urethra, periurethral striated muscle, bulbocavernosus muscle, external anal sphincter, pubococcygeus, or other) – state whether sites are single or multiple, unilateral or bilateral; also state number of samples per site.
   b) Recording electrode – define the precise anatomical location of the electrode; for needle electrodes, include site of needle entry, angle of entry, and needle depth; for vaginal or urethral surface electrodes,

state method of determining position of electrode.

c) Reference electrode position. (Note: ensure that there is not electrical interference with any other machines, e.g., x-ray apparatus.)

4. Types of electrode:
   a) Needle electrodes:
      Design (concentric, bipolar, monopolar, single fiber, other)
      Dimensions (length, diameter, recording area)
      Electrode material (e.g., platinum)
   b) Surface electrodes:
      Type (skin, plug, catheter, other)
      Size and shape
      Electrode material
      Mode of fixation to recording surface
      Conducting medium (e.g. saline, jelly)
5. Amplifier (make and specifications)
6. Signal processing (data: raw, averaged, integrated, or other).
7. Display equipment (make and specifications to include method of calibration, time base, full scale deflection in microvolts, and polarity):
   a) Oscilloscope
   b) Chart recorder
   c) Loudspeaker
   d) Other
8. Storage (make and specifications)
   a) Paper
   b) Magnetic tape recorder
   c) Microprocessor
   d) Other
9. Hard copy production (make and specifications)
   a) Chart recorder
   b) Photographic/video reproduction of oscilloscope screen
   c) Other

### Description of EMG Findings

#### *Individual Motor Unit Action Potentials*

Normal motor unit potentials have a characteristic configuration, amplitude, and duration. Abnormalities of the motor unit may include an increase in the amplitude, duration, and complexity of waveform (polyphasicity) of the potentials. A polyphasic potential is defined as one having more than five deflections. The EMG findings of fibrillations, positive sharp waves, and bizarre, high-frequency potentials are thought to be abnormal.

#### *Recruitment patterns*

In normal subjects, there is a gradual increase in "pelvic floor" and "sphincter" EMG activity during bladder filling. At the onset of micturition, there is a complete absence of activity. Any sphincter EMG activity during voiding is abnormal unless the patient is attempting to inhibit micturition. The finding of increased sphincter EMG activity during voiding, accompanied by a bladder contraction and flow changes is called detrusor sphincter dyssynergia which is a condition where a detrusor contraction occurs concurrently with inappropriate contraction of the urethral and or periurethral striated muscle often times resulting in urinary retention.

A thorough review of some neurophysiologic terminology and techniques is omitted here because it is beyond the scope of this text but may be found in Abrams et al. (1986).

## B.8 Lower Urinary Tract Rehabilitation Techniques

Lower urinary tract rehabilitation comprises non-surgical, non-pharmacological treatment for lower urinary tract dysfunction. Most of the conditions for which rehabilitation techniques are employed have both a subjective and an objective component. In many instances, treatment may relieve symptoms but not the underlying disease. Therefore, symptoms should be quantified before and after treatment, and the way in which the underlying pathophysiology is altered should be clearly stated.

### Pelvic Floor Training

Pelvic floor training is defined as repetitive selective voluntary contractions and relaxations of specific pelvic floor muscles. This necessitates muscle awareness in order to be sure that the correct muscles are being utilized and to avoid unwanted contractions of adjacent muscle groups.

*Standard of Diagnosis and Implementation*

The professional status of the individual who establishes the diagnosis must be stated as well as the diagnostic techniques employed. Also the professional status of the person who institutes, supervises and assesses treatment should be stated.

*Techniques*

The technique used for obtaining selective pelvic floor contractions and relaxations should be stated. Registration of electromyographic (EMG) activity from the muscles of the pelvic floor, urethral or anal sphincter, or the anterior abdominal wall may be necessary to obtain this muscle awareness. Alternatively or additionally, registration of abdominal, vaginal, urethral and anal pressure may be used for the same purpose.

One should specify whether treatment is given on an inpatient or outpatient basis and should specify the patient position, duration of each contraction, interval between contractions, number of contractions per exercise, number of exercises per day and the length of treatment.

Any adjunctive equipment used to enhance muscle awareness should be detailed as to its mechanism of action and how it is used. Examples of equipment in current use are:

Perineometers and other pressure recording devices.
EMG equipment
Ultrasound equipment
Faradic stimulators
Interferential current equipment
Vaginal cones

Patient compliance should be documented and has three major components:

1. Appropriate comprehension of the instructions and the technique.
2. Ability to perform the exercises.
3. Compliance and completion of the training program.

Objective documentation of both the patient's ability to perform the exercises and the result of the training program is mandatory.

The parameters employed for objective documentation during training should be the same as those used for teaching muscle awareness.

*Applications*

Pelvic floor training can be used as a treatment on its own, as an adjunctive therapy or for prophylaxis. Examples of indications for therapeutic pelvic floor training are incontinence and genital prolapse. Examples of indications for prophylactic pelvic floor training are postpartum therapy and following pelvic surgery.

## Biofeedback

Biofeedback is a technique by which information about a normally unconscious physiological process is presented to the patient and the therapist as a visual, auditory or tactile signal. The signal is derived from a measurable physiological parameter which is subsequently used in an educational process to accomplish a specific therapeutic result. The signal is displayed in a quantitive way and the patient is taught how to alter it and thus control the basic physiological process.

*Techniques*

The physiological parameter (e.g. pressure, flow, EMG) being monitored, the method of measurement and the mode by which it is displayed should be qualified (e.g. light, sound, electric stimulus). The specific instructions given to the patient should be stated.

The patient position, duration and interval of sessions, number of sessions per day, week, or month, and length of the treatment program should be defined.

*Applications*

The indications, intended mode of action and therapeutic goals should be defined. The aim of biofeedback is to improve a specific lower urinary tract dysfunction by increasing patient awareness and alteration of a measurable physiological parameter. Biofeedback can be applied in functional voiding disorders where the underlying pathophysiology can be monitored and subsequently altered by the patient. The following are examples of indications and techniques for biofeedback treatment:

Motor urgency and urge incontinence: display of detrusor pressure and control of detrusor contractions

Dysfunctional voiding: display of sphincter EMG and relaxation of the external sphincter

Pelvic floor relaxation: display of pelvic floor EMG and pelvic floor training.

## Behavioral Modification

Behavioral modification comprises analysis and alteration of the relationship between the patient's symptoms and her environment for the treatment of maladaptive voiding patterns. This may be achieved by modification of the behavior or the environment of the patient.

### *Technique*

A thorough analysis of possible interactions between the patient's symptoms, her general condition and her environment is essential for behavioral modification. One should clearly specify the following:

1. The assessment and quantification of complaints by symptom analysis, visual analogue score, fluid intake chart, frequency/volume chart (voiding diary), pad weighing test, and urodynamic studies (when applicable).
2. The general patient assessment including an evaluation of their general performance status (e.g. Kurtzke disability scale), mobility, concurrent medical disorders (e.g. constipation, congestive heart failure, diabetes mellitus, chronic bronchitis, hemiplegia, current medication (e.g. diuretics), psychological state, and mental state (e.g. dementia, confusion).
3. An assessment of their environment including access to toilet facilities, their living conditions, working conditions, social relations access to health care and availability of suitable incontinence aids.

For behavioral modification, various therapeutic concepts and techniques may be employed and these should be clearly specified. Examples of these are:

1. Conditioning techniques such as
   a) timed voiding
   b) double or triple voiding, bladder drill, biofeedback, and the use of enuresis alarms;
2. Fluid intake regulation (e.g. restriction);
3. Measures to improve patient mobility (e.g. physiotherapy, wheelchair);
4. Changes of medication (e.g. diuretics, anticholinergics);
5. Treatment of concurrent medical and psychiatric disorders;
6. Psychoanalysis or hypnotherapy (e.g. idiopathic detrusor instability);
7. Environmental changes (e.g. provision of incontinence pads, condom urinals, commode, furniture protection, etc.).

Treatment is often empirical, and may require a combination of the above-mentioned concepts and techniques. The results of treatment should be objectively documented using the same techniques as used for the initial assessment of micturition complaints.

### *Applications*

Behavior modification may be used for the treatment of maladaptive voiding patterns in patients when the etiology and pathophysiology of their symptoms cannot be identified (e.g. sensory urgency), the symptoms are caused by a psychological or functional problem, or the symptoms have failed to respond to conventional therapy or they are unfit for definitive treatment of their condition.

Behavioral modification may be employed alone or as an adjunct to any other form of treatment for lower urinary tract dysfunction.

## Electrical Stimulation

Electrical stimulation is the application of electrical current to stimulate the pelvic viscera or their nerve supply. The aim of electrical stimulation may be to induce a therapeutic response directly or to modulate lower urinary tract, bowel or sexual dysfunction.

### *Techniques*

When one uses electrical stimulation one should clearly state the method of stimulation (surface electrodes, percutaneous electrodes or implantable electrodes), whether stimulation is temporary or permanent and what organ, nerve or site is being stimulated.

The stimulation parameters should be defined as to the frequency, voltage, current, pulse width, and shape (e.g. rectangular, biphasic, capacitatively coupled) used. With monopolar stimulation, it should be stated whether the active electrode is anodic or cathodic. One should also define the duration of pulse trains and the shape of pulse trains (e.g. surging trains). Stimulation should be defined as continuous, phasic (regular automatic on/off) or intermittent (variable duration and time intervals). The number, duration and intervals between periods of stimulation should be stated.

The design of electronic equipment, electrodes and related electrical stimulation characteristics should be stated.

The type of electrode (monopolar or bipolar), surface area of electrodes, maximum charge density per pulse at active electrode surface, impedance of implanted systems, and power source should be controlled and defined.

For transurethral intravesical stimulation the filling medium, filling volume and number of intravesical electrodes should be stated.

## *Units of Measurement and Symbols*

Parameters related to electrical stimulation, units of measurement and the corresponding symbols are listed in Table B.1.

## *Applications*

The aims of treatment should be clearly stated. These may include control of voiding, continence, defecation, erection, ejaculation or relief of pain. It should be specified whether electrical stimulation aims at a functional result dependent on the continuous use of electrical current or modulation,

**Table B.1**

| Quantity | Unit | Symbol | Definition |
|---|---|---|---|
| Electric current | ampere | A | 1 A of electric current is the transfer of 1 C of electric charge per second |
| Direct current (d.c.) | | | Steady unidirectional electric current |
| Galvanic current | | | Unidirectional electric current derived from a chemical battery |
| Alternating current (a.c.) | | | Electric current that physically changes direction of flow in a sinusoidal manner. |
| Faradic current | | | Intermittent oscillatory current similar to alternating current (a.c.) e.g. as produced by an induction coil |
| Voltage | volt | V | 1 V potential difference between 2 points requires 1 J of energy to transfer 1 C of charge from one point to the other (potential difference) |
| Resistance | ohm | Ω | 1 Ω of resistance between 2 points allows 1 V of potential difference to cause a flow of 1 A of direct current (d.c.) between them. |
| Impedance | ohm | Ω | Analogue of resistance for alternating current (a.c.); vector sum of ohmic resistance and reactance (inductive and/or capacitative resistance) |
| Charge | coulomb | C | 1 C of electric charge is transferred through a conductor in 1 s by 1 A of electric current |
| Capacity | farad | F | A condensor (capacitor) has 1 F of electric capacity (capacitance) if transfer of 1 C of electric charge causes 1 V of potential difference between its elements |
| Frequency | hertz | $Hz(s^{-1})$ | Number of cycles (phases) of a periodically repeating oscillation per second |
| Pulse width | time | ms | Duration of 1 pulse (phase) of a phasic electric current or voltage |
| Electrode surface area | area | $mm^2$ | Active area of electrode surface |
| Charge density per pulse | coulomb/ area/time | $\mu C/mm^2/ms^1$ | Electric charge delivered to a given electrode surface area in a given time (one pulse width) |

reflex facilitation, reflex inhibition, re-education or conditioning with a sustained functional result even after withdrawal of stimulation.

Electrical stimulation is applicable in neurogenic or non-neurogenic lower urinary tract, bowel or sexual dysfunction. Techniques and equipment vary widely with the type of dysfunction and the goal of electrical stimulation. If electrical stimulation is employed for control of a neuropathic dysfunction, and the chosen site of stimulation is the reflex arc (peripheral nerves, spinal nerves or spinal cord), this reflex arc must be intact. Consequently electrical stimulation is not applicable for complete "lower motor neuron" lesions except when direct stimulation of the effector organ is chosen.

When ablative surgery is performed (i.e. dorsal rhizotomies, ganglionectomies, sphincterotomy or levatorotomies) in conjunction with an implant to achieve the desired functional effect, one should specify the techniques used to reduce pain or mass reflexes during stimulation, the number and spinal level of interrupted afferents, site of interruption of afferents (i.e., dorsal rhizotomy (intradural or extradural), ganglionectomy), and techniques used to reduce stimulated sphincter dyssynergia.

If electrical stimulation is combined with ablative surgery, other functions (e.g. erection or continence) may be impaired.

When the aim of electrical stimulation is to achieve voiding, one should state whether this is obtained by stimulation of the afferent fibers to induce bladder sensation and thus facilitate voiding or by stimulation of efferent fibers or detrusor muscle to induce a bladder contraction (electromicturition).

Electrical stimulation may aim to inhibit overactive detrusor function or to improve urethral closure. State whether overactive detrusor function is abolished or reduced by reflex inhibition (pudendal to pelvic nerve) or by blockade of nerve conduction. When electrical stimulation is applied to improve urethral closure, state whether this is by a direct effect on the urethra during stimulation or re-education and conditioning to restore pelvic floor tone.

When electrical stimulation is applied to control pelvic pain, the nature and etiology of the pain should be stated. When pelvic pain is caused by pelvic floor spasticity, electrical stimulation may be effective by relaxation of the pelvic floor muscles.

Defecation may be obtained by electrical stimulation – either intentionally or as a side effect of electromicturition.

At present, the mechanism of action of electrically induced control of pelvic pain, erection, ejaculation and defecation are not fully understood. The clinical applications of these techniques have not yet been fully established.

## Voiding Maneuvers

Voiding maneuvers are employed to obtain or facilitate bladder emptying. For lower urinary tract rehabilitation, voiding maneuvers may be used alone or in combination with other techniques (e.g. biofeedback, behavioral modification). The aim is to achieve complete bladder emptying at low intravesical pressures. The techniques employed may be invasive (e.g. catheters) or non-invasive such as triggering reflex detrusor contractions or increasing intra-abdominal pressure.

When reporting on voiding maneuvers, the professional status of the individual(s) who establishes the diagnosis and initiates treatment should be stated as well as the diagnostic techniques employed.

## Catheterization

Catheterization is a technique for bladder emptying employing a catheter to drain the bladder or a urinary reservoir. Catheter use may be intermittent or indwelling.

### *Intermittent Catheterization*

Intermittent catheterization is defined as drainage or aspiration of the bladder or a urinary reservoir with subsequent removal of the catheter. The following types of intermittent catheterization are defined:

1. Intermittent self-catheterization performed by the patient herself.
2. Intermittent catheterization by an attendant (e.g. doctor, nurse or relative)
3. Clean intermittent catheterization: use of a clean technique. This implies ordinary washing techniques and use of disposable or cleansed reusable catheters
4. Aseptic intermittent catheterization: use of a sterile technique. This implies genital disinfection and the use of sterile catheters and gloves.

**Table B.2** The principal units used in urodynamics

| Quantity | Acceptable unit | Symbol |
|---|---|---|
| Volume | milliliter | ml |
| Time | second | s |
| Flow rate | milliliters/second | ml/s |
| Pressure | centimeters of water | $cmH_2O$ |
| Length | meters or submultiples | m, cm, mm |
| Velocity | meters/second or submultiples | m/s, cm/s |
| Temperature | degree Celsius | °C |

The SI unit is the pascal (Pa), but it is only practical at present to calibrate our instruments in $cmH_2O$. One centimeter of water pressure is approximately equal to 100 pascals. (1 $cmH_2O$ = 98.07 Pa 0.098 kPa).

The preparation used for genital disinfection, lubricant, type of catheter, number of catheterizations per day and length of treatment (e.g. week, months, permanent) should be specified.

### *Indwelling Catheter*

An indwelling transurethral or suprapubic catheter remains in the bladder, urinary reservoir or urinary conduit for a period of time longer than one emptying. The type of catheter, lubricant, method of catheter fixation (e.g. balloon skin suture, tape), mode of drainage (continuous or intermittent) should be defined. The intervals between catheter change and duration of catheterization should be stated.

### Bladder Reflex Triggering

Bladder reflex triggering comprises various maneuvers performed by the patient or the therapist in order to elicit reflex detrusor contractions by exteroceptive stimuli. The most commonly used maneuvers are: suprapubic tapping, thigh scratching and anal or rectal manipulation.

For each maneuver the investigator should specify the details of the maneuver and the frequency, intervals and duration of practice.

Bladder reflex triggering maneuvers are indicated only in patients with an intact sacral arc (suprasacral spinal cord lesions).

### Bladder Expression

Bladder expression comprises various maneuvers aimed at increasing intravesical pressure in order to facilitate bladder emptying. The most commonly used maneuvers are abdominal straining, Valsalva's maneuver and Credé's maneuver. The details of the maneuver, frequency, interval and duration of practice should be stated.

Bladder expression is best used in patients where the urethral closure mechanism can be easily overcome.

## B.9 Units of Measurement

In the urodynamic literature, pressure is measured in $cmH_2O$ and not in mmHg. When Laplace's law is used to calculate tension in the bladder wall, it is often found that pressure is then measured in dyne/$cm^2$. This lack of uniformity in the systems used leads to confusion when other parameters, that are a function of pressure, are computed, e.g., "compliance" (contraction force/velocity), etc. From these few examples, it is evident that standardization is essential for meaningful communication. Many journals now require that the results be given in SI Units. This section is designed to give guidance in the application of the SI system to urodynamics and defines the units involved. The principal units to be used are listed in Table B.2.

## B.10 Symbols

If is often helpful to use symbols and abbreviations. Table B.3 has been devised to standardize a code of symbols for use in urodynamics. The rationale of the system is to have a basic symbol representing the physical quantity with qualifying subscripts. This list of basic symbols conforms to international usage. The qualifying subscripts relate to the basic symbols for commonly used urodynamic parameters.

## References

Abrams P, Blaivas JG, Stanton SL et al: Sixth report on the standardization of terminology of lower urinary tract function. Procedures related to neurophysiological investigations: electromyography, nerve conduction studies, reflex latencies, evoked potential and sensory testing. Scand J Urol Nephrol 20:161, 1986.

Andersen JT, Blaivas JG, Cardozo L, Thüroff J: Seventh

**Table B.3** List of symbols

| Basic symbol | | Urological qualifiers | | Value | |
|---|---|---|---|---|---|
| Pressure | P | Bladder | ves | Maximum | max |
| Volume | V | Urethra | ura | Minimum | min |
| Flow rate | Q | Ureter | ure | Average | ave |
| Velocity | v | Detrusor | det | Isovolumetric | isv |
| Time | t | Abdomen | abd | Isotonic | ist |
| Temperature | T | External Stream | ext | Isobaric | isb |
| Length | l | | | Isometric | ism |
| Area | A | | | | |
| Diameter | d | | | | |
| Force | F | | | | |
| Energy | E | | | | |
| Power | P | | | | |
| Compliance | C | | | | |
| Work | W | | | | |
| Energy per unit volume | e | | | | |

Examples:
$P_{det\ max}$ = maximum detrusor pressure.
$e_{ext}$ = kinetic energy per unit volume in external stream.

report on the standardization of terminology of lower urinary tract function: lower urinary tract rehabilitation techniques: Int Urogynecol J 3:75, 1992.

Bates P, Bradley WE, Glen E et al: First report on the standardization of terminology of lower urinary tract function. Urinary incontinence. Procedures related to the evaluation of urine storage – cystometry, urethral closure pressure profile, units of measurement. Br J Urol 48:39, 1976.

Bates P, Glen E, Griffiths D et al: Second report on the standardization of terminology of lower urinary function. Procedures related to the evaluation of micturition – flow rate, pressure measurement, symbols. Scand J Urol Nephrol 11:197, 1977.

Bates P, Bradley WE, Glen E, et al: Third report on the standardization of terminology of lower urinary tract function. Procedures related to the evaluation of micturition: pressure flow relationships, residual urine. Br J Urol 52:348, 1980.

Bates P, Bradley WE, Glen E et al: Fourth report on the standardization of terminology of lower urinary tract function. Terminology related to neuromuscular dysfunction of lower urinary tract. Br J Urol 53:333, 1981.

# Appendix C
# Recording Forms for Urodynamics and Evaluation of Urinary Dysfunction

The forms in this section offer an example of data recording forms that we use in our investigation of women with lower urinary tract dysfunction. They may serve as a format for the investigation of women with these problems or they may be modified for other individual purposes.

URO I
INITIAL HISTORY AND
PHYSICAL EXAMINATION
(Form 1)

PETER K. SAND. M.D.
SECTION OF UROGYNECOLOGY
EVANSTON CONTINENCE CENTER
EVANSTON HOSPITAL
NORTHWESTERN UNIVERSITY
(708) 570-2750

Name: ______________________ FIRST ______________________ LAST

DATE ______________

PATIENT NO. ______________

Urine C & S Negative ☐ Positive ☐

**DRUG ALLERGIES**

**I HISTORY**

Age ________ LMP ________ Weight ________
Gravida ________ Para ________ Abortions ________
Age of Menarche ________ Age of Menopause ________
Menopausal Status: Pre ☐ Peri ☐ Post ☐
ABDOMINAL ANTERIOR REPAIR ☐ : ________ MMK ☐ : ________
HYSTERECTOMY ☐ : ____ STAMEY ☐ ____ PEREYRA ☐ ________
POSTERIOR REPAIR: ________ BURCH ☐ ________ SLING ☐ ________
VAGINAL HYSTERECTOMY ☐ : ________

**II SYMPTOMS**

☐ Dysuria ________ + ☐ Freq. q. ____ hrs. ☐ Urgency ________ +
☐ Nocturia x ________ Incontinence: ☐ Stress ________ +
☐ Post Void Fullness ________ + ☐ Urge ________ +

**III NEUROLOGICAL EVALUATION** **Normal** ☐ **Normal Except for** ☐

Rectal Evaluation (check if abnormal)
Contractions — Voluntary ☐ with Cough ☐ With hold ☐
Tone: Normal ☐ Abnormal ☐
Reflexes (check if abnormal)
Babinski ☐
Pattellar ☐ Ankle ☐ Clitoral ☐ Bulbocavernosis ☐
Proprioception ☐
Sensory: L5 ☐ S1 ☐ S2 ☐ S3 ☐ S4 ☐ | Abnormal on
Motor: L5 ☐ S1 ☐ S2 ☐ S3 ☐ S4 ☐ | Right ☐ Left ☐
Other:

**IV PHYSICAL EXAMINATION** **None** ☐

| | 2° | 3° | 4° |
|---|---|---|---|
| Cystocele | ☐ | ☐ | ☐ |
| Rectocele | ☐ | ☐ | ☐ |
| Uterine / Vault Prolapse | ☐ | ☐ | ☐ |
| Enterocele | ☐ | ☐ | ☐ |

Caruncle ☐ Fistula ☐ Type:
Other Positive Findings:

| | Normal | Describe if Abnormal |
|---|---|---|
| Vulva | ☐ | |
| Vagina | ☐ | |
| Urethra | ☐ | |
| Cervix | ☐ | |
| Fundus | ☐ | |
| Adnexa | ☐ | |
| Rectal | ☐ | |

**V Q-TIP TEST**

Resting Angle + ☐ - ☐
Straining Angle + ☐ - ☐

**VI UROFLOWMETRY**

| **VII UROLOG** | Flow Rate (cc/sec) Maximum/Mean | / |
|---|---|---|
| FREQUENCY | Urine Volume (cc) In/Voided | / |
| Day | Flowtime (sec) | |
| Night | Time to Maximum Flow (sec) | |
| VOLUME | Residual Urine (cc) | |
| Day | Normal Voiding for patient? | Yes ☐ No ☐ |
| Night | Interpretation | N ☐ Ab ☐ |

**VIII URETHRAL CALIBRATION**

Calibration to ________ F Dilated to ________ F

**IX DIAGNOSIS** **Normal** ☐

**X X-RAYS** **VCUG** ☐ **TRATNER** ☐ **IVP** ☐ **UTZ** ☐

**XI MEDICATIONS** **None** ☐

| Code | Drug | Dose | Freq. | Dur/Treatment | Rx'd |
|---|---|---|---|---|---|
| | Nitrofurantoin | 50 mg. | tid | 3 days | |
| | Vaginal Estrogen | | | | |
| | Pyridium | 200 mg. | tid | prn | |
| | | | | | |

**XII COMMENTS**

**TREATMENT PLAN:**

**RETURN APPOINTMENT:**

**Other Studies:** **Dictated** ☐

540-46

________________________ **M.D.**

**Fig. C.1.** Form 1. Initial history and physical examination form.

**URO II**
**RETURN VISIT SUMMARY**
**(Form 2)**

**PETER K. SAND. M.D.**
**SECTION OF UROGYNECOLOGY**
**EVANSTON CONTINENCE CENTER**
**EVANSTON HOSPITAL**
**NORTHWESTERN UNIVERSITY**
**(708) 570-2750**

DATE: ____________

NAME ____________ (Last) ____________ (First) PATIENT NO. ____________

**I INTERVAL HISTORY LMP ________ CYCLE DAY NO. ______**

Dysuria: ☐ ____ Freq ☐ q ____ hrs. Urgency ☐ ____
Nocturia: ☐ X ____ Incontinence: Stress ☐ ____
Post Void Fullness ☐ ____ Urge ☐ ____

**II CURRENT MEDICATIONS** None ☐

| DRUG | DOSE | FREQ | DUR OF USE | SUBJECTIVE RESPONSE* |
|---|---|---|---|---|
| | | | | 1 ___ 5 ___ 10 |
| | | | | 1 ___ 5 ___ 10 |
| | | | | 1 ___ 5 ___ 10 |

* < 5 = worse, 5 = no response, > 5 = improved, 10 = no symptoms

**III SUBJECTIVE RESPONSES TO PREVIOUS TREATMENTS** None ☐

| TREATMENT | RESPONSE | COMMENTS |
|---|---|---|
| ☐ Dilatations | 1 ____ 5 ____ 10 | |
| | 1 ____ 5 ____ 10 | |

**IV UROFLOWMETRY**

NOT DONE ☐

| | |
|---|---|
| Flow Rate (cc/sec) Maximum/Mean | / |
| Urine Volume (cc) In/Voided | / |
| Flowtime (sec) | |
| Time to Maximum Flow (sec) | |
| Residual Urine (cc) | |
| Normal Voiding for Patient? | YES ☐ NO ☐ |
| Interpertation | N ☐ Ab ☐ |

**V CYSTO URETHROSCOPY** Anesthesia: Topical: ☐ Local ☐ None ☐

| Urethro-Vesical Junction | Partial Closure | Closes | No Change | Opens |
|---|---|---|---|---|
| Response to Hold | ☐ | ☐ | ☐ | ☐ |
| Response to Cough | ☐ | ☐ | ☐ | ☐ |
| Response to Valsalva | ☐ | ☐ | ☐ | ☐ |

Mobility: Fixed ☐ Minimal ☐ Moderate ☐ Extreme ☐
Palpation of Urethra with Scope in Place: Normal ☐ Diverticula ☐

| Description Normal ☐ | Bladder Trigone | UV Junction | URETHRA Proximal | URETHRA Mid | URETHRA Distal |
|---|---|---|---|---|---|
| Erythema | ☐ | ☐ | ☐ | ☐ | ☐ |
| Granularity | ☐ | ☐ | ☐ | ☐ | ☐ |
| Shaggy Fronds | ☐ | ☐ | ☐ | ☐ | ☐ |
| Polyps | ☐ | ☐ | ☐ | ☐ | ☐ |
| Cysts | ☐ | ☐ | ☐ | ☐ | ☐ |
| Exudate | ☐ | ☐ | ☐ | ☐ | ☐ |
| Diverticulum | ☐ | ☐ | ☐ | ☐ | ☐ |
| Paleness | ☐ | ☐ | ☐ | ☐ | ☐ |
| Squamous Metaplasia | ☐ | ☐ | ☐ | ☐ | ☐ |

CYSTOSCOPY WNL ☐

**VI SUPINE $H_2O$ CYSTOMETRY**

1st Sensation ________ cc Fullness ________ cc
Max Volume ________ cc Vesical Contraction:
DI Volume ________ cc ☐ None ☐ Voluntary ☐ Involuntary
☐ Inhibited ☐ Uninhibited

**VII STANDING $H_2O$ CYSTOMETRY** **Flowrate: cc/min.**

| | | |
|---|---|---|
| 1st Sensation | cc | Vesical Contraction None ☐ |
| | | ☐ Voluntary ☐ Involuntary |
| Fullness | cc | ☐ Inhibited ☐ Uninhibited |
| Maximum Volume | cc | Pressure CM $H_2O$ |
| DI Volume | cc | Induced By: Filling ☐ ☐ |

**VIII STRESS TESTING** Volume ________ cc
Supine: ☐ Pos ☐ Neg Standing: ☐ Pos ☐ Neg

**IX DIAGNOSIS**

**X X-RAYS VCUG ☐ TRATNER ☐ IVP ☐ UTZ ☐**

**XI MEDICATIONS** **None ☐**

| Code | Drug | Dose | Freq. | Dur/Treatment | Rx'd |
|---|---|---|---|---|---|
| | Nitrofurantoin | 50 mg. | tid | 3 days | |
| | Vaginal Estrogen | | | | |
| | Pyridium | 200 mg. | tid | prn | |
| | | | | | |

**XII COMMENTS**

**TREATMENT PLAN:**

**RETURN VISIT:**

**Dictated ☐**

540-47

____________ **M.D.**

**Fig. C.2.** Form 2. Return visit summary form, for endoscopy, cystometry, uroflowmetry and stress testing.

**RETURN VISIT SUMMARY**
**(Form 3)**

**PETER K. SAND, M.D.**
**SECTION OF UROGYNECOLOGY**
**EVANSTON CONTINENCE CENTER**
**EVANSTON HOSPITAL**
**NORTHWESTERN UNIVERSITY**

DATE: ____________________

NAME ____________________ ____________________ PATIENT NO. ____________________
Last First

**I INTERVAL HISTORY LMP ________ CYCLE DAY NO. ______**

Dysuria: ☐ ____ Freq ☐ q ____ hrs. Urgency ☐ ____
Nocturia: ☐ X ____ Incontinence: Stress ☐ ____
Post Void Fullness ☐ ____ Urge ☐ ____

**II SUBJECTIVE RESPONSES TO PREVIOUS TREATMENTS** None ☐

| TREATMENT | RESPONSE | RESPONSE ☐ |
|---|---|---|
| ☐ Dilatations | 1 ____ 5 ____ 10 | 1 ____ 5 ____ 10 |
| | 1 ____ 5 ____ 10 | 1 ____ 5 ____ 10 |

| **III UROFLOWMETRY** | | **† SPONT.** | **† INST.** |
|---|---|---|---|
| Voiding Mechanism | Vesical Contraction | | ☐ |
| | Urethra | | R ☐ C ☐ NC ☐ |
| | Voluntary Strain | | ☐ |
| | Flow Rate (cc/sec) Maximum/Mean | / | / |
| | Urine Volume (cc) In/Voided | / | / |
| | Flowtime (sec) | | |
| | Time to Maximum Flow (sec) | | |
| | Residual Urine (cc) | | |
| Maximum Intravesical Pressure (cm/$H_2O$) | | | |
| Resistance = $P/F^2$ | | | |
| Time: UP ↓ to VP ↑ (sec) | | | ⊞ ⊟ |
| Normal Voiding for patient? | | YES ☐ NO ☐ | YES ☐ NO ☐ |
| Interpertation | | N ☐ Ab ☐ | N ☐ Ab ☐ |

**IV URETHROSCOPY** **Anesthesia: Topical ☐ Local ☐**

| Urethro-Vesical Junction | Closes | No Change | Opens |
|---|---|---|---|
| Response to Hold | ☐ | ☐ | ☐ |
| Response to Cough | ☐ | ☐ | ☐ |
| Response to Valsalva | ☐ | ☐ | ☐ |

Mobility: Fixed ☐ Minimal ☐ Moderate ☐ Extreme ☐
Palpation of Urethra with Scope in Place: Normal ☐ Diverticula ☐

| Description | Bladder Trigone | UV Junction | URETHRA Proximal | URETHRA Mid | URETHRA Distal |
|---|---|---|---|---|---|
| Red | ☐ | ☐ | ☐ | ☐ | ☐ |
| Granular | ☐ | ☐ | ☐ | ☐ | ☐ |
| Shaggy Fronds | ☐ | ☐ | ☐ | ☐ | ☐ |
| Polyps | ☐ | ☐ | ☐ | ☐ | ☐ |
| Cysts | ☐ | ☐ | ☐ | ☐ | ☐ |
| Exudate | ☐ | ☐ | ☐ | ☐ | ☐ |
| Diverticulum | ☐ | ☐ | ☐ | ☐ | ☐ |
| Paleness | ☐ | ☐ | ☐ | ☐ | ☐ |
| Metaplasia | ☐ | ☐ | ☐ | ☐ | ☐ |
| | ☐ | ☐ | ☐ | ☐ | ☐ |

Cystoscopy

**V TREATMENT PROCEDURES** **None ☐**

Anesthesia: Local ☐ Topical ☐

Dilatation: Previous Present
☐ Calibration To ____________ ____________ F Bleeding ☐
Dilation To ____________ ____________ F Pain ☐

☐ CRYOSURGERY FREEZE ______ S REFREEZE ______ S
TEMPERATURE ____________ °C
Pelvic Floor Stimulation: ____ Acute ____ Chronic
Frequency ____ Hz Work ____ sec Rest ____ sec
Maximal Amperage ____ mA or % Time ____ min
Periurethral Injection
☐ Kenalog ____ mg ☐ Marcaine ____ ml ☐ GAX Collagen ____ ml

**VI LABORATORY**
Urine C&S ordered ☐ :
Negative ☐ Positive ☐ on ____________ (date)

**VII X-RAYS VCUG ☐ UTZ ☐ TRATNER ☐ IVP ☐**

**VIII DIAGNOSIS codes:** **No Change ☐**

1. ____________________
____________ Code: ____________
2. ____________________
____________ Code: ____________
3. ____________________
____________ Code: ____________
4. ____________________
____________ Code: ____________

**IX MEDICATIONS** **None ☐**

| Code | Drug | Dose | Freq. | Dur/Treatment | Rx'd |
|---|---|---|---|---|---|
| | Nitrofurantoin | 50 mg. | tid | 3 days | |
| | Vaginal Estrogen | | | | |
| | Pyridium | 200 mg. | tid | 3 days prn | |
| | | | | | |

**COMMENTS**

**PLAN:**

**RETURN VISIT:** **Dictated ☐**

+ R = RELAXES C = CONTRACTS NC = NO CHANGE RETURN VISIT: ______________________________ M.D.

**Fig. C.3.** Form 3. Return vist summary form for treatment follow-up.

EVANSTON CONTINENCE CENTER
EVANSTON HOSPITAL
NORTHWESTERN UNIVERSITY
2650 RIDGE AVE., SUITE 435
EVANSTON, ILLINOIS 60201
(708) 570-2750

**URODYNAMICS VISIT SUMMARY**
**(Form 4)**

New ☐ PRE-OP ☐
Returning ☐ POST-OP ☐

DATE: ____________

Name ____________ ____________
Last First

PATIENT NO. ____________

**I INTERVAL HISTORY LMP ____________ CYCLE DAY NO. ______**

Dysuria: ☐ ______ + Freq ☐ q ______ hrs. Urgency ☐ ______ +
Nocturia: ☐ x ______ Incontinence: Stress ☐ ______ +
Post Void Fullness ☐ ______ + Urge ☐ ______ +

**II CURRENT MEDICATIONS** None ☐

| DRUG | DOSE | FREQ. | DUR. OF USE | SUBJECTIVE RESPONSE* |
|---|---|---|---|---|
| | | | | 1 ___ 5 ___ 10 |
| | | | | 1 ___ 5 ___ 10 |
| | | | | 1 ___ 5 ___ 10 |

* < 5 = worse, 5 = no response, > 5 = better, 10 = cured

**III SUBJECTIVE RESPONSES TO PREVIOUS TREATMENTS** None ☐

| TREATMENT | RESPONSE | COMMENTS |
|---|---|---|
| Dilatation | 1 ______ 5 ______ 10 | |
| | 1 ______ 5 ______ 10 | |

**IV UROFLOWMETRY**

| | | †SPONT. | †INST. |
|---|---|---|---|
| Voiding Mechanism | Vesical Contraction | | ☐ |
| | Urethra | | ⁝ R ☐ C ☐ NC ☐ |
| | Voluntary Strain | | ☐ |
| Flow Rate (cc/sec) Maximum/Mean | | / | / |
| Urine Volume (cc) In/Voided | | / | / |
| Flowtime (sec) | | | |
| Time to Maximum Flow (sec) | | | |
| Residual Urine (cc) | | | |
| Intravesical Pressure at Max. flow (cm/$H_2O$) | | | |
| Resistance = P/F² | | | |
| Time: UP ↓ to VP ↑ (sec) | | | ⊞ ⊟ ____ |
| Normal Voiding for patient? | | YES ☐ NO ☐ | YES ☐ NO ☐ |
| Interpretation | | N ☐ Ab ☐ | N ☐ Ab ☐ |

**V ELECTROMYOGRAPHIC STIMULATION** **STIMULATION ____________ V**

Anal Sphincter response to urethral stimulation:
Normal ☐ Abnormal ☐ Latency ________ Msec Voltage ________ mV

Perineal Relaxation:
No Effect ☐ Response: Abolished ☐ Decreased ☐ Voltage ________ mV

Interpretation: Normal ☐ Abnormal ☐

**VI URODYNAMICS: UCPP AND URETHROVESICAL PRESSURE DYNAMICS**

| | SITTING | | | | SITTING WITH PESSARY | | | STANDING | | UNITS |
|---|---|---|---|---|---|---|---|---|---|---|
| | EMPTY | FULL | FULL | FULL | FULL | FULL | FULL | FULL | FULL | |
| Length Functional | | | | | | | | | | CM |
| Total | | | | | | | | | | |
| Pressure Closure | | | | | | | | | | CM $H_2O$ |
| UCPP Closure Area | | | | | | | | | | CM² |
| Urethral CP + FL | CP FL | CP FL | CP FL | CP FL | CP FL | CP FL | CP FL | CP FL | CP FL | †† |
| Valsalva | | | | | | | | | | CM $H_2O$ |
| Leak With Valsalva | ⊞ ⊟ | ⊞ ⊟ | ⊞ ⊟ | ⊞ ⊟ | ⊞ ⊟ | ⊞ ⊟ | ⊞ ⊟ | ⊞ ⊟ | ⊞ ⊟ | |
| Cough / Pressure Transmission Ratio * | $Q_1$ $Q_2$ $Q_3$ M | $Q_1$ $Q_2$ $Q_3$ M | $Q_1$ $Q_2$ $Q_3$ M | $Q_1$ $Q_2$ $Q_3$ M | $Q_1$ $Q_2$ $Q_3$ M | $Q_1$ $Q_2$ $Q_3$ M | $Q_1$ $Q_2$ $Q_3$ M | $Q_1$ $Q_2$ $Q_3$ M | $Q_1$ $Q_2$ $Q_3$ M | % |
| Cough Profile | ⊞ ⊟ | ⊞ ⊟ | ⊞ ⊟ | ⊞ ⊟ | ⊞ ⊟ | ⊞ ⊟ | ⊞ ⊟ | ⊞ ⊟ | ⊞ ⊟ | |
| Intravesical Pressure | | | | | | | | | | CM $H_2O$ |
| Urethral instability | | | | | | | | | | |
| | | | | | | | | | | |

† SPONTANEOUS/INSTRUMENTED ⁝ R = RELAXES C = CONTRACTS NC = NO CHANGE

*$Q_1$ = 1st Quartile $Q_2$ = 2nd Quartile $Q_3$ = 3rd Quartile M = Maximum

#540-51

**Fig. C.4.** Form 4. Urodynamics visit summary form.

EVANSTON CONTINENCE CENTER
EVANSTON HOSPITAL
NORTHWESTERN UNIVERSITY
2650 RIDGE AVE., SUITE 435
EVANSTON, ILLINOIS 60201
(708) 570-2750

**URODYNAMICS VISIT SUMMARY**
**(Form 4)**

DATE: ____________

Name ____________ ____________
Last First

PATIENT NO. ____________

| **VII CYSTOMETRICS and EMG ($H_2O$)** | | **SITTING** | **STANDING** |
|---|---|---|---|
| VOLUME | FIRST SENSATION | ____ cc | ____ cc |
| | FULLNESS | ____ cc | ____ cc |
| | MAXIMUM | ____ cc | ____ cc |
| VOLUNTARY VOIDING TERMINAL CONTRACTION None ☐ | Inhibited | ☐ | ☐ |
| | Uninhibited | ☐ | ☐ |
| | | ____ $cmH_2O$ | ____ $cmH_2O$ |
| Urethral Sphincter Response | Relaxes | †P ☐ †E ☐ | P ☐ E ☐ |
| | Contracts | P ☐ E ☐ | P ☐ E ☐ |
| | No Change | P ☐ E ☐ | P ☐ E ☐ |
| Urethral Pressure Change ($cmH_2O$) | | ⊞ ⊟ | ⊞ ⊟ |
| Time From Up ↓ to VP ↑ (sec) | | ⊞ ⊟ | ⊞ ⊟ |
| Anal Sphincter Response | Relaxes | E ☐ | E ☐ |
| | Contracts | E ☐ | E ☐ |
| | No Change | E ☐ | E ☐ |
| OTHER VESICAL CONTRACTIONS None ☐ | Inhibited | ☐ $cmH_2O$ | ☐ $cmH_2O$ |
| | Partial Inhib. | ☐ | ☐ |
| | Uninhibited | ☐ | ☐ |
| Induced by: | Jolt | ☐ | ☐ |
| | Cough | ☐ | ☐ |
| | Filling | ☐ | ☐ |
| | Valsalva | ☐ | ☐ |
| | Running Water | ☐ | ☐ |
| Bladder Volume | | ____ cc | ____ cc |
| Urethral Sphincter Response | Relaxes | P ☐ E ☐ | P ☐ E ☐ |
| | Contracts | P ☐ E ☐ | P ☐ E ☐ |
| | No Change | P ☐ E ☐ | P ☐ E ☐ |
| Urethral Pressure Change ($cmH_2O$) | | ⊞ ⊟ | ⊞ ⊟ |
| Time From Up ↓ to VP ↑ (sec) | | ⊞ ⊟ | ⊞ ⊟ |
| Anal Sphincter Response | Relaxes | E ☐ | E ☐ |
| | Contracts | E ☐ | E ☐ |
| | No Change | E ☐ | E ☐ |

†P = Pressure Response E = EMG Response

**VIII TREATMENT PROCEDURES** None ☐

☐ Anesthesia: Local ☐ Topical ☐

| | | Previous | Present | | |
|---|---|---|---|---|---|
| ☐ | Calibration To | ____ | ____ | F | Bleeding ☐ |
| | Dilation To | ____ | ____ | F | Pain ☐ |

☐ CRYOSURGERY FREEZE ____ S REFREEZE ____ S

TEMPERATURE ____ °C

**IX LABORATORY**

Urine C&S ordered ☐ :
Negative ☐ Positive ☐ on ____ (date)

**X X-RAYS** **VCUG** ☐ **TRATNER** ☐ **UTZ** ☐ **IVP** ☐

**XI DIAGNOSIS codes:** **No Change** ☐

1. ____ Code: ____
2. ____ Code: ____
3. ____ Code: ____
4. ____ Code: ____
5. ____ Code: ____
6. ____ Code: ____
7. ____ Code: ____
8. ____ Code: ____

**XII MEDICATIONS** None ☐

| Code | Drug | Dose | Freq. | Duration/Treatment | Rx'd |
|---|---|---|---|---|---|
| | Nitrofurantoin | 50 mg. | tid | 3 days | |
| | Vaginal Estrogen | | | | |
| | Pyridium | 200 mg. | tid | 3 days/prn | |
| | | | | | |
| | | | | | |

**XIII TREATMENTS**

1. ____ Code: ____
2. ____ Code: ____
3. ____ Code: ____
4. ____ Code: ____

**COMMENTS AND RECOMMENDATIONS**

**DICTATED** ☐

#540-52 **RETURN APPOINTMENT DATE** ____ ____ **M.D.**

**Fig. C.4.** (*continued*)

**Peter K. Sand, MD**
Director, Section of Urogynecology
Director, Evanston Continence Center
The Evanston Hospital
Northwestern University
(708) 570-2750

**PATIENT'S RESPONSE CHART**
**(Form 5)**

NAME ______________ ______________ DATE: ______________
Last First

PATIENT NO. ______________

**INSTRUCTIONS**

You are under treatment for your urinary complaints. We are anxious to learn more from you regarding your urinary problem and any change which may occur. We are also interested in any other symptom that is currently present or may develop in your general condition. The accurate completion of this form will enable us to help you in the best way possible. Below is a list of symptoms. Each is followed by 4 columns with dates marked at the top. On the date indicated, please circle the correct choice for each item.

**THE NUMBERS REFER TO THESE PHRASES:**

0 - NONE
1 - A LITTLE
2 - SOME
3 - QUITE A BIT
4 - UNBEARABLE

| Reporting Date | ______ | ______ | ______ | ______ |
|---|---|---|---|---|
| 1) Nausea | 0 1 2 3 4 | 0 1 2 3 4 | 0 1 2 3 4 | 0 1 2 3 4 |
| 2) Vomiting | 0 1 2 3 4 | 0 1 2 3 4 | 0 1 2 3 4 | 0 1 2 3 4 |
| 3) Diarrhea | 0 1 2 3 4 | 0 1 2 3 4 | 0 1 2 3 4 | 0 1 2 3 4 |
| 4) Loss of appetite | 0 1 2 3 4 | 0 1 2 3 4 | 0 1 2 3 4 | 0 1 2 3 4 |
| 5) Dryness of mouth | 0 1 2 3 4 | 0 1 2 3 4 | 0 1 2 3 4 | 0 1 2 3 4 |
| 6) Dizziness | 0 1 2 3 4 | 0 1 2 3 4 | 0 1 2 3 4 | 0 1 2 3 4 |
| 7) Weakness | 0 1 2 3 4 | 0 1 2 3 4 | 0 1 2 3 4 | 0 1 2 3 4 |
| 8) Change of vision | 0 1 2 3 4 | 0 1 2 3 4 | 0 1 2 3 4 | 0 1 2 3 4 |
| 9) Sleeplessness | 0 1 2 3 4 | 0 1 2 3 4 | 0 1 2 3 4 | 0 1 2 3 4 |
| 10) Sleepiness | 0 1 2 3 4 | 0 1 2 3 4 | 0 1 2 3 4 | 0 1 2 3 4 |
| 11) Palpitations | 0 1 2 3 4 | 0 1 2 3 4 | 0 1 2 3 4 | 0 1 2 3 4 |
| 12) Trembling | 0 1 2 3 4 | 0 1 2 3 4 | 0 1 2 3 4 | 0 1 2 3 4 |
| 13) Nervousness | 0 1 2 3 4 | 0 1 2 3 4 | 0 1 2 3 4 | 0 1 2 3 4 |
| 14) Tension | 0 1 2 3 4 | 0 1 2 3 4 | 0 1 2 3 4 | 0 1 2 3 4 |
| 15) Depression | 0 1 2 3 4 | 0 1 2 3 4 | 0 1 2 3 4 | 0 1 2 3 4 |
| 16) Uncomfortably strong need to pass urine (urge) | 0 1 2 3 4 | 0 1 2 3 4 | 0 1 2 3 4 | 0 1 2 3 4 |
| 17) Burning when passing urine | 0 1 2 3 4 | 0 1 2 3 4 | 0 1 2 3 4 | 0 1 2 3 4 |
| 18) Sensation of continued need to pass urine after emptying bladder | 0 1 2 3 4 | 0 1 2 3 4 | 0 1 2 3 4 | 0 1 2 3 4 |
| 19) Loss of urine with coughing or straining | 0 1 2 3 4 | 0 1 2 3 4 | 0 1 2 3 4 | 0 1 2 3 4 |
| 20) Loss of urine before reaching toilet | 0 1 2 3 4 | 0 1 2 3 4 | 0 1 2 3 4 | 0 1 2 3 4 |
| 21) Lower abdominal pressure | 0 1 2 3 4 | 0 1 2 3 4 | 0 1 2 3 4 | 0 1 2 3 4 |
| 22) Lower abdominal pain | 0 1 2 3 4 | 0 1 2 3 4 | 0 1 2 3 4 | 0 1 2 3 4 |
| 23) Backache | 0 1 2 3 4 | 0 1 2 3 4 | 0 1 2 3 4 | 0 1 2 3 4 |
| 24) Painful intercourse | 0 1 2 3 4 | 0 1 2 3 4 | 0 1 2 3 4 | 0 1 2 3 4 |
| 25) Indicate number of headaches in last 24 hours. | ______ | ______ | ______ | ______ |
| 26) Indicate number of hours between times you pass urine. | ______ | ______ | ______ | ______ |
| 27) Indicate number of times you pass urine at night after going to sleep. | ______ | ______ | ______ | ______ |
| 28) Indicate number of times you pass urine during first hour after going to bed. | ______ | ______ | ______ | ______ |
| **PHYSICIAN USE ONLY:** RESPONSE TO TREATMENT | ______ | ______ | ______ | ______ |

< 5 = worse, 5 = no response, > 5 = improved, 10 = no symptoms

**Fig. C.5.** Form 5. Patient's response chart for subjective evaluation during treatment.

Peter K Sand, MD
Director, Section of Urogynecology
Director, Evanston Continence Center
The Evanston Hospital
Northwestern University
(708) 570-2750

---

## MEDICAL HISTORY QUESTIONNAIRE

NAME . . . . . . . . . . . . . . . . . . . . . . . . . . . . . . . DATE . . . . . . . . . . . . . . . . . . . . . . . . . . . .

In order to help us provide you with the best medical care, please complete this form in as much detail as possible. Please bring the completed form with you at the time of your first visit. DO NOT MAIL IT.

Please write, in your own words, the nature of your current gynecologic or urologic medical problem (use the other side if necessary:

. . . . . . . . . . . . . . . . . . . . . . . . . . . . . . . . . . . . . . . . . . . . . . . . . . . . . . . . . . . . . . . . . . . . . . .

. . . . . . . . . . . . . . . . . . . . . . . . . . . . . . . . . . . . . . . . . . . . . . . . . . . . . . . . . . . . . . . . . . . . . . .

**PLEASE FILL IN THE FOLLOWING INFORMATION:** Age . . . . . . . . . . . . . . Birthdate . . . . . . . . .

Number of pregnancies . . . . . . . . . . . . . . . . . . . .
Number of children born alive . . . . . . . . . . . . . . .
Number of miscarriages . . . . . . . . . . . . . . . . . . .
Number of abortions . . . . . . . . . . . . . . . . . . . . .
Birth control method . . . . . . . . . . . . . . . . . . . . .
DES exposure . . . . . . . . . . . . . . . . . . . . . . . . . .
Have you gone through the menopause? Yes □, No □
If yes, age . . . . . . . . . . . . . . . . . . . . . . . . . . .

Age when periods first started . . . . . . . . . . . . . .
Date most recent menstrual period started . . . . .
Number of days from the start of one period to the start of the next period . . . . . . . . . . . . . . . . . .
Are your periods regular? Yes □, No □
How long do they last? . . . . . . . . . . . . . . . . . .

**PAST MEDICAL HISTORY: Check if your answer is yes**

As a child did you have:

□ Rheumatic fever
□ Scarlet fever
□ Rubella (measles)
□ Other
□ Bladder infections
□ Kidney infections

As an adult have you had:

□ Heart disease
□ Heart murmur
□ Kidney disease
□ Kidney infection
□ Bladder infection
□ Liver disease
□ Tuberculosis
□ Diabetes
□ Pneumonia
□ Cancer
□ Asthma
□ Jaundice
□ High blood pressure
□ Serious injuries or accidents
□ Thyroid disease

**SURGICAL HISTORY**

Have you had any operations? Yes □, No □ If yes, please list type and date or age . . . . . . . . . . . . . . . . . .

. . . . . . . . . . . . . . . . . . . . . . . . . . . . . . . . . . . . . . . . . . . . . . . . . . . . . . . . . . . . . . . . . . . . . . .

Have you had any blood transfusions? Yes □, No □
Previous Rhogam injections? Yes □, No □
Any reaction? Yes □, No □

**Fig. C.6.** Medical history questionnaire.

**REVIEW OF SYSTEMS: Please check if you have recently had:**

- ☐ Fever, chills
- ☐ Sweating at night
- ☐ Skin rashes
- ☐ Skin infections
- ☐ Change in any mole
- ☐ Severe headaches
- ☐ Dizziness
- ☐ Ear pain
- ☐ Ear infections
- ☐ Ear discharge
- ☐ Ringing in ears
- ☐ Decreased hearing
- ☐ Breast pain
- ☐ Breast lumps
- ☐ Nipple discharge
- ☐ Breast size change
- ☐ Breast x-ray, if so date . . . . . . . . . . . .
- ☐ Asthmas
- ☐ Chest x-ray, if so date . . . . . . . . . . . .
- ☐ Chest pain
- ☐ Fainting
- ☐ Swelling of legs
- ☐ Varicose veins
- ☐ Blood clots
- ☐ Heart murmur
- ☐ Pain in legs with exercise
- ☐ Joint pain
- ☐ Floating stools
- ☐ Bad food digestion
- ☐ Hemorrhoids
- ☐ Change in bowel habits
- ☐ Enlarged thyroid
- ☐ Intolerance to heat
- ☐ Intolerance to cold
- ☐ Involuntary loss of urine
- ☐ Excessive urination
- ☐ Excessive water drinking
- ☐ Excessive eating
- ☐ Psychiatric treatment
- ☐ Weakness
- ☐ Fatigue
- ☐ Recent weight loos
- ☐ Recent weight gain
- ☐ Change in appetite
- ☐ Loss of hair
- ☐ Low blood count (anemia)
- ☐ Easy bruising
- ☐ Prolonged bleeding
- ☐ Gland enlargement in neck, axilla or groin
- ☐ Frequent bloody noses
- ☐ Sores in mouth
- ☐ Bleeding gums
- ☐ False teeth
- ☐ Hoarseness
- ☐ Sinus infections
- ☐ Throat infections
- ☐ Cough
- ☐ Coughing up blood
- ☐ Sputum
- ☐ Difficulty breathing
  - ☐ with laying down
  - ☐ with exercise
  - ☐ during sleep
- ☐ Nausea
- ☐ Vomiting
- ☐ Difficulty swallowing
- ☐ Vomiting blood
- ☐ Constipation
- ☐ Hernia
- ☐ Diarrhea
- ☐ Black stools
- ☐ Joint tenderness
- ☐ Joint swelling
- ☐ Convulsions
- ☐ Stroke
- ☐ Difficulty speaking
- ☐ Nervousness
- ☐ Tremors
- ☐ Difficulty walking
- ☐ Depression
- ☐ Thoughts of suicide
- ☐ Itching
- ☐ Other

**Fig. C.6.** *(continued)*

## MEDICINES

Do you smoke? Yes □, No □ How many packs per day? . . . . . . . . . . . . . . . . .
Do you use alcohol? Yes □, No □ Marijuana? Yes □, No □ Cocaine? Yes □, No □ Other? . . . . . . . . . . . . .
Do you have any drug allergies? Yes □, No □ If yes, which drugs? . . . . . . . . . . . . . . . . . . . . . . . . . . . . . .
Please list all medicines which you are currently taking (include contraceptives, hormones and vitamins: . . . . . .
. . . . . . . . . . . . . . . . . . . . . . . . . . . . . . . . . . . . . . . . . . . . . . . . . . . . . . . . . . . . . . . . . . . .

## GYNECOLOGIC HISTORY

Do you have any of the following? Please check if you do

□ Bleeding between periods; if yes, duration . . . . . . . . . . . . . . . . . . . . .
□ Bleeding after intercourse; if yes, duration . . . . . . . . . . . . . . . . . . . . .
□ Heavy menstrual periods; if yes, duration . . . . . . . . . . . . . . . . . . . . . . .
□ Pain with periods; if yes, duration . . . . . . . . . . . . . . . . . . . . . . . . . . .
□ Uncontrolled loss of urine with coughing or at other times: if yes, for how long? . . . . . . . . . . . . . . . . . .

Date of last Pap smear: . . . . . . . . . . . . . . . . . . . . . . . . . . . . . . . . . . Normal: Yes □, No □
Date of last mammogram: . . . . . . . . . . . . . . . . . . . . . . . . . . . . . . . . Normal: Yes □, No □
Have you had any treatment to your cervix? Yes □, No □

□ Cautery
□ Cryosurgery
□ Other

If yes, when? . . . . . . . . . . . . . . . . . . . . . . . . . . . . . . . . . . . . . . . . .

Have you had any infection in your female organs? Yes □, No □ If yes, when? . . . . . . . . . . . . . . . . . . . . .
Have you ever had herpes? Yes □, No □
Have you ever had venereal warts or condylomata? Yes □, No □
Are you sexually active at this time? Yes □, No □
How long have you been with your current sexual partner? . . . . . . . . . . . . . . . . . . . . . . . . . . . . . . . . .
Is your sex life satisfactory for you? Yes □, No □
Do you have any questions about sex you would like to ask? Yes □, No □

## FAMILY HISTORY

Has anyone in your family had any of these diseases? If so, please give relationship

High blood pressure . . . . . . . . . . . . . . . . . . . . . .
Stroke . . . . . . . . . . . . . . . . . . . . . . . . . . . . . .
Heart disease . . . . . . . . . . . . . . . . . . . . . . . . .
Diabetes . . . . . . . . . . . . . . . . . . . . . . . . . . . . . . .
Breast cancer . . . . . . . . . . . . . . . . . . . . . . . . . .
Other cancer . . . . . . . . . . . . . . . . . . . . . . . . . . .
List other diseases . . . . . . . . . . . . . . . . . . . . . . . . . . . . . . . . . . . . . . . . . . . . . . . . . . . . . . . . . . . . .
. . . . . . . . . . . . . . . . . . . . . . . . . . . . . . . . . . . . . . . . . . . . . . . . . . . . . . . . . . . . . . . . . . . .

## SOCIAL HISTORY

Current marital status: married □, single □, divorced □, widowed □, separated □
Number of people living in your household? . . . . . . . . . . . . . . . . . . . . . . .
Your occupation . . . . . . . . . . . . . . . . . . . . . . . . . . . . . . . . . . . . . . . . .
Your husband's occupation . . . . . . . . . . . . . . . . . . . . . . . . . . . . . . . . .

## HEALTH HABITS

How many hours do you sleep at night? . . . . . . . . . . . . . . . . . . . . . . . . . . . . . . . . . . . . . . . . . . .
Do you eat regular meals including breakfast? . . . . . . . . . . . . . . . . . . . . . . . . . . . . . . . . . . . . . . .
Do you eat whole grain bread and cereal, fresh fruits and vegetables daily? . . . . . . . . . . . . . . . . . . . . . . .
Do you exercise regularly? Yes □, No □ If yes, what type of exercise do you do? . . . . . . . . . . . . . . . . . . . .
. . . . . . . . . . . . . . . . . . . . . . . . . . . . . . . . . . . . . . . . . . . . . . . . . . . . . . . . . . . . . . . . . . . .
How often do you exercise? . . . . . . . . . . . . . . . . . . . . . . . . . . . . . . . . . . . . . . . . . . . . . . . . . .
What do you do to relax? . . . . . . . . . . . . . . . . . . . . . . . . . . . . . . . . . . . . . . . . . . . . . . . . . . . .
Do you consider yourself healthy? . . . . . . . . . . . . . . . . . . . . . . . . . . . . . . . . . . . . . . . . . . . . . .

THANK YOU

**Fig. C.6.** (*continued*)

Peter K Sand, MD
Director, Section of Urogynecology
Director, Evanston Continence Center
The Evanston Hospital
Northwestern University
(708) 570-2750

## UROGYNECOLOGY HISTORY QUESTIONNAIRE

NAME . . . . . . . . . . . . . . . . . . . . . . . . . . . . . . . . . . . . . . . . . . . . . . . . . . . . . . . . . . . . . .

INSTRUCTIONS TO PATIENT, Check the box if your answer is *"YES"*

1. Have you had treatment for urinary tract disease such as (please check): stones □, kidney disease □, infections □, tumors □, injuries □?
2. Have you ever had paralysis □, polio □, multiple sclerosis □, pernicious anemia □? (If yes, check proper ones)
3. Have you had an operation on your spine □, brain □, or bladder □?
4. Have you had a bladder infection during the last year? □
5. If yes, did it occur more than twice during the last year? □
6. Did the bladder infection follow intercourse at any time? □
7. Is your urine every bloody? □
8. Have you ever been treated by urethral dilation? □
9. If yes, when? . . . . . . . . . . . . . . . . . . . . . . . . . . .
   How many times? . . . . . . . . . . . . . . . . . . . . . . . .
10. Did urethral dilation help you? □
11. Did you have trouble holding urine as a child? □
12. As a child, did you wet the bed beyong age 5? □
13. If yes, at what age did you stop? . . . . . . . . . . . . . . . .
14. Do you wet the bed now? □
15. What is the volume of urine you usually pass when you urinate? large □, medium □, small □, very small □
16. Do you notice any dribbling of urine when you stand after passing urine? □
17. Do you lose urine by spurts during severe coughing □, sneezing □, vomiting □, laughing □?
18. If yes, in which position(s) does it occur? (please check) standing □, sitting □, laying down □
19. Do you lose urine without coughing, sneezing, laughing, or vomiting? □
20. If yes, when does it occur? (please check) walking □, running □, straining □, laying down □, any change of position □, after intercourse □, during intercourse □?
21. If you lose urine, how long has this been happening? ..............years
22. When you are passing urine, can you ususally stop the flow? □
23. Did your urine difficulty start during pregnancy □, or after delivery of an infant □? (If yes check proper one)
24. Did it follow an operation? □
25. If yes, check the yes, check the type of operation:
    - □ Hysterectomy (removal of womb), through the abdomen, radical □
    - □ Hysterectomy (removal of womb), through the vagina
    - □ Removal of tumor through the abdomen
    - □ Vaginal repair operation (bladder or rectum)
    - □ Suspension of uterus
    - □ Abdominal incontinence surgery
    - □ Cesarean section
    - □ Other (describe) . . . . . . . . . . . . . . . . . . . .
      . . . . . . . . . . . . . . . . . . . . . . . . . . . . . . . .
26. Did it follow x-ray treatment? □
27. If your menstrual periods have stopped, did the menopause make your condition worse? □
28. Do you lose control and pass a large amount of urine when you cough □, sneeze □, laugh □, lift □, □ strain □, vomit □, during intercourse □, after intercourse □?
29. Do you have difficulty holding urine if you suddenly stand up after sitting or lying down? □
30. Do you find it necessary to wear protection because you get wet from the urine you lose? □
31. If yes, at what age did you start using this protection?
    . . . . . . . . . . . . . . . . . . . . . . . . . . . . . . . . . . years
32. When do you wear protection? Occasionally □, all the time □, only during the day □, only at night □
33. Is your urinary problem bad enough that you would request surgery to fix it ? □
34. When you lose your urine accidentally, are you ever unaware that it is passing? □
35. Do you always have an uncomfortably strong need to pass urine before you empty your bladder? □

**Fig. C.7.** Urogynecology history form.

36. Do you lose urine before reaching to toilet? □

37. If yes, is this urine less painful? □

38. Do you have to hurry to the toilet or can you take your time? (Please check) hurry □, take time □

39. Can you overcome the uncomfortably strong need to pass urine? Usually □, occasionally □, rarely □

40. Do you have an uncomfortably strong need to pass urine with a full bladder? □

42. How many times do you void during the night after going to bed? ..............................

43. How many time do you void during the first hour after going to bed? ...........................

44. Does an uncomfortably strong need to pass urine wake you? □

45. Are you usually awake and simply pass urine while up? □

46. After passing urine, can you usually go back to sleep? □

47. How much fluid do you usually drink before going to bed? ......................cups

48. Do you have discomfort in the area above or to the side of your bladder? □

49. Do you have pain while you pass urine? □

50. Is it painful during the entire time you pass urine? □

51. Is it painful only at the end of passing urine? □

52. Do you always feel that your bladder is empty after passing urine? □

53. Do you usually have painful passing of urine after intercourse? □

54. Do you need to pass urine more frequently after intercourse? □

55. Does your bladder discomfort stop completely after passing urine? □

56. How often do you pass urine during the day? Every ............ hours

57. Is it still necessary for you to pass urine frequently? □

58. Does the sound, the sight, or the feel of running water cause you to lose urine? □

59. Do you need to pass urine more frequently when riding in a car? □

60. Is your clothing slightly damp □, wet □, soaking wet □, or do you leave puddles on the floor □?

61. Is you loss of urine a continual drip so that you are constantly wet? □

62. Are you ever suddenly aware that you are losing or about to lose control of your urine? □

63. How often does this occur? ................/day ............../week

64. Do you usually have difficulty starting your urine stream? □

65. Do you find it frequently necessary to have your urine removed by means of a catheter because you are unable to pass it? □

## FAMILY INCONTINENCE HISTORY

Does (did) your natural mother □, sister □, aunt □ or grandmother □ have problems with urine loss as a child or an adult? □

Did she have surgery to correct this problem? mother □, sister □, aunt □, grandmother □

At what age did her problem start? mother ..........., sister ..........., aunt .........., grandmother ...........

How old were you when her problem started? ........

Did she wet the bed as a child? mother □, sister □, aunt □, grandmother □

At what age did she stop? ......................

## SUMMARY

In the space below summarize your urinary history problems(s) as briefly as possible:

..........................................

..........................................

..........................................

..........................................

..........................................

..........................................

..........................................

..........................................

..........................................

..........................................

..........................................

..........................................

..........................................

..........................................

..........................................

..........................................

..........................................

..........................................

..........................................

..........................................

**Fig. C.7.** *(continued)*

Peter K Sand, MD
Director, Section of Urogynecology
Director, Evanston Continence Center
The Evanston Hospital
Northwestern University
(708) 570-2750

---

## VOIDING DIARY/UROLOG

This chart is a record of your voiding (urinating) and leakage (incontinence) of urine. Please complete this according to the following instructions prior to your visit to our office. Choose a *24 hour* period to keep this record when you can conveniently measure every voiding, and begin your record with the first voiding upon arising as in the example below.

*Example*

### VOIDING DIARY

| (1) TIME | (2) AMOUNT VOIDED | (3) ACTIVITY | (4) LEAK VOLUME | (5) URGE PRESENT | (6) AMOUNT/TYPE OF INTAKE |
|---|---|---|---|---|---|
| 6:45 am | 550 cc | Awakening | | | |
| 7: am | | Turned on $H_2O$ | 2 | Yes | 2 cups coffee |
| | | | | | 6 oz OJ |
| | | | | | |

(1) Record time of all voidings, leakage, intake of liquids.

(2) Measure all intake and output in *cc's* or *oz's.*

(3) Describe activity you were performing at time of leakage. If you were not actively doing anything, record whether you were sitting, standing or lying.

(4) Estimate the amount of leakage according to the following scale:

1 = damp, few drops only
2 = wet underwear or pad
3 = soaked or emptied bladder

(5) If the urge to urinate accompanied (or preceded) the urine leakage write YES. If you felt no urge when the leakage occurred write NO.

(6) Record the amount and type of *all liquid* intake using either cc's or oz's (1 cup = 8 oz = 240 cc).

**Fig. C.8.** Voiding diary/urolog instructions.

## VOIDING DIARY

| TIME | AMOUNT VOIDED | ACTIVITY | LEAK VOLUME | URGE PRESENT | AMOUNT/TYPE OF INTAKE |
|---|---|---|---|---|---|
| | | | | | |
| | | | | | |
| | | | | | |
| | | | | | |
| | | | | | |
| | | | | | |
| | | | | | |
| | | | | | |
| | | | | | |
| | | | | | |
| | | | | | |
| | | | | | |
| | | | | | |
| | | | | | |
| | | | | | |
| | | | | | |
| | | | | | |
| | | | | | |
| | | | | | |
| | | | | | |
| | | | | | |
| | | | | | |
| | | | | | |
| | | | | | |
| | | | | | |
| | | | | | |
| | | | | | |
| | | | | | |

**Fig. C.8.** *(continued)*

Peter K Sand, MD
Director, Section of Urogynecology
Director, Evanston Continence Center
The Evanston Hospital
Northwestern University
(708) 570-2750

## BLADDER RETRAINING

You currently have a suprapubic catheter draining your bladder. Because there is nothing obstructing your urethra, you will be able to urinate even with this catheter in place. Approximately 3 days after surgery, we will clamp off the suprapubic catheter during the day and let your bladder fill. When you feel the need to urinate, you will sit on the toilet and empty your bladder into the collecting device placed under the seat. If you do not feel the need to urinate by 4 hours, try to urinate at that time. Do not worry if no urine comes out. The *voided volume* will then be measured and marked on this sheet along with the date and time. After this the catheter will be unclamped for 10 minutes and the *residual volume* (urine left in the bladder after urinating) will be collected in the bag and measured. This residual volume will also be recorded. This process will occur only during wakeful hours. The catheter will be left open to drain during the night while you are asleep.

When the voided amounts are 3 times the volume of the residual amounts and the residuals are less than 100 cc for 2 days, you should notify your physician and the suprapubic catheter will be removed.

| DATE | TIME | VOIDED VOLUME | RESIDUAL VOLUME | DATE | TIME | VOIDED VOLUME | RESIDUAL VOLUME |
|---|---|---|---|---|---|---|---|
| | | | | | | | |
| | | | | | | | |
| | | | | | | | |
| | | | | | | | |
| | | | | | | | |
| | | | | | | | |
| | | | | | | | |
| | | | | | | | |
| | | | | | | | |
| | | | | | | | |
| | | | | | | | |
| | | | | | | | |
| | | | | | | | |
| | | | | | | | |
| | | | | | | | |
| | | | | | | | |
| | | | | | | | |

**Fig. C.9.** Bladder retraining form and instructions.

Peter K Sand, MD
Urogynecology
The Evanston Hospital

## VOIDING CHART

| DATE | TIME | VOIDED VOLUME | RESIDUAL VOLUME | DATE | TIME | VOIDED VOLUME | RESIDUAL VOLUME |
|---|---|---|---|---|---|---|---|
| | | | | | | | |
| | | | | | | | |
| | | | | | | | |
| | | | | | | | |
| | | | | | | | |
| | | | | | | | |
| | | | | | | | |
| | | | | | | | |
| | | | | | | | |
| | | | | | | | |
| | | | | | | | |
| | | | | | | | |
| | | | | | | | |
| | | | | | | | |
| | | | | | | | |
| | | | | | | | |
| | | | | | | | |
| | | | | | | | |
| | | | | | | | |
| | | | | | | | |
| | | | | | | | |
| | | | | | | | |
| | | | | | | | |
| | | | | | | | |
| | | | | | | | |

**Fig. C.10.** Voiding chart for monitoring urinary retention during self-catheterization.

## UROGYNECOLOGY VISIT SUMMARY

| | | | |
|---|---|---|---|
| NAME (FIRST) | | | (LAST) |
| HOME TELEPHONE | | | WORK TELEPHONE |
| ADDRESS | | | |
| DATE OF BIRTH | | | SOCIAL SECURITY # |
| REFERRED BY | | | ADDRESS |
| CITY | STATE | ZIP | TELEPHONE |
| PHARMACY | | | PHARMACY TELEPHONE |

| DATE | PROCEDURE | VISIT SUMMARY (ONE LINE PER VISIT) | DICT | INITIALS |
|---|---|---|---|---|
| | | Urine C & S ☐ | | |
| | | | | |
| | | | | |
| | | | | |
| | | | | |
| | | | | |
| | | | | |
| | | | | |
| | | | | |
| | | | | |
| | | | | |
| | | | | |
| | | | | |
| | | | | |
| | | | | |
| | | | | |
| | | | | |
| | | | | |
| | | | | |
| | | | | |
| | | | | |

**Fig. C.11.** Urogynecology visit summary form, running visit log.

DATE:

**PREOPERATIVE HISTORY & PHYSICAL**
**EVANSTON CONTINENCE CENTER**

Name______________________________ D.O.B.___/___/_____ MR#______

Diagnosis:______________________ Procedures:____________________

Special Requests:______________________________________________

****ALLERGIES**

| Medications | Dose | Schedule |
|---|---|---|
| | | |
| | | |
| | | |
| | | |

AGE____ G___ P__ Menopause: Pre___ LMP___/___/__ Post___ ERT? Y N

History of Present Illness:

Urogynecology Workup:

Past Medical History: Card/Pul/GU/HTN/DM/Thyroid/Hepatitis/CTD
(Circle if positive)

**Fig. C.12.** Preoperative history and physical examination form.

**Past Surgical History:**

GYN: ________________________________

General: ______________________________

______________________________

**Social History:** Tobacco________ Alcohol______ Drugs________

**Family History:** ________________________________

________________________________

________________________________

________________________________

## REVIEW OF SYSTEMS:

HEENT +/-
Cardiorespiratory +/-
Gastrointestinal +/-
Genitourinary +/-
Musculoskeletal +/-
CNS +/-

## PHYSICAL EXAM:

| Weight | Height | BP / | Pulse | Resp |
|---|---|---|---|---|

**General** Normal/Abnormal
**Skin:** Normal/Abnormal
**HEENT:** Normal/Abnormal
**Cor:** Normal/Abnormal
**Lungs:** Normal/Abnormal
**Breasts:** Normal/Abnormal
**Abdomen:** Normal/Abnormal
**Neuro:** Normal/Abnormal

**Extremities:** Normal/Abnormal

## PELVIC:

**Introitus:**
**Vagina:**
**Cervix:**
**Uterus:**
**Adnexa:**
**Rectum:**

**Impression:** (See Page 1) **Plan:** (See Page 1)

______________________ Peter K. Sand, M.D.

______________________ John W. Utrie, Jr., D.O.

**Fig. C.12.** (*continued*)

# Appendix D
# Self Test

This section is designed to test the skills you have gained reviewing the prior chapters of this text. Appendix D is divided into different sections by the type of urodynamic study being reviewed. Questions are asked about each urodynamic tracing which are either multiple choice or true/false queries. The answers to these questions, a brief explanation of the answer and the chapter that deals with the facts in question may be found at the end of this Appendix.

## D.1 Leak Point Pressure Testing

1. In Fig. D.1 a 42-year-old incontinent woman holds her breath and gradually strains as hard as she can in the standing position with a bladder volume of 250 ml. Three such efforts are made by the patient and in none of these leak point pressure measurements does the patient lose any urine involuntarily. What is the proper leak point pressure for this patient?
   a. 245 $cmH_2O$ without leakage (250 ml)
   b. 165 $cmH_2O$ without leakage (250 ml)
   c. None
   d. 0 $cmH_2O$
   e. 115 $cmH_2O$ (250 ml)

2. In Fig. D.2 a 65-year-old woman with genuine stress incontinence is undergoing leak point pressure measurements in the standing position at a bladder volume of 250 ml. On the first two Valsalva efforts the patient fails to leak urine involuntarily, but does lose urine coincident with the last two Valsalva manuevers. During these two straining efforts the urethral closure pressure is seen to fall below zero coincident with the loss of urine as one would usually expect. These points of urinary leakage are marked by the two small arrows. Please calculate the abdominal leak point pressure in this patient at 250 ml in the standing position.
   a. 150 $cmH_2O$
   b. 95 $cmH_2O$
   c. 145 $cmH_2O$
   d. 125 $cmH_2O$
   e. 104 $cmH_2O$

3. When calculating abdominal leak point pressures the urethral pressure rise from the baseline urethral pressure is calculated to give the pressure rise increment or leak point pressure, True or False?
   a. True
   b. False

## D.2 Urethrocystometry Studies

4. Fig. D.3 shows the standing urethrocystometry study of a 45-year-old woman who complains of urgency, frequency and stress incontinence. The patient notes first sensation at 165 ml, fullness at 207 ml and has a maximum cystometric capacity of 425 ml. What does this study demonstrate?
   a. Detrusor hyperreflexia at 207 ml
   b. A normal urethrocystometry study
   c. Urethral syndrome
   d. Urinary retention
   e. Detrusor instability

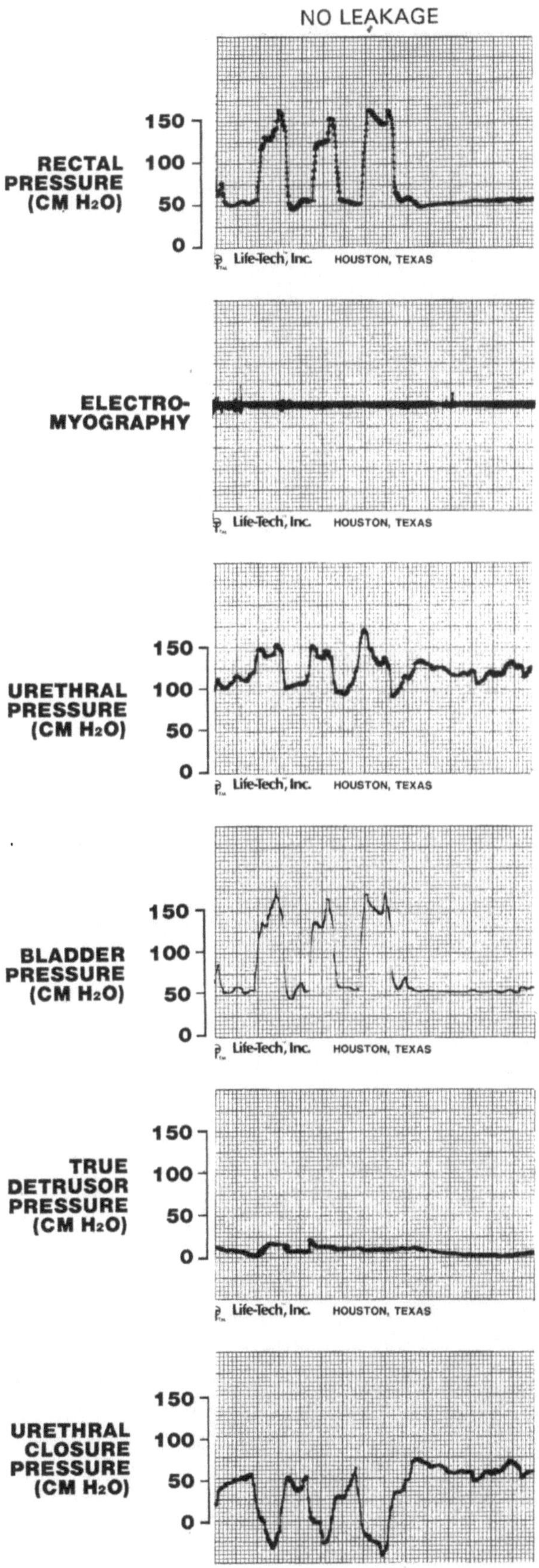


**Fig. D.1.** Leak point pressure measurements without leakage.

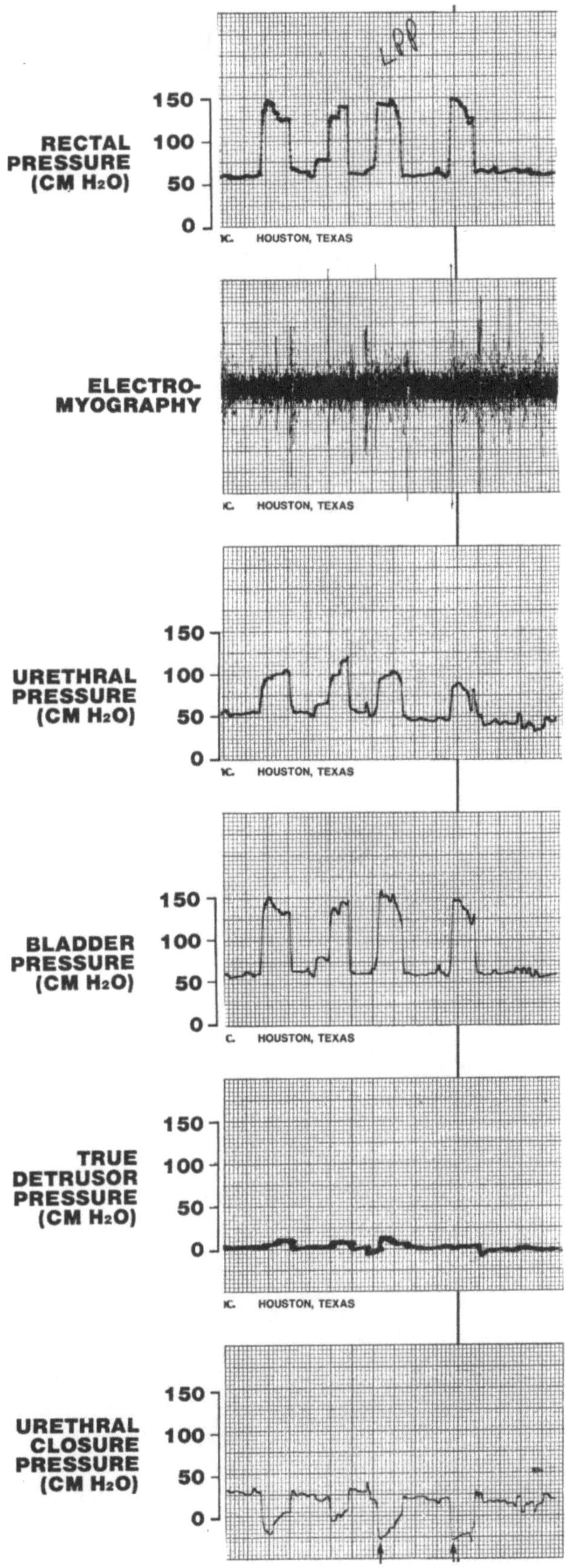


**Fig. D.2.** Leak point pressure measurements with leakage.

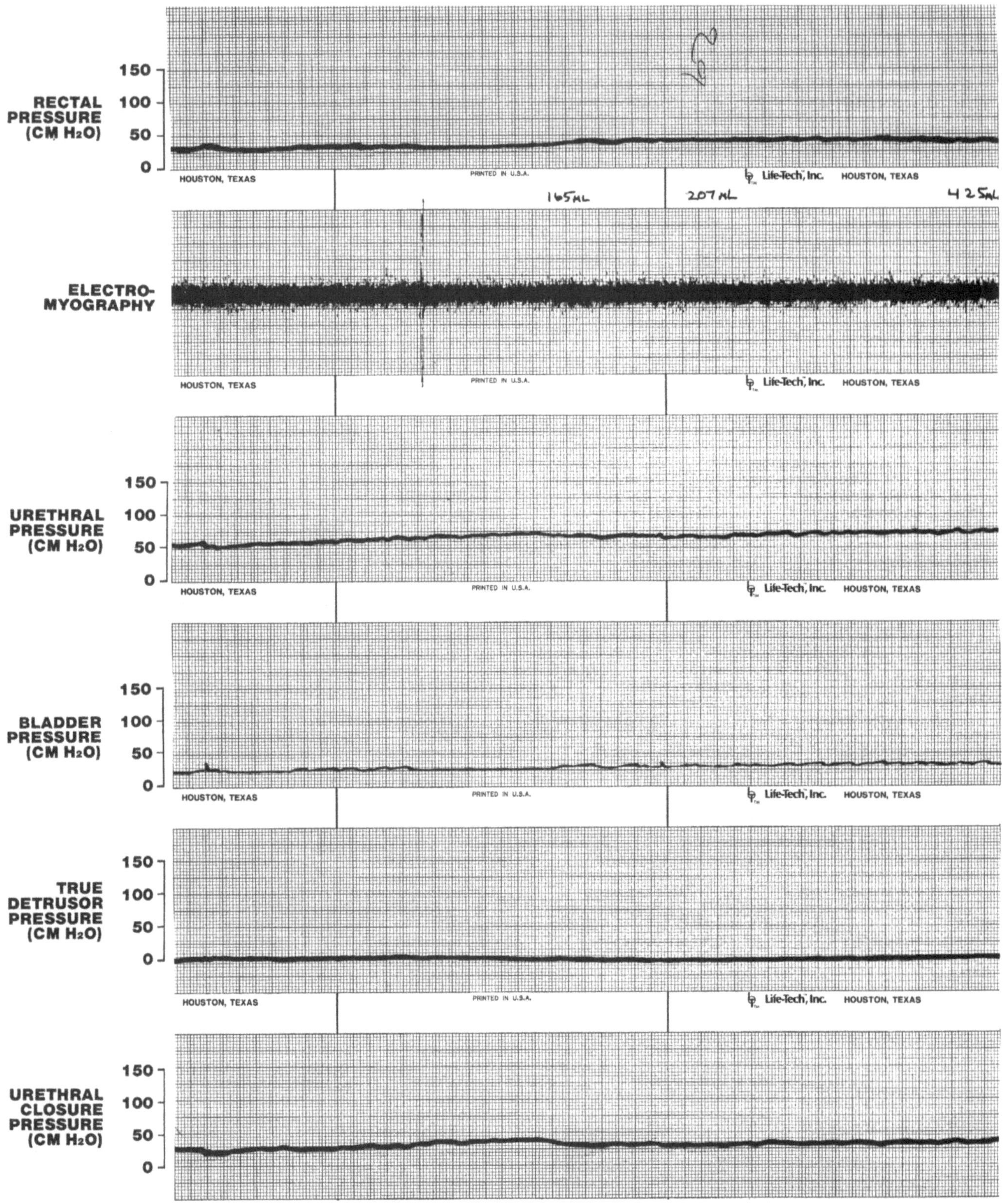


**Fig. D.3.** Standing urethrocystometry.

5. Fig. D.4 shows the sitting urethrocystometry study of a 76-year-old nulliparous female who recently had the onset of severe urge incontinence and insensible urine loss following the removal of a Foley catheter. It was placed for urinary retention occurring after a CVA which left her with a right-sided hemiparesis. Which of the following is not demonstrated on this tracing?
   a. Vascular pulsations in the urethral pressure
   b. Detrusor hyperreflexia
   c. Pressure equalization during a detrusor contraction
   d. Genuine stress incontinence
   e. A detrusor contraction > 100 $cmH_2O$

6. Fig. D.5 shows the standing urethrocystometry study of a 47-year-old multiparous female who had undergone pelvic irradiation therapy 3 years earlier for a Stage 2 cervical carcinoma. She currently complains of urinary frequency, urgency, suprapubic pressure, nocturia ×5 and insensible urine loss almost constantly. Filling her bladder to a maximum cystometric capacity of 175 ml in this study leads to continuous involuntary dripping of urine. What is the diagnosis?
   a. A low compliance bladder
   b. Interstitial cystitis
   c. Uninhibited urethral relaxation
   d. Sensory urge incontinence
   e. Vesicovaginal fistula

7. Fig. D.6 shows the standing urethrocystometry study of a 41-year-old G2P2 woman who complains of an almost constant feeling that she is going to involuntarily leak urine but never is incontinent. Her voiding diary shows that she voids every 15–45 min during the day but wakens only once during the night to void. She feels extreme urgency at the points marked by arrows. What on this study could explain these symptoms?
   a. Detrusor instability
   b. Detrusor hyperreflexia
   c. A low compliance bladder
   d. Ureterovaginal fistula
   e. Urethral instability

8. Fig. D.7 shows the sitting urethrocystometry study of a 74-year-old G5P2 woman who complains of urinary incontinence with position changes and walking. Although not marked on the tracing, she reaches a maximum cystometric capacity of 535 ml. Can a diagnosis be made from this study to explain her symptoms?
   a. Detrusor instability
   b. Overflow incontinence
   c. No
   d. Detrusor sphincter dyssynergia
   e. Diabetes mellitus

9. Fig. D.8 shows an isolated segment of a standing urethrocystometry study, between a bladder volume of 450 and 500 ml, in a 34-year-old G3P2 female complaining of urinary incontinence only while playing tennis. She leaks urine involuntarily during this segment of the tracing from:
   a. Genuine stress incontinence
   b. Overflow incontinence
   c. Sensory urge incontinence
   d. Detrusor instability
   e. None of the above

10. Urethrocystometry is a study of the storage phase of the micturition cycle. Performance of urethrocystometry can enable us to diagnose all of the following conditions, except:
   a. Detrusor overactivity
   b. Interstitial cystitis
   c. Low bladder compliance
   d. Urethral instability
   e. Uninhibited urethral relaxation

## D.3 Urethral Closure Pressure Profiles

11. Fig. D.9 shows a resting and a Valsalva urethral closure pressure profile from a 14-year-old nulliparous female complaining of insensible urine loss. These profiles are best described as:
   a. Normal
   b. Showing genuine stress incontinence
   c. Demonstrating stress induced detrusor instability
   d. Representing a spastic high pressure urethra
   e. Diagnostic of intrinsic sphincteric deficiency

12. What is the resting urethral closure pressure (CP) and functional length (FL) in the resting urethral closure pressure profile pictured in Fig. D.9? (Note that each small box on the *x* axis is equal to 1 mm)
   a. CP 112 $cmH_2O$ and FL 21 mm
   b. CP 53 $cmH_2O$ and FL 36 mm
   c. CP 56 $cmH_2O$ and FL 36 mm
   d. CP 212 $cmH_2O$ and FL 16 mm
   e. CP 112 $cmH_2O$ and FL 36 mm

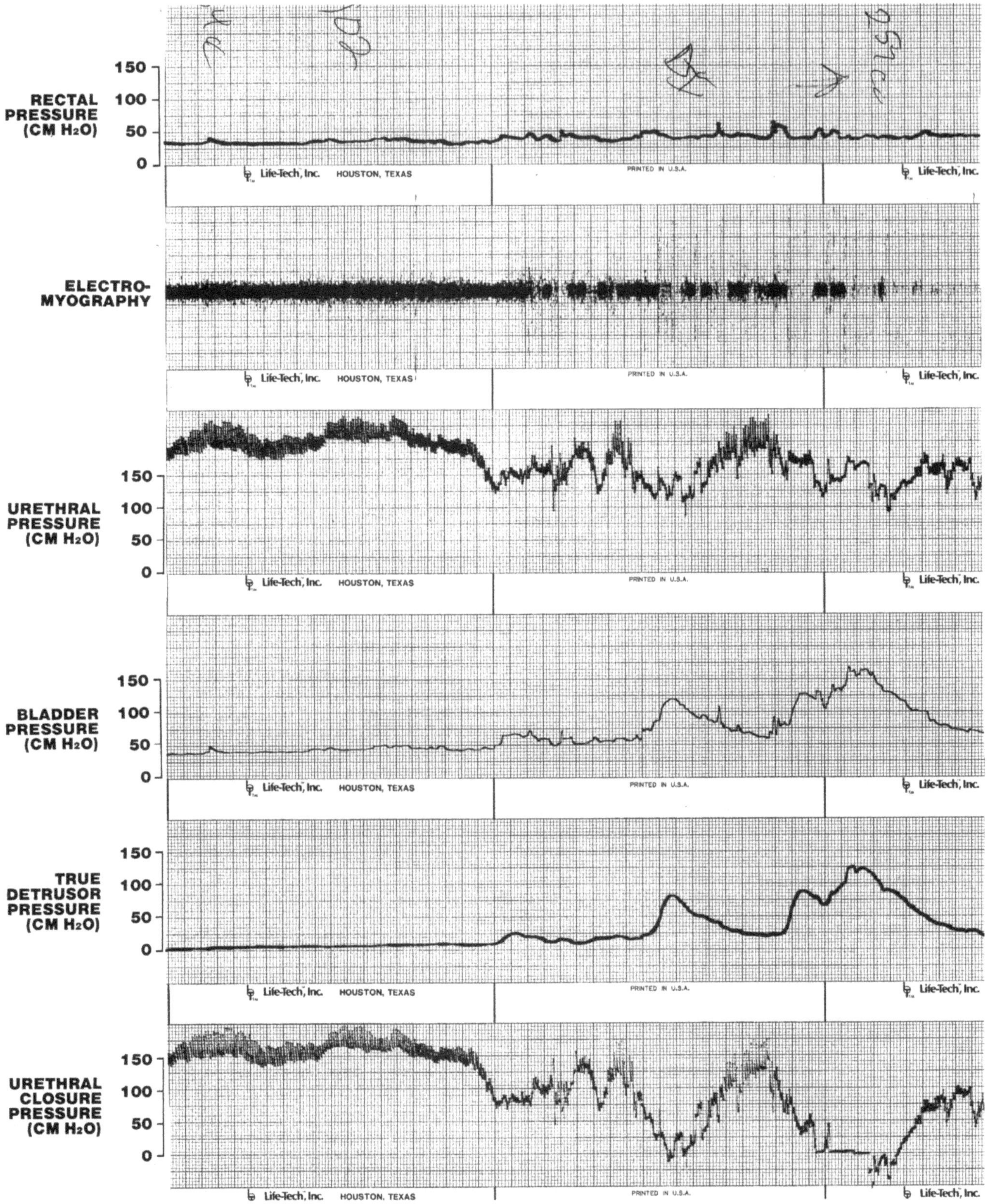


**Fig. D.4.** Sitting urethrocystometry study.

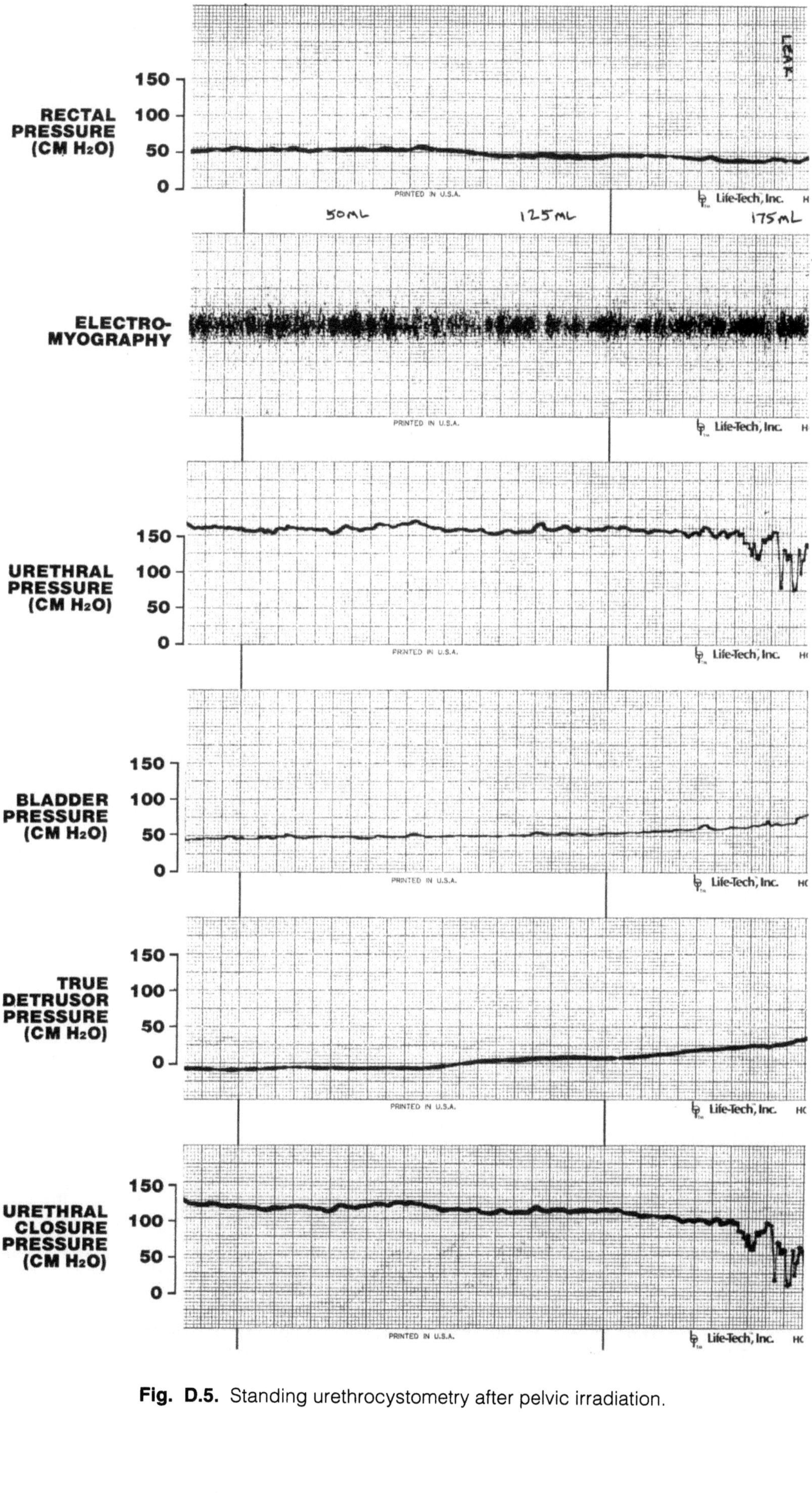


**Fig. D.5.** Standing urethrocystometry after pelvic irradiation.

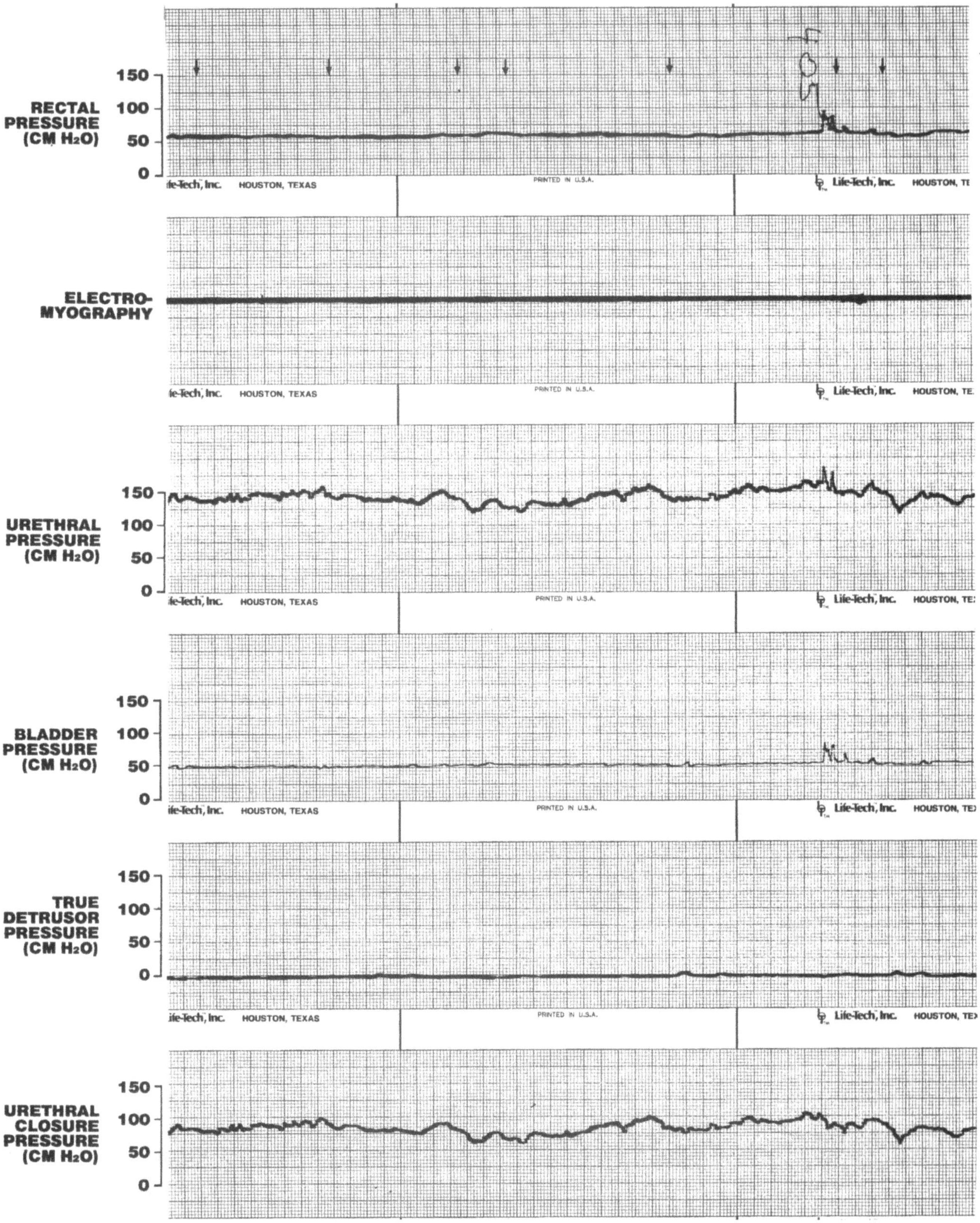


**Fig. D.6.** Standing urethrocystometry with complaints of urgency.

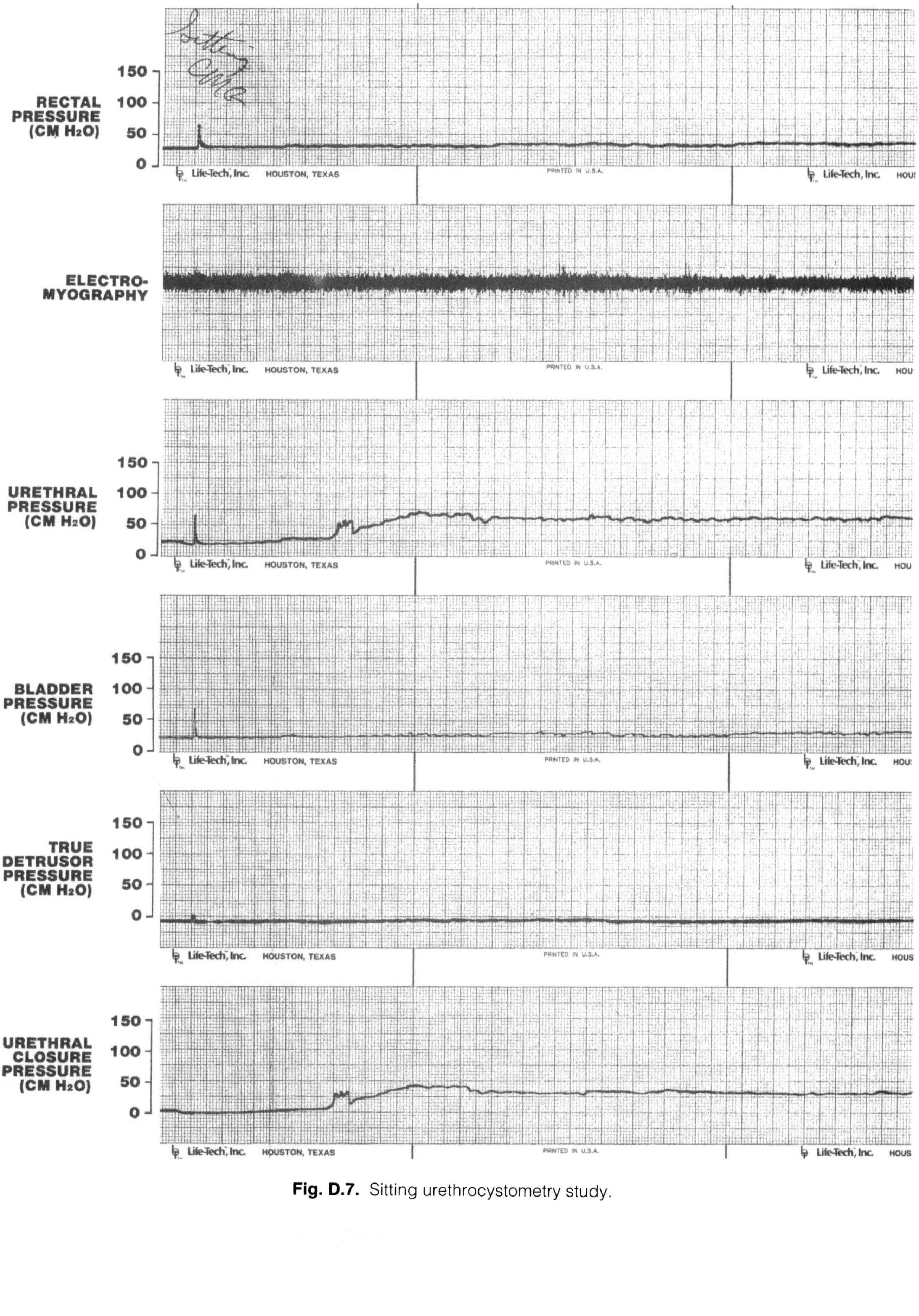


**Fig. D.7.** Sitting urethrocystometry study.

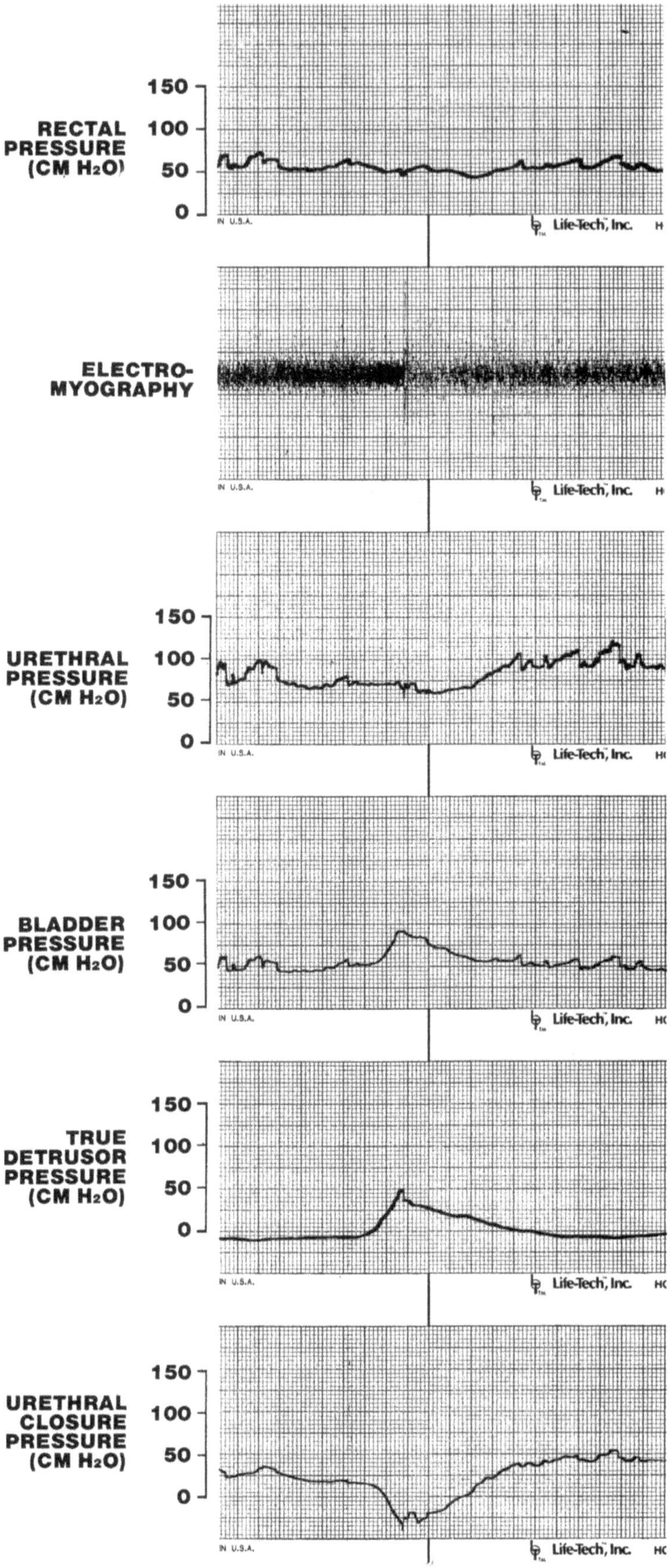


**Fig. D.8.** Leakage during a standing urethrocystometry study.

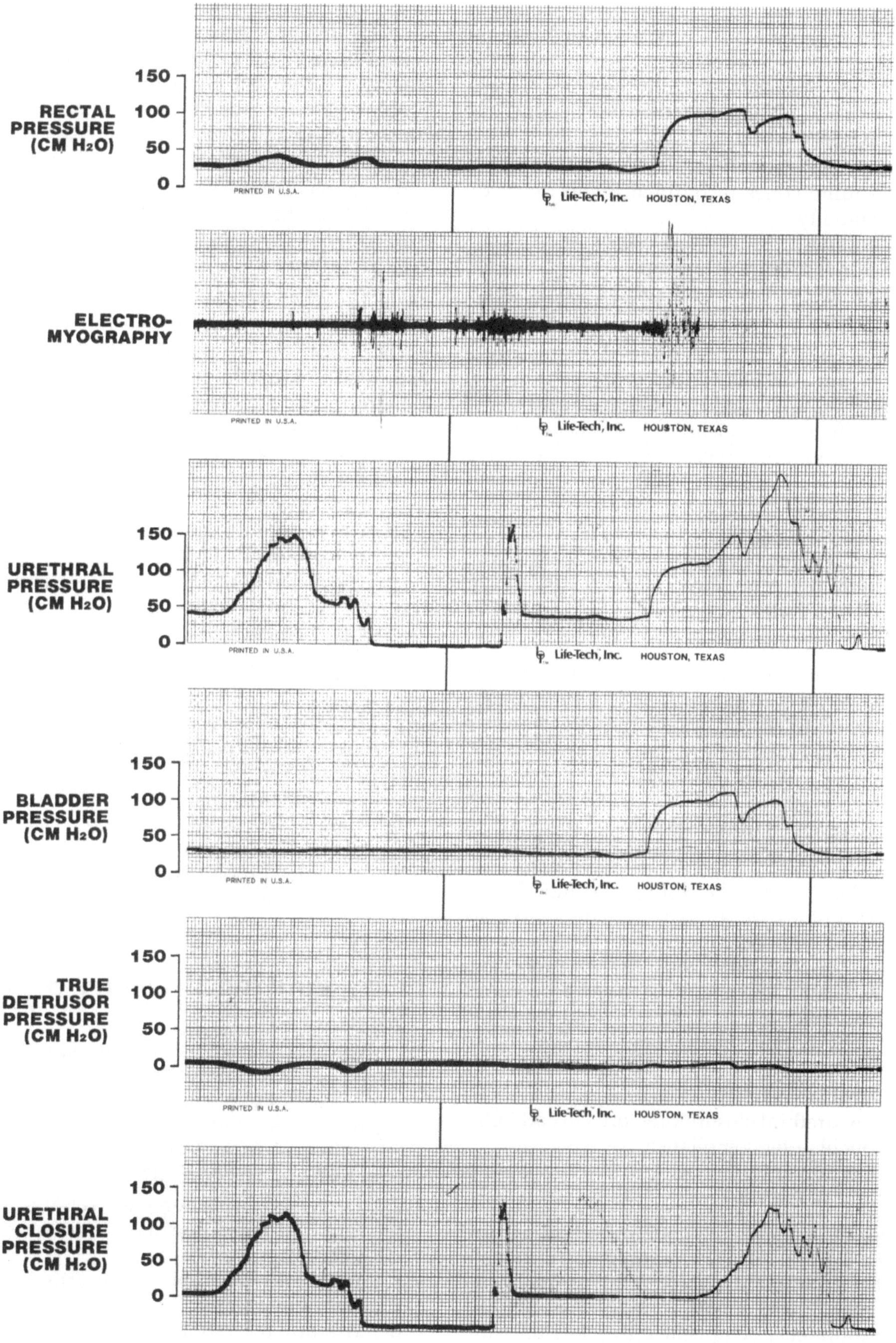


**Fig. D.9.** Resting and Valsalva urethral closure pressure profiles.

13. Fig. D.10 shows the Valsalva urethral closure pressure profiles of a 74-year-old G6P5 female with longstanding complaints of stress and urge incontinence. She leaks urine during both of these profiles done at a bladder volume of 500 ml. What is the diagnosis?
  a. Detrusor instability
  b. Genuine stress incontinence and detrusor instability
  c. Genuine stress incontinence
  d. Normal profiles at any age
  e. Normal profiles for the patient's age

14. Fig. D.11 shows a resting urethral closure pressure profile from a 38-year-old primiparous female who complains of urinary urgency, frequency, nocturia, and dyspareunia for the last three months since noticing a bulge beneath her urethra. Examination reveals a 3×2 cm fluctuant mass under the midurethra. This profile shows a bimodal pattern suggesting a:
  a. Urethral caruncle
  b. Urethral fistula
  c. Urethral diverticulum
  d. Genuine stress incontinence
  e. Low pressure urethra

15. In the case described in question 14, which of the following studies would be helpful in establishing the underlying diagnosis?
  a. Voiding cystourethrogram
  b. Tratner catheter urethrogram
  c. Urethroscopy
  d. Endovaginal ultrasound
  e. All of the above

16. Fig. D.12 shows the resting urethral closure pressure profiles of a G4P2 female who had undergone a prior Stamey bladder neck suspension and Marshall–Marchetti–Krantz procedure for stress incontinence. Both of these procedures failed to correct her symptoms. What do these profiles show that might help explain these failures?
  a. Detrusor instability
  b. Low urethral closure pressure (18 $cmH_2O$)
  c. Low bladder compliance
  d. Overflow incontinence
  e. None of the above

17. Fig. D.13 shows the cough urethral closure pressure profiles of a 78-year-old G7P7 female who had undergone a successful vaginal wall sling procedure 6 months earlier for genuine stress incontinence complicated by a low pressure urethra and detrusor instability. The patient is demonstrated to have positive pressure transmission as calculated at the pen written arrows in the original tracing. Calculations of the pressure transmission ratios are seen at the top of the tracing for the best point in each of these three profiles. Calculate the pressure transmission ratios for the next cough (curved arrow) in each profile.
  a. 56/78=72%, 86/80=108%, 50/102=49%
  b. 78/65=120%, 98/49=200%, 68/60=113%
  c. 78/65=120%, 78/62=126%, 68/31=219%
  d. 78/65=120%, 86/80=108%, 50/102=49%
  e. 56/78=72%, 98/49=200%, 50/75=67%

18. Fig. D.14 shows the resting urethral closure pressure profiles of a 38-year-old G3P3 female with complaints of urinary urgency, frequency and stress incontinence. Please calculate the closure pressure, functional length and total length of both of these profiles.
  a. CP 78 $cmH_2O$, FL 29 mm, TL 41 mm; CP 64 $cmH_2O$, FL 30 mm, TL 45 mm
  b. CP 64 $cmH_2O$, FL 24 mm, TL 35 mm; CP 54 $cmH_2O$, FL 28 mm, TL 41 mm
  c. CP 78 $cmH_2O$, FL 21 mm, TL 41 mm; CP 48 $cmH_2O$, FL 30 mm, TL 45 mm
  d. CP 53 $cmH_2O$, FL 23 mm, TL 31 mm; CP 51 $cmH_2O$, FL 65 mm, TL 69 mm
  e. CP 64 $cmH_2O$, FL 34 mm, TL 62 mm; CP 59 $cmH_2O$, FL 46 mm, TL 53 mm

19. Urethral closure pressure profiles may be useful in establishing all but which one of the following diagnoses?
  a. Low pressure urethra
  b. Genuine stress incontinence
  c. Urethral syndrome
  d. Negative pressure transmission
  e. Positive pressure transmission

## D.4 Voiding Pressure Studies

20. Fig. D.15 shows the voiding study of a 42-year-old woman complaining of urge incontinence who was found to have detrusor hyperreflexia secondary to a back injury. She voided 160 ml over 30 s. What is her voiding mechanism and is it normal?
  a. Detrusor contraction with Valsalva, normal
  b. Urethral relaxation with detrusor contraction, normal
  c. Urethral relaxation with detrusor contraction, abnormal
  d. Urethral relaxation with Valsalva, normal
  e. Detrusor contraction with Valsalva, abnormal

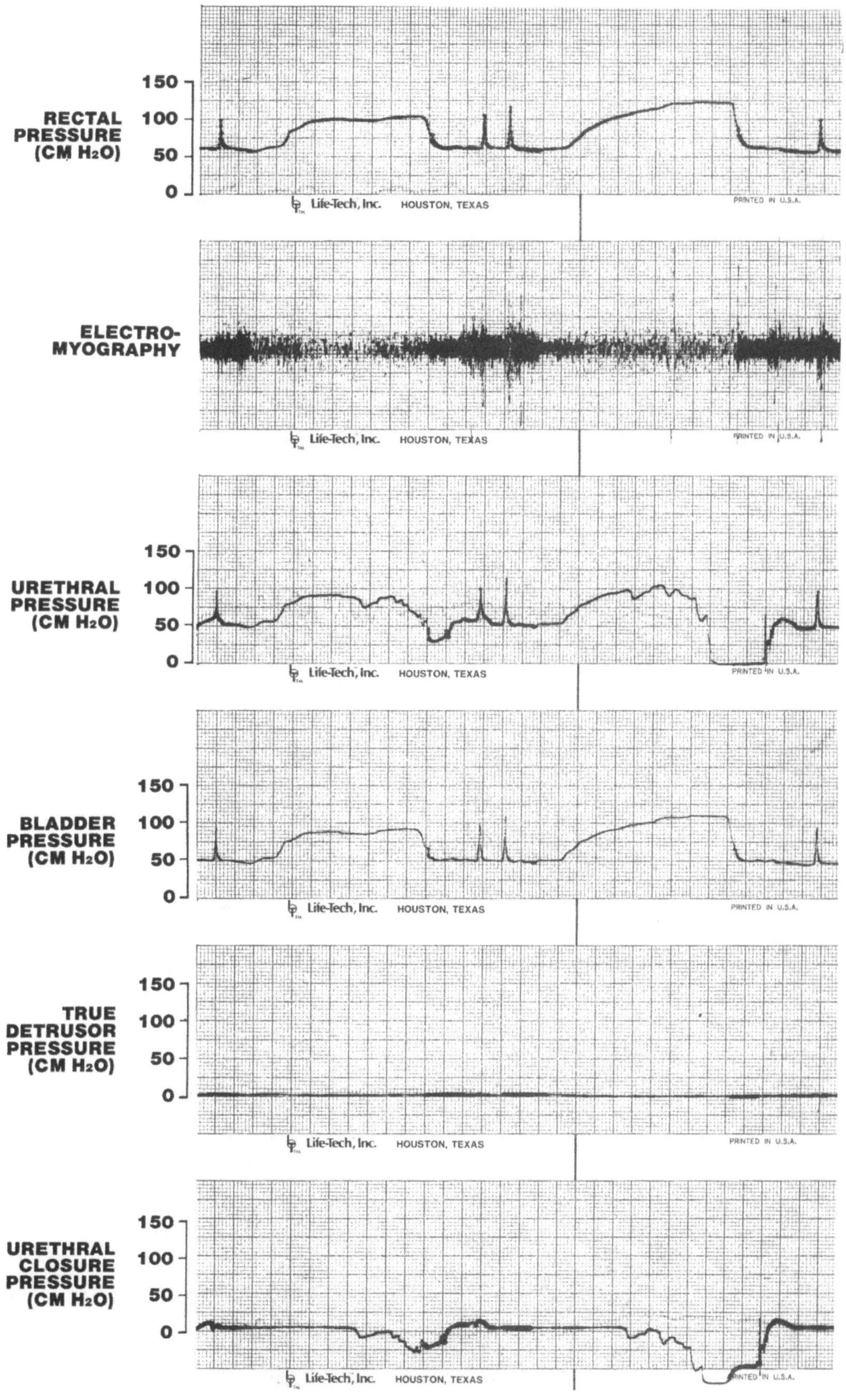


**Fig. D.10.** Valsalva urethral closure pressure profiles with leakage.

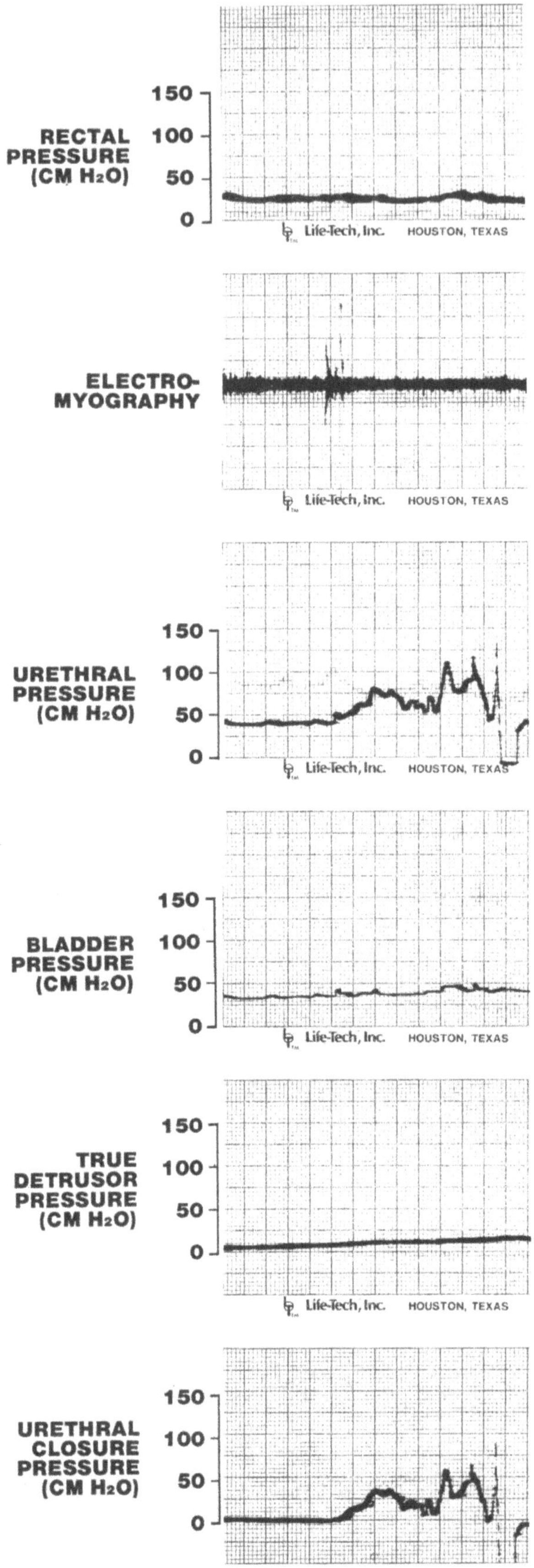


**Fig. D.11.** Urethral closure pressure profiles with a suburethral mass.

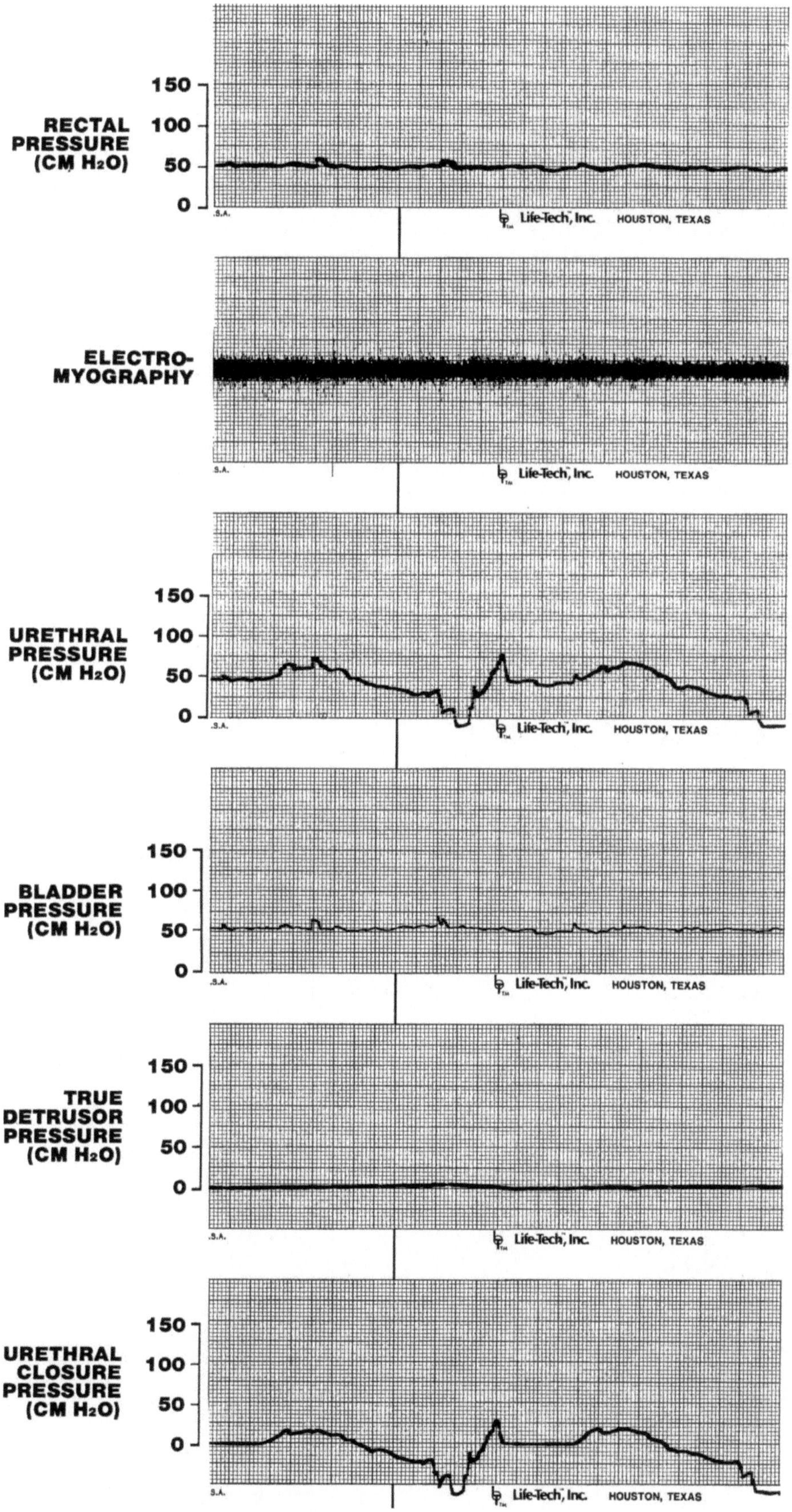


**Fig. D.12.** Urethral closure pressure profiles after failed surgery.

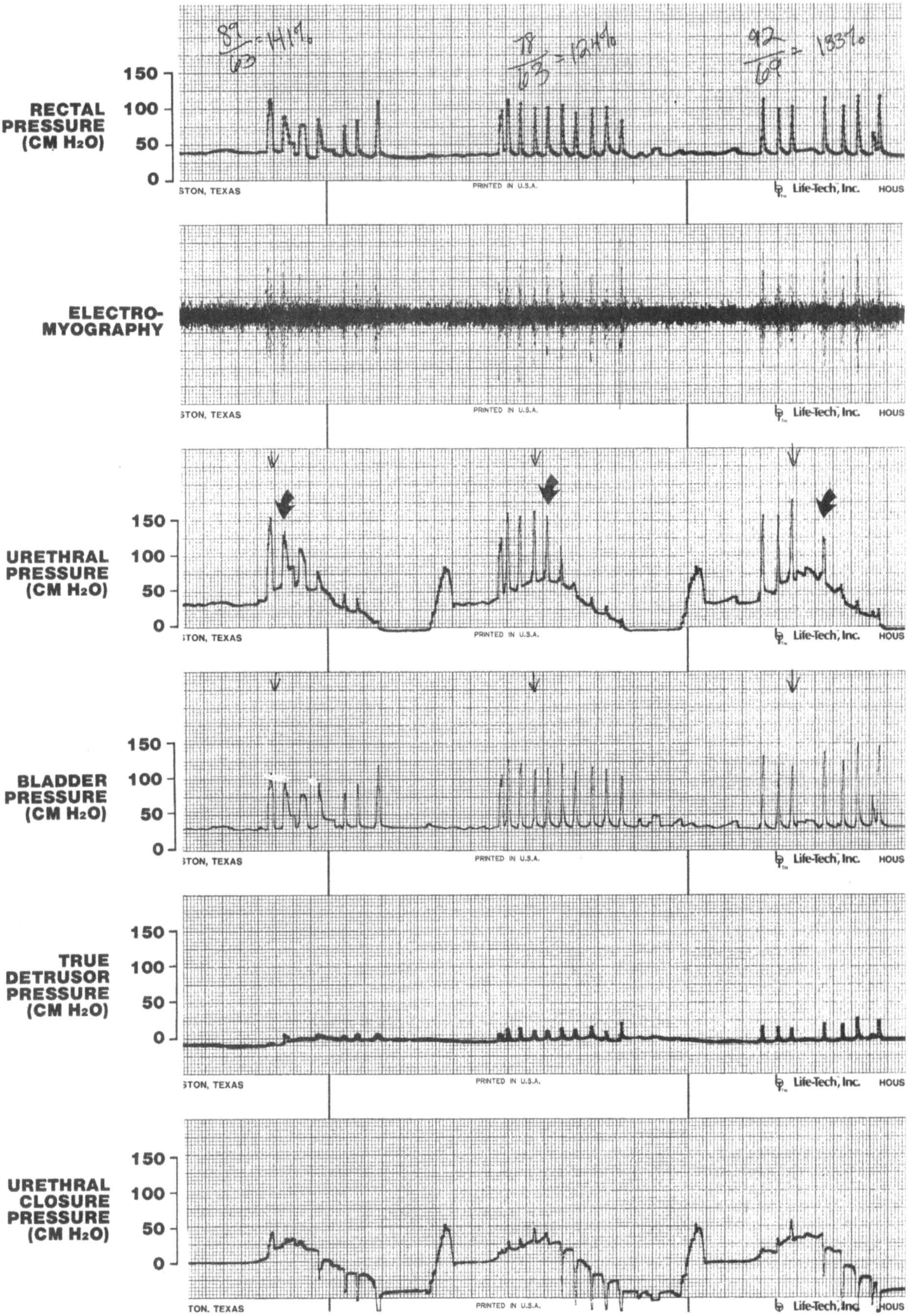


**Fig. D.13.** Cough urethral closure pressure profiles after successful surgery.

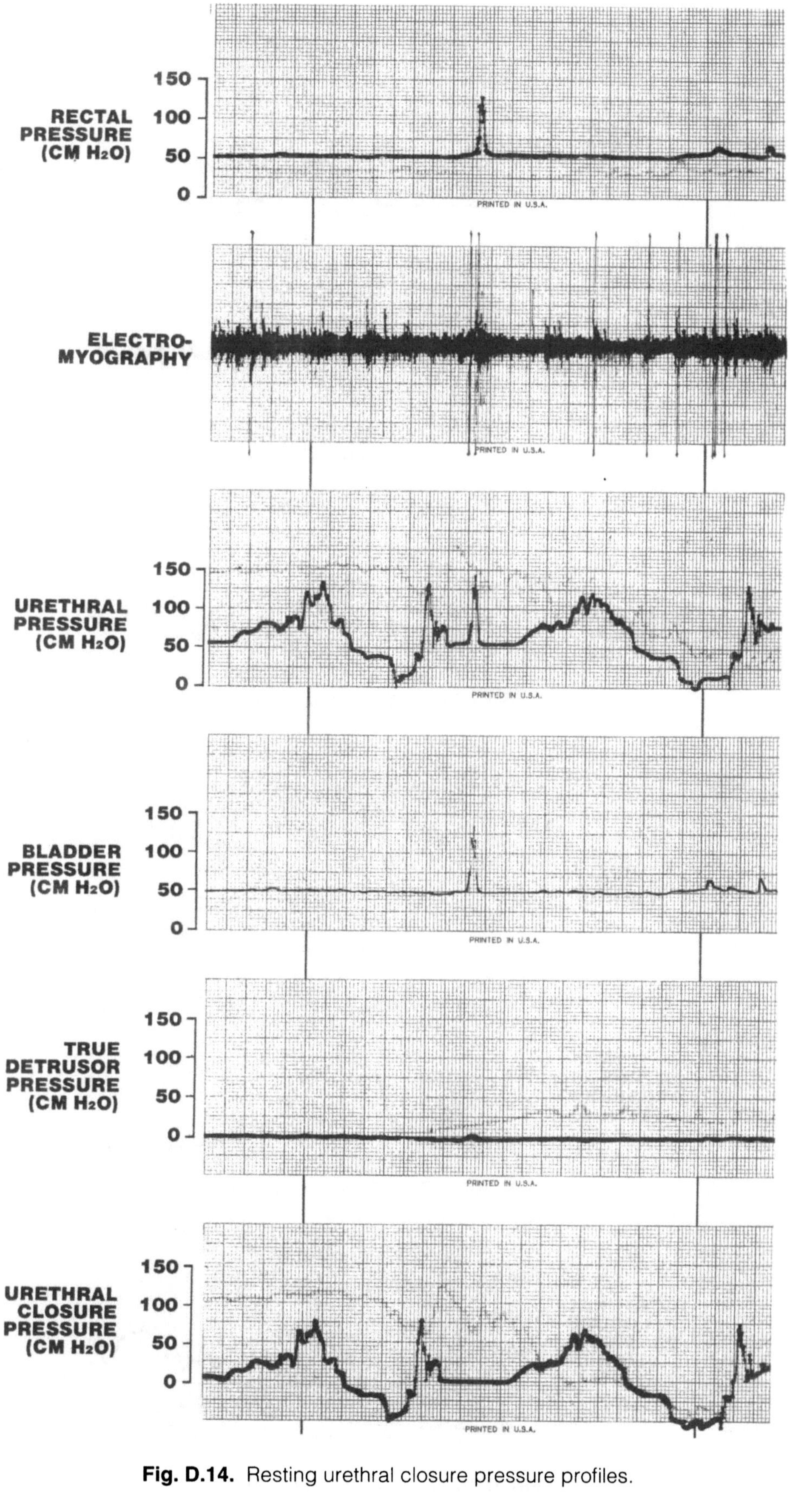


**Fig. D.14.** Resting urethral closure pressure profiles.

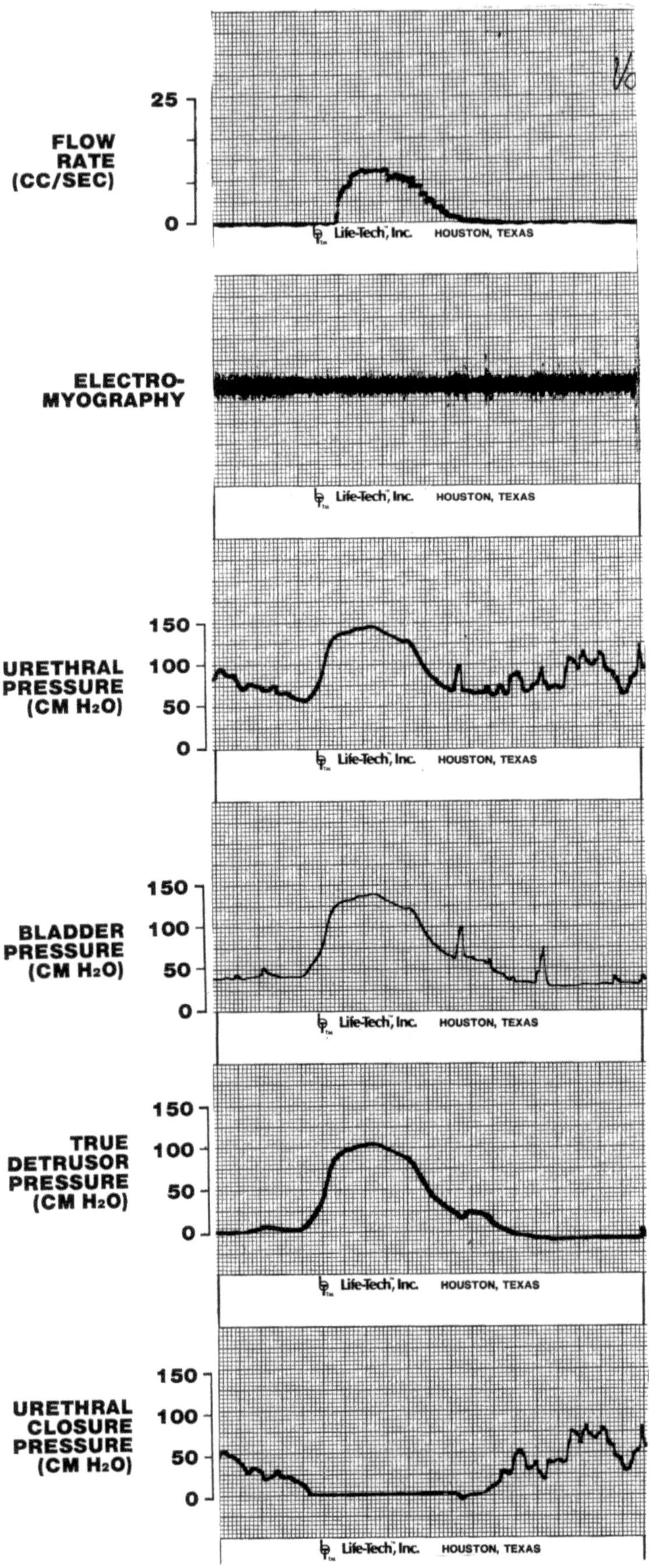


**Fig. D.15.** Voiding pressure study.

21. Fig. D.16 shows the voiding pressure study of a 50-year-old nulliparous female complaining of stress incontinence complicated by the presence of a 20 cm ovarian cyst. Her screening uroflow study showed her to void 400 ml with a residual of 110 ml with a normal flow rate. On this instrumented uroflowmetry study with surface EMG patches the patient voids 400 ml with a 20 ml residual and a maximum flow rate of 19 ml/s. What is her voiding mechanism and is it normal?

a. Urethral contraction with detrusor contraction, abnormal
b. Valsalva with detrusor contraction, abnormal
c. Urethral and detrusor relaxation, abnormal
d. Urethral relaxation and detrusor contraction, normal
e. Detrusor and sphincter relaxation, abnormal

22. Fig. D.17 shows the voiding pressure study of a 78-year-old G8P7 woman with a history of complete uterine procidentia for 10 years with known urinary retention. Here she attempts to void by what mechanism?

a. Urethral relaxation with Valsalva
b. Urethral relaxation with detrusor contraction
c. Urethral relaxation alone
d. Urethral and bladder contraction
e. None of the above

23. In Fig. D.17 what diagnosis best describes the cause of the patient's urinary retention?

a. Detrusor sphincter dyssynergia
b. Detrusor overactivity
c. Acontractile bladder
d. Urethral areflexia
e. Dementia

24. Fig. D.18 shows the voiding pressure study of a 69-year-old G3P1 female who is known to have genuine stress incontinence and a low pressure urethra. She voids 400 ml over 88 s with a maximum flow rate of about 20 ml/s by what mechanism?

a. Urethral relaxation with detrusor contraction
b. Urethral contraction alone
c. Detrusor contraction with Valsalva
d. Urethral relaxation with Valsalva
e. Urethral relaxation alone

25. Fig. D.19 shows the voiding pressure study of a 38-year-old G2P2 woman with urodynamic findings of genuine stress incontinence and detrusor instability. She voids in a continuous, yet obstructive fashion by urethral relaxation with a detrusor contraction. A stop test is done after she voids 250 ml. What is the actual pressure of her voiding detrusor contraction?

a. 200 $cmH_2O$
b. 104 $cmH_2O$
c. 36 $cmH_2O$
d. 141 $cmH_2O$
e. 10 $cmH_2O$

26. Fig. D.20 shows the voiding pressure study of a 43-year-old G2P1 woman with uterovaginal prolapse and potential genuine stress incontinence (Chapter 28) who voids in an obstructive, intermittent flow pattern? What is her voiding mechanism?

a. Valsalva alone
b. Urethral relaxation alone
c. Urethral relaxation with detrusor contraction
d. Urethral relaxation, detrusor contraction and Valsalva
e. Detrusor contraction alone

27. Fig. D.21 shows the voiding pressure study of a 67-year-old G3P3 woman who has had persistent urinary retention since undergoing extensive reconstructive surgery for a vaginal vault inversion with a suburethral sling for her genuine stress incontinence and low pressure urethra. She voids here in an obstructive and retentive fashion by urethral relaxation with a detrusor contraction. Her voiding abnormality is best classified as:

a. Detrusor areflexia
b. Detrusor sphincter dyssynergia
c. Urethral syndrome
d. Valsalva voiding
e. Underactive detrusor

28. Fig. D.22 shows the voiding pressure study of a 34-year-old G2P2 female with genuine stress incontinence who voids in an obstructive and intermittent fashion. Electromyographic recordings in this tracing are from perianal surface electrodes and show some artifact from getting wet. What is her voiding mechanism?

a. Urethral relaxation alone
b. Detrusor sphincter dyssynergia
c. Urethral relaxation with Valsalva
d. Urethral relaxation with detrusor contraction
e. None of the above

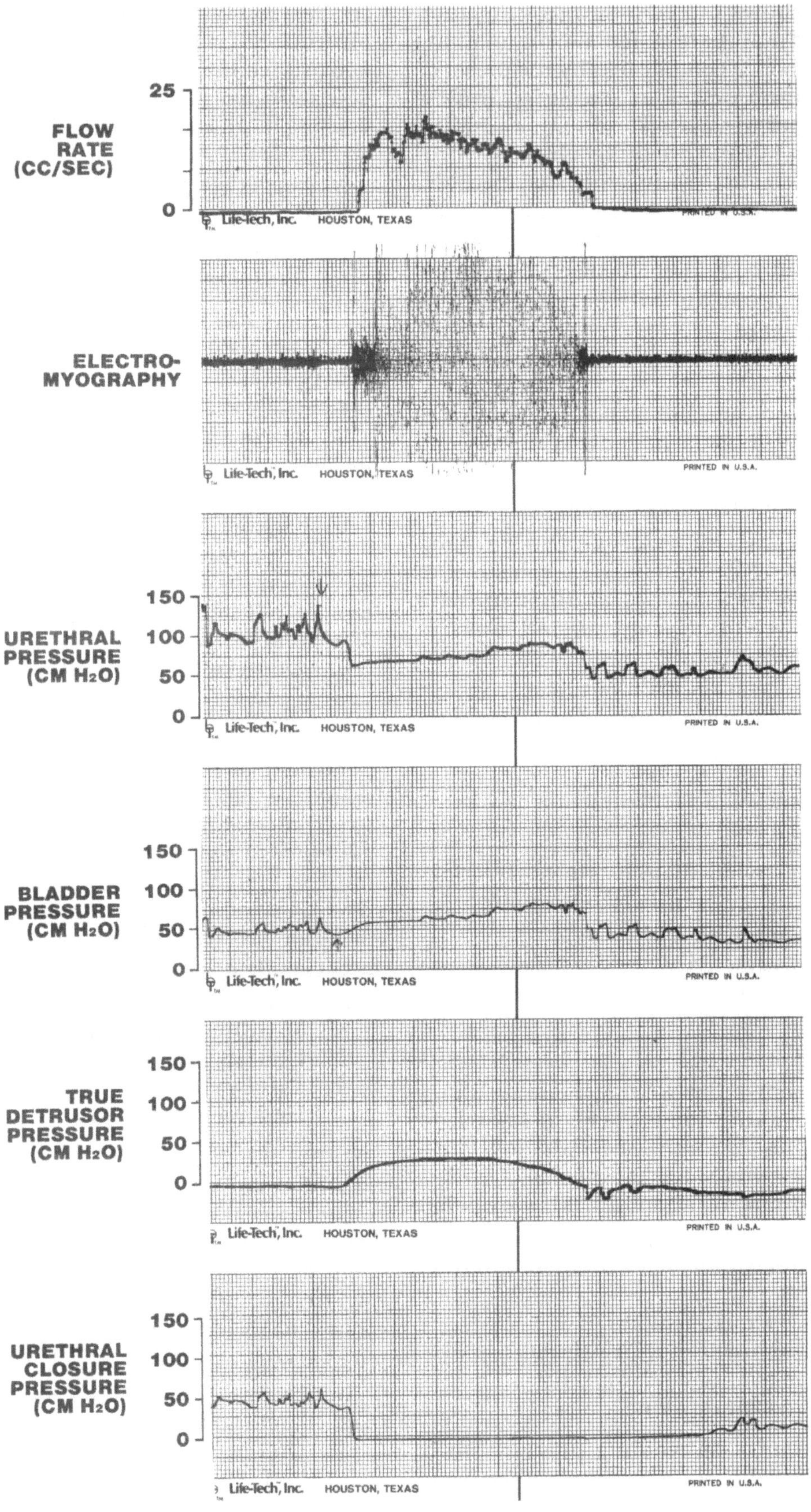


**Fig. D.16.** Voiding pressure study in a patient with a pelvic mass.

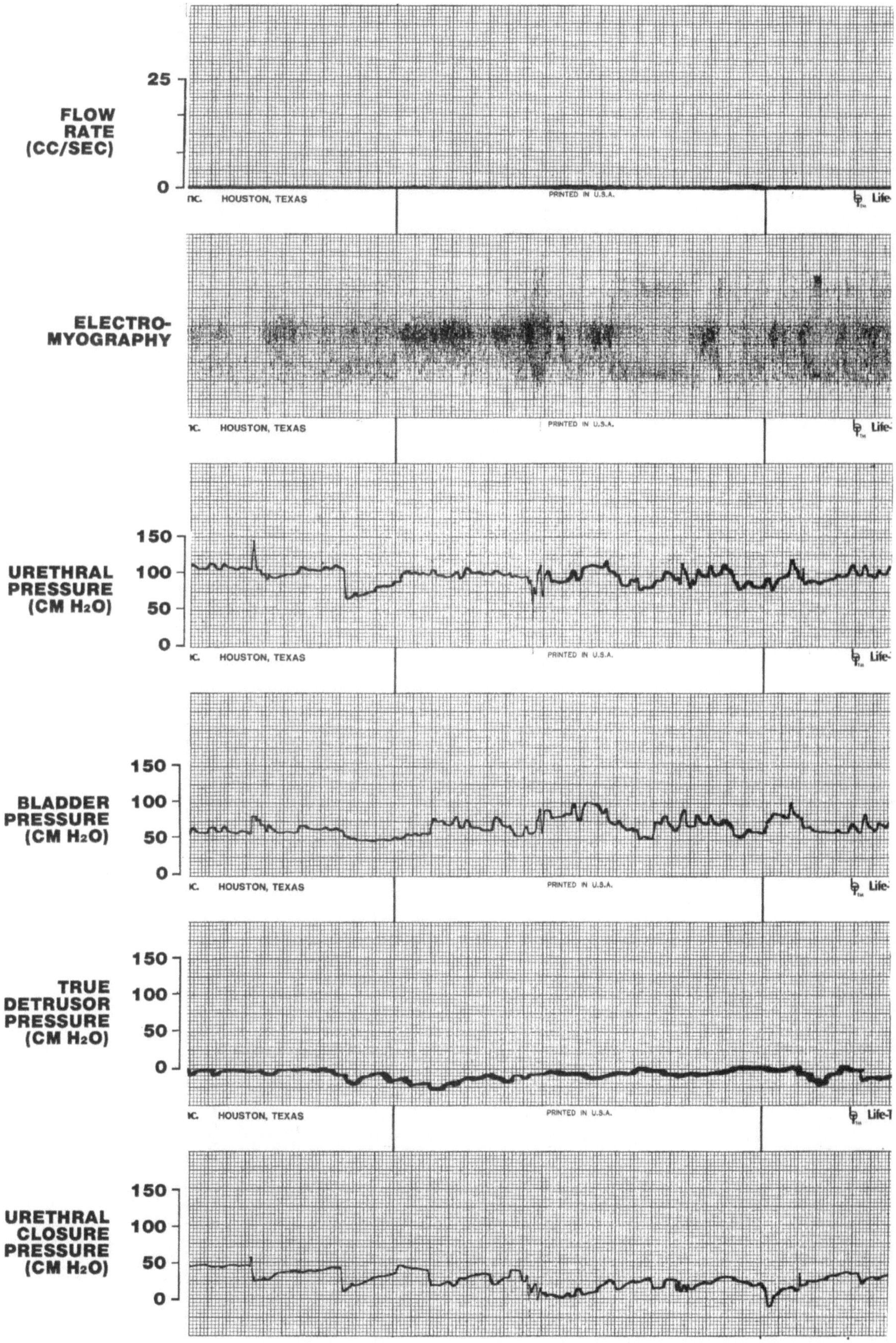


**Fig. D.17.** Voiding pressure study with retention and prolapse.

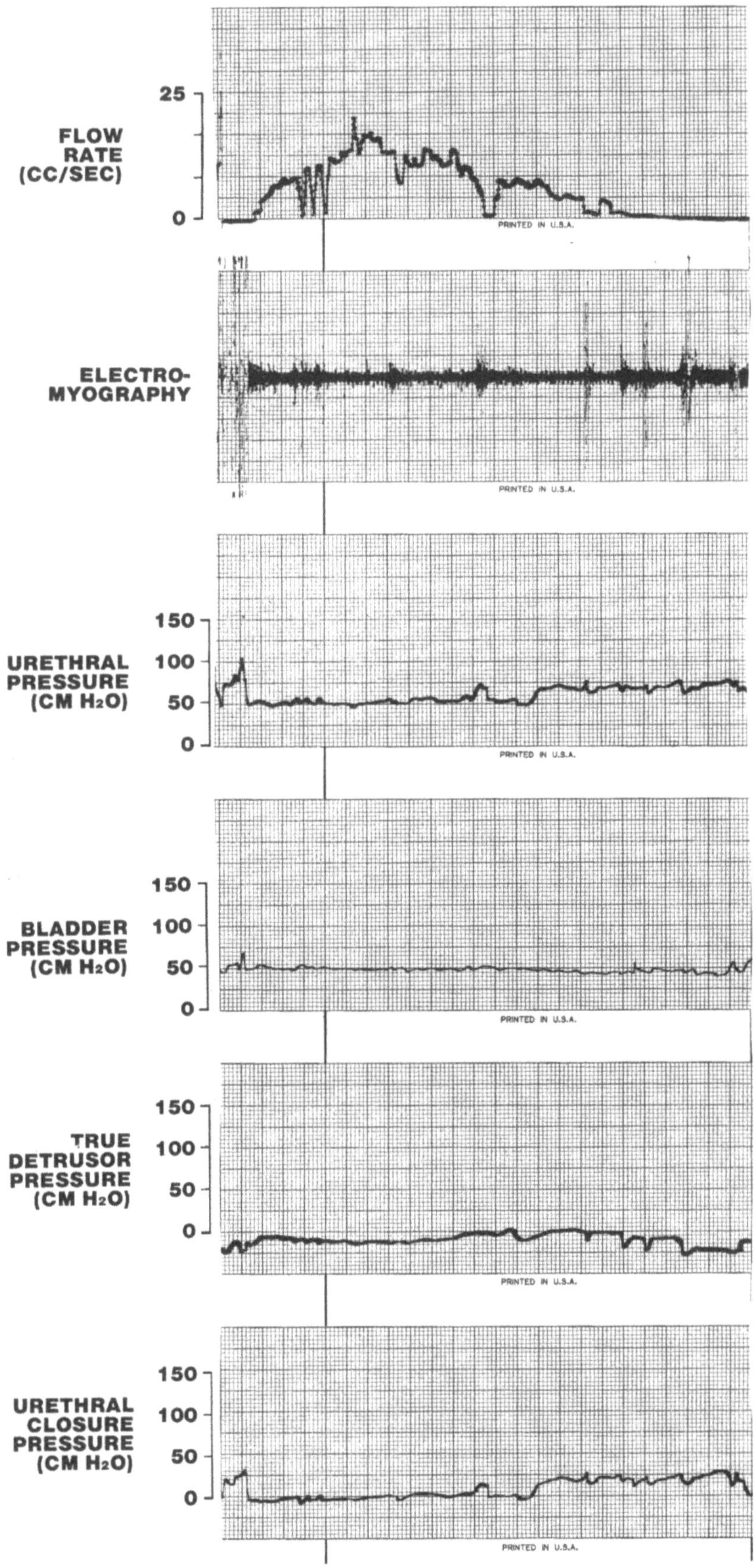


**Fig. D.18.** Voiding pressure study without retention.

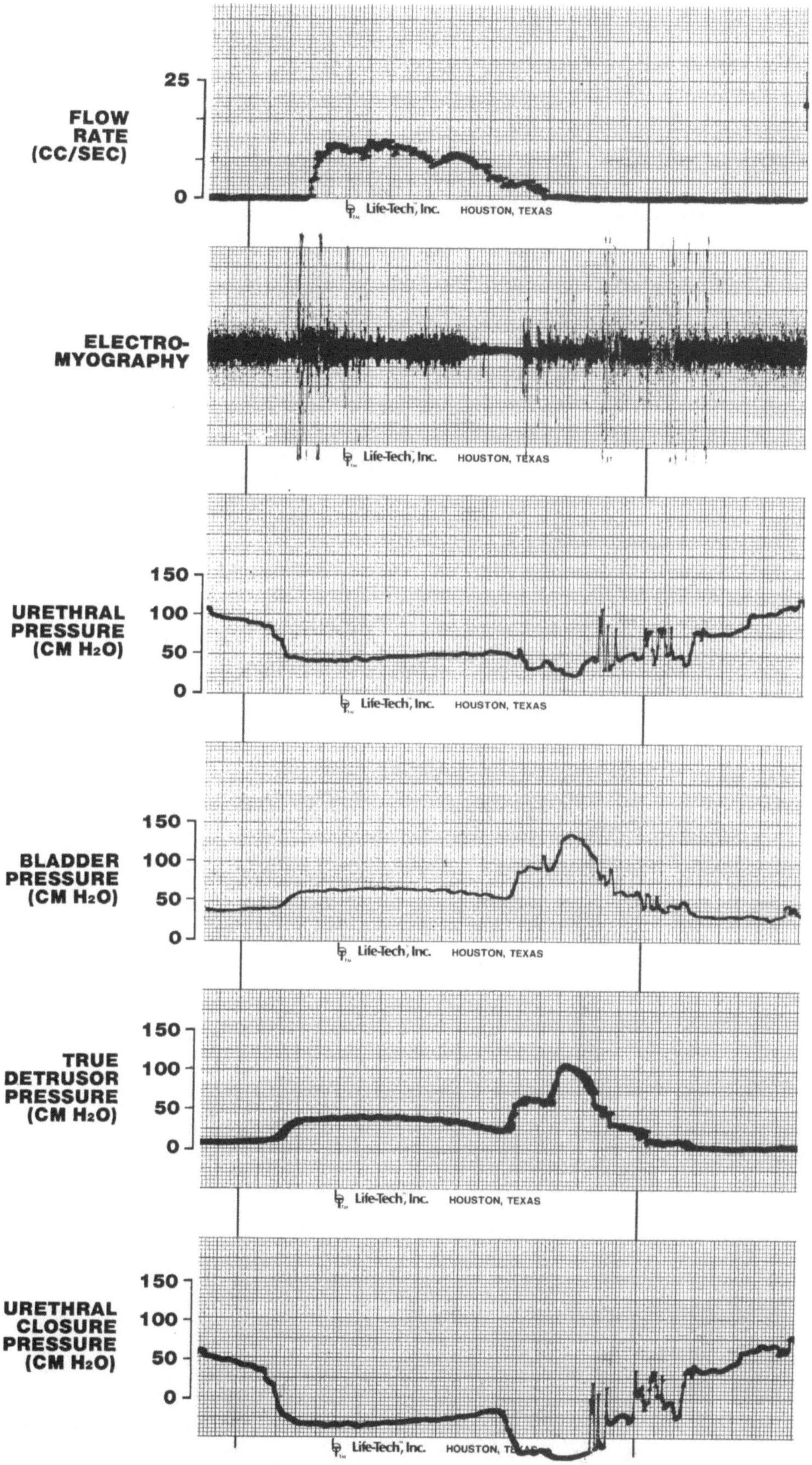


**Fig. D.19.** Voiding pressure study with a stop test.

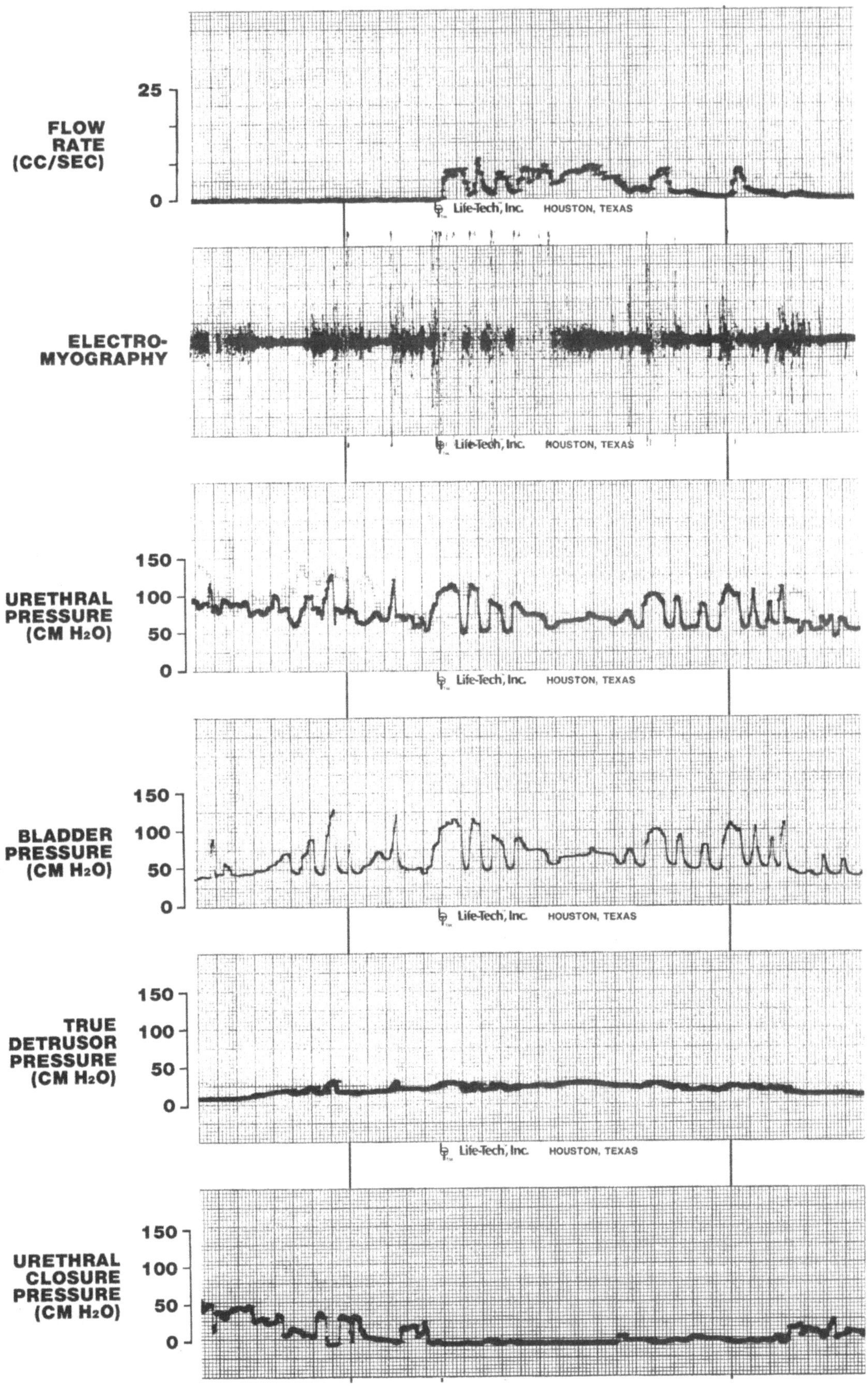


**Fig. D.20.** Obstructive voiding pressure study with intermittent flow.

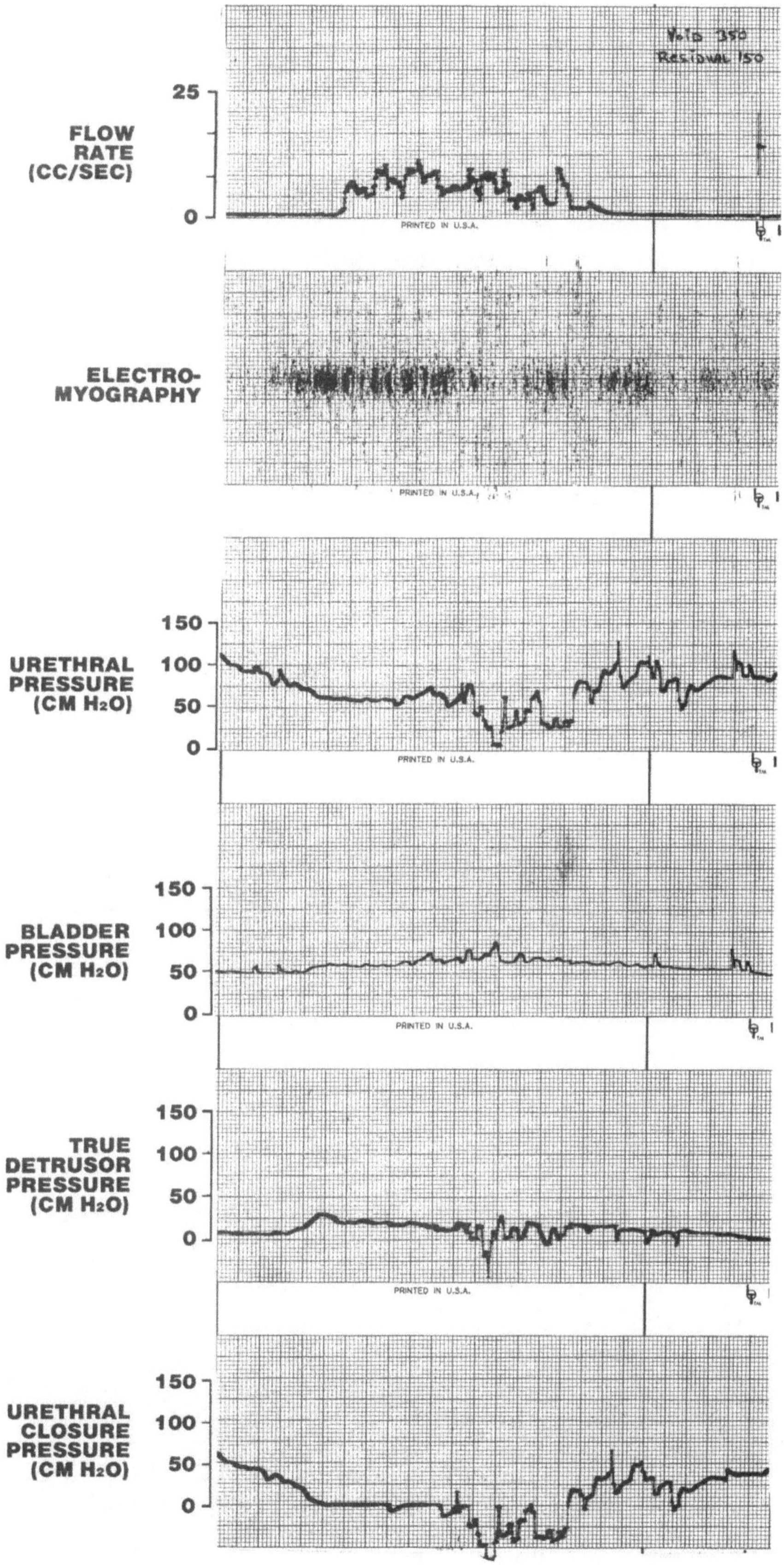


**Fig. D.21.** Voiding pressure study with retention.

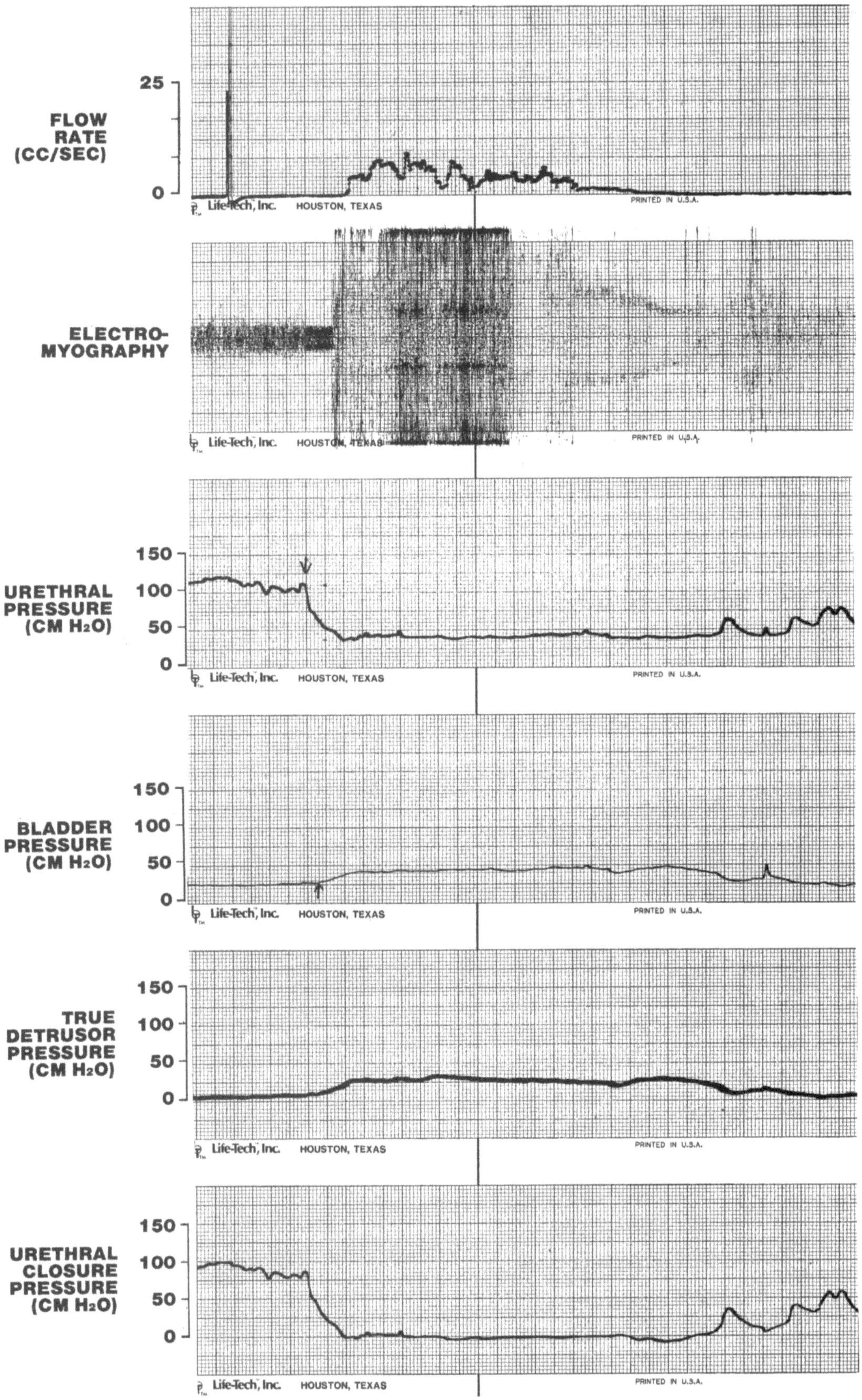


**Fig. D.22.** Voiding pressure study with wet EMG electrodes.

29. Fig. D.23 shows the voiding pressure study of a 49-year-old G4P2 woman with detrusor hyperreflexia due to multiple sclerosis. She also has intermittently worsening retention depending on exacerbations of multiple sclerosis. What is her voiding mechanism here as she voids 75 ml with a 300 ml residual?

a. Urethral relaxation
b. Valsalva with detrusor contraction
c. Detrusor sphincter dyssynergia after urethral relaxation
d. Valsalva alone
e. Detrusor contraction alone

## D.5 Urodynamic Case Study

30. Figs. D.24–D.26 show the urodynamic study of a 58-year-old G6P5 woman who has a large cystocele (central defect) that protrudes beyond the introitus with a similar sized enterocele after having had a prior vaginal hysterectomy for menorrhagia. She denies any urinary tract complaints. In Fig. D.24 urethral closure pressure profiles are performed in the sitting position with a full bladder (590 ml). She does not lose urine involuntarily during coughing in this setting. Do you think she has genuine stress incontinence (GSI)? Does she have a low pressure urethra (LPU)?

a. GSI no; LPU yes
b. GSI yes; LPU no
c. GSI no; LPU no
d. GSI yes; LPU yes
e. Cannot answer either from this tracing

31. Fig. D.25 shows the same profiles from the same patient as in Fig. D.24 repeated after insertion of a ring pessary to support the prolapse. She loses urine involuntarily during the second cough urethral closure pressure profile. She now has genuine stress incontinence.

a. True
b. False

32. Fig. D.26 shows the standing urethrocystometry study of the same patient. She notes first sensation at 170 ml and reaches a maximum cystometric capacity of 590 ml. Besides her cystocele and enterocele, which of these urodynamic diagnoses best describes the findings in Figs. D.24–D.26?

a. Uninhibited urethral relaxation and detrusor instability
b. Genuine stress incontinence and detrusor instability
c. Detrusor instability alone
d. Potential genuine stress incontinence
e. Genuine stress incontinence with a low pressure urethra

## D.6 Answers

1. b. 165 $cmH_2O$ without leakage. Leak point pressure is measured from baseline atmospheric pressure (0) to the point where leakage first occurs. If there is no leakage, then the highest abdominal (or bladder) pressure reached is the leak point pressure without leakage (Chapter 43).

2. c. 145 $cmH_2O$. Leakage occurs at 145 $cmH_2O$ the first time and at 150 $cmH_2O$ the second time. The abdominal leak point pressure is the lowest pressure at which involuntary leakage occurs (Chapter 43).

3. b. False. The abdominal leak point pressure is a measure of the change in abdominal pressure and not the urethral pressure (Chapter 43).

4. b. A normal urethrocystometry study. There are no increases in detrusor pressure throughout the study to a maximum cystometric capacity of 425 ml. Urethral syndrome and urinary retention cannot be diagnosed by filling phase cystometry alone (Chapter 20).

5. d. Genuine stress incontinence. This urethrocystometry study demonstrates repetitive, high pressure, involuntary detrusor contractions in a woman with a preceding CVA. These findings suggest a direct neurological cause of her urge incontinence – detrusor hyperreflexia. There is no evidence of genuine stress incontinence and the patient has a very high baseline urethral pressure of about 200 $cmH_2O$ (Chapter 24).

6. a. A low compliance bladder. Although all of these could cause irritative symptoms and leakage, the slow gradual rise in true detrusor pressure associated with urinary leakage distinguishes a loss of compliance from the tonic contractions of detrusor instability (Chapter 27).

7. e. Urethral instability. This is a relatively normal urethrocystometry study to a maximum cystometric capacity of 405 ml but the patient continually feels urgency with decreases in urethral pressure at the arrows. Treatment with an alpha-blocker relieved these symptoms without causing genuine stress incontinence (Chapter 32).

8. c. No. This is a normal urethrocystometry study with a normal bladder capacity and a somewhat reduced urethral closure pressure. The

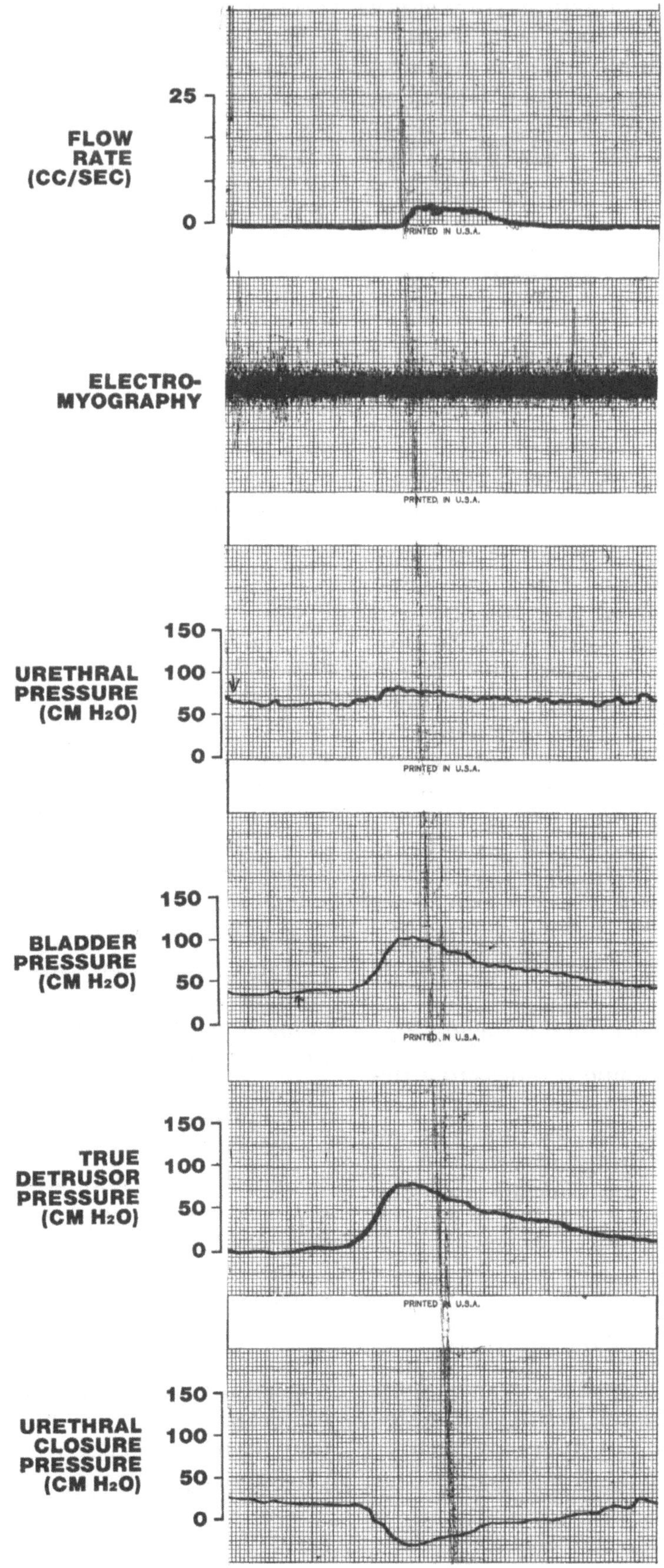


**Fig. D.23.** Voiding pressure study in a patient with multiple sclerosis.

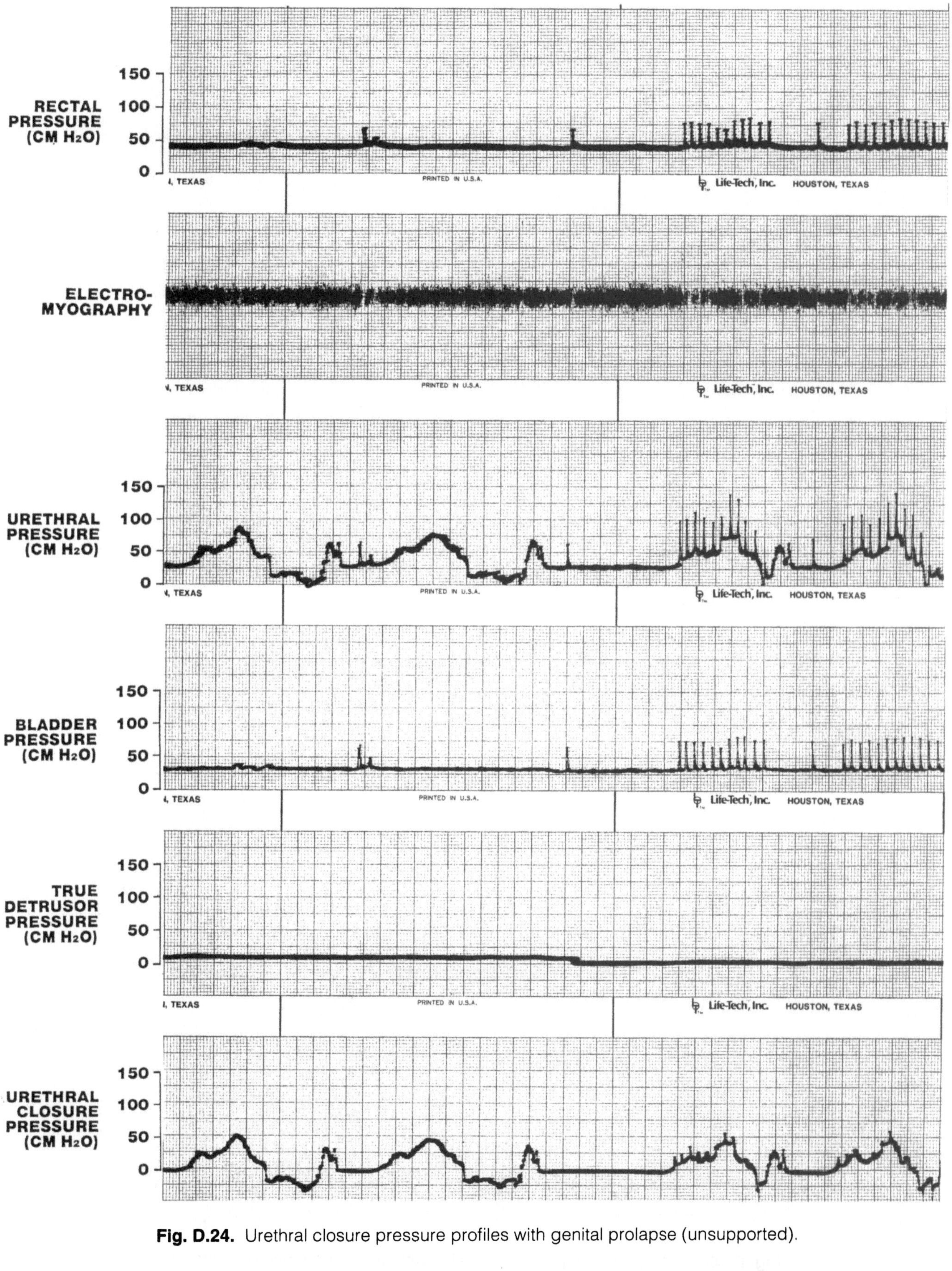


**Fig. D.24.** Urethral closure pressure profiles with genital prolapse (unsupported).

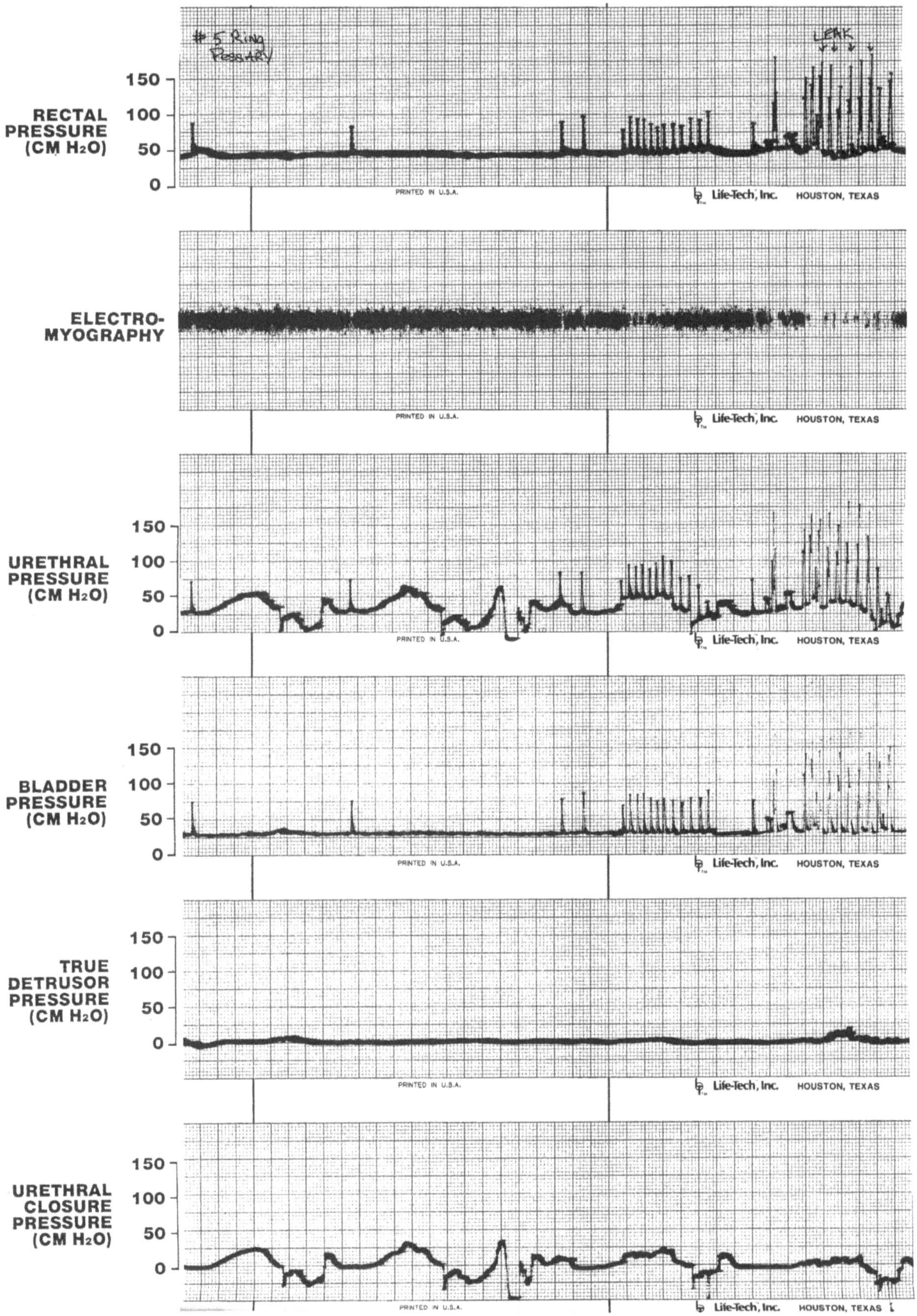


**Fig. D.25.** Urethral closure pressure profiles with genital prolapse (supported).

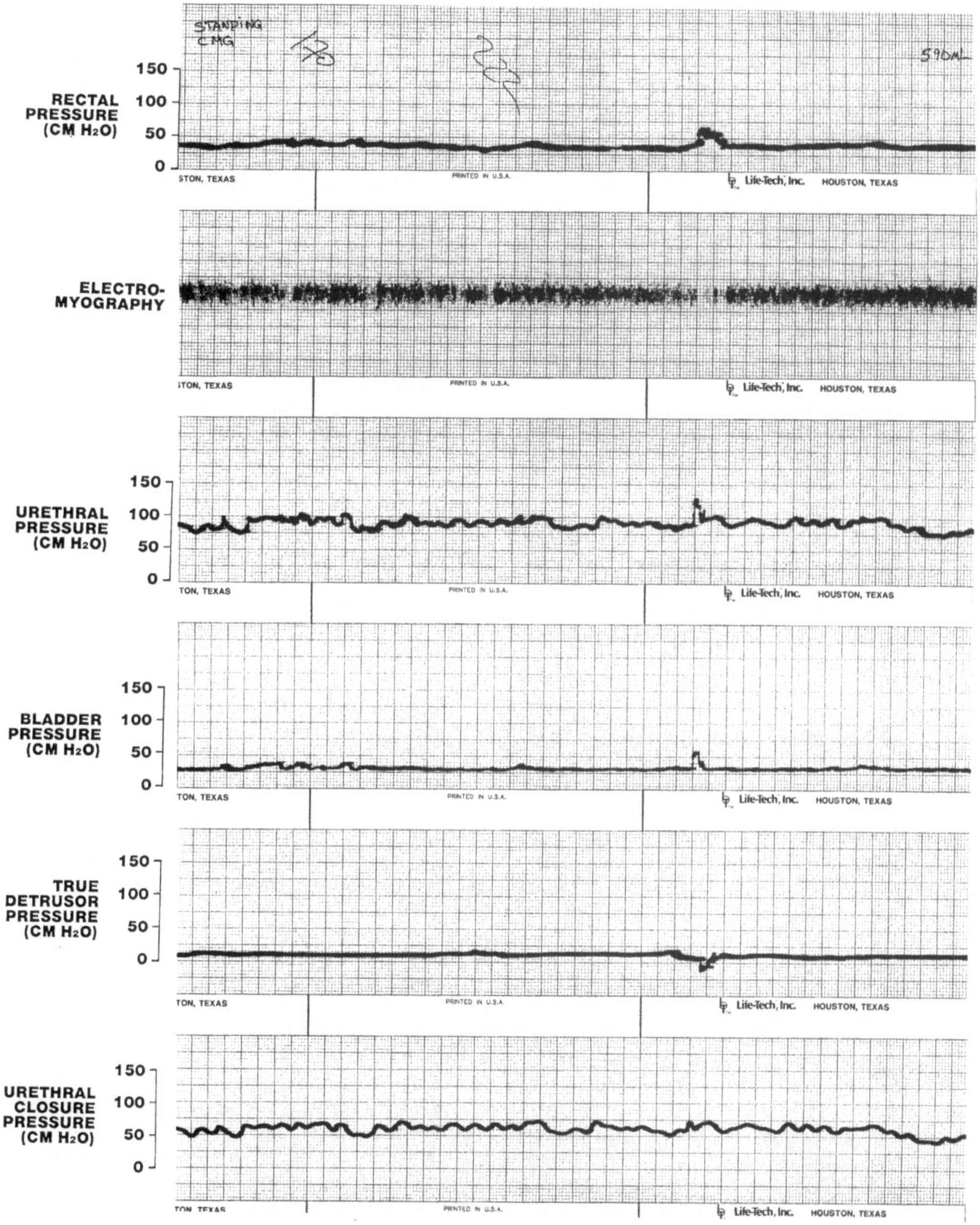


**Fig. D.26.** Standing urethrocystometry with genital prolapse.

patient has genuine stress incontinence but there is no sign of it in this study (Chapter 20).

9. d. Detrusor instability. This is a 42 $cmH_2O$ involuntary detrusor contraction during bladder filling. Note that the 58 $cmH_2O$ rise in the true detrusor pressure is from decreased abdominal pressure plus the bladder pressure rise (Chapter 24).

10. b. Interstitial cystitis. Interstitial cystitis is a syndrome, which although very controversial is diagnosed on cystoscopy with or without biopsy. Urethrocystometry is used to diagnose conditions where symptoms develop during bladder filling due to dysfunction of the urethra, bladder or their surrounding musculature and supporting structures (Chapter 20).

11. a. Normal. These are normal urethral closure pressure profiles for a 14-year-old girl, but we are used to seeing pathologic studies and studies in older women whose urethral pressure decreases with aging (Chapter 15).

12. e. CP 112 $cmH_2O$, FL 36 mm (Chapter 15).

13. c. Genuine stress incontinence. These Valsalva profiles demonstrate pressure equalization with zero closure pressure or less throughout the length of the urethra during increased abdominal pressure. The patient may have detrusor instability, but it is not found in this study (Chapter 17).

14. c. Urethral diverticulum. Both diverticulae and fistulae can cause negative urethral pressure zones due to the defect in the urethral wall (Chapter 31).

15. e. All of the above. Visualizing the diverticular sac with radiopaque dye, with ultrasound or seeing the neck of the diverticulum on urethroscopy can all aid in the diagnosis of a urethral diverticulum (Chapter 31).

16. b. Low urethral closure pressure (18 $cmH_2O$). Low urethral closure pressure has been shown to be an independent risk factor for failure of routine anti-incontinence operations. Diagnosis of a CP less than or equal to 20 $cmH_2O$ at cystometric capacity in this patient led to the performance of a suburethral sling procedure with cure of her genuine stress incontinence (Chapter 29).

17. d. 78/65=120%, 86/80=108%, 50/102=49%. Pressure transmission ratios are measured as the increment in pressure increase in urethral pressure from a cough divided by the bladder pressure increment. Determining the actual "take-off" point of the pressure increment is sometimes difficult (Chapter 23).

18. a. CP 78 $cmH_2O$, FL 29 mm, TL 41 mm; CP 64 $cmH_2O$, FL 30 mm, TL 45 mm (Chapter 15).

19. c. Urethral syndrome. Urethral closure pressure profiles are utilized to diagnose deficiencies in the sphincteric function of the urethra and not inflammatory, infectious or functional disorders (Chapter 15).

20. c. Urethral relaxation with detrusor contraction, abnormal. The voiding study is obstructive with a maximum flow rate of about 10 ml/s. The urethral pressure channel exhibits a pressure rise during voiding due to a common cavity effect from bladder neck funneling during urethral relaxation (Chapter 21).

21. d. Urethral relaxation and detrusor contraction, normal. The surface electrodes get wet during voiding creating a pseudo-detrusor sphincter dyssynergia pattern. A maximum flow rate of 19 ml/s is in the lower range of normal, but more importantly, the flow pattern is normal (Chapters 21 and 26).

22. a. Urethral relaxation with Valsalva. This patient relaxes her urethra and then intermittently strains. This can be "seen" indirectly on the urethral and bladder pressure tracings. There is no detrusor activity and the patient is unable to void (Chapter 25).

23. c. Acontractile bladder. There is no detrusor contraction so there can be no detrusor sphincter dyssynergia (Chapter 25).

24. e. Urethral relaxation alone. Examination of the bladder pressure channel shows a flat tracing without measureable contraction. A stop test might be able to reveal an unobserved contraction secondary to low urethral resistance (Chapter 38).

25. b. 104 $cmH_2O$. Detrusor voiding pressure is measured as the maximal rise in true detrusor pressure during the isometric contraction of the stop test after the urethra has closed and voiding has ceased. It is not measured from the bladder pressure channel because this may reflect additional changes from abdominal pressure increases (Chapter 38).

26. d. Urethral relaxation, detrusor contraction and Valsalva. Many women with prolapse and bladder neck incompetence will add Valsalva to their normal voiding mechanism. Habituation to this voiding pattern may interfere with postoperative voiding (Chapter 21).

27. b. Detrusor sphincter dyssynergia. This tracing shows intermittent bursts of EMG activity during voiding consistent with detrusor–sphincter dyssynergia, but this is not associated with significant increases in urethral pressure in

this tracing. This might be due to movement of the catheter into the distal urethra during voiding. If for this reason you picked e. underactive detrusor, then you probably understand these concepts (Chapter 26).

28. d. Urethral relaxation with detrusor contraction. The wet surface electrodes cause a dramatic increase in the EMG recording pattern after initial urethral relaxation (downward arrow). A bladder contraction begins 3 s later and then the EMG artifact occurs from the wet electrodes shorting out. There is no true detrusor sphincter dyssynergia (Chapter 21).

29. c. Detrusor sphincter dyssynergia after urethral relaxation. After initial urethral relaxation (downward arrow), the detrusor pressure rises accompanied by an increase in urethral pressure and no decrease in skeletal muscle activity as measured by the EMG activity (Chapter 26).

30. e. Cannot answer either from this tracing. Whereas the answer appears to be GSI no; LPU no, one cannot evaluate urethral function adequately until any potential mechanical obstruction is removed by supporting the prolapse (Chapter 28).

31. a. True. The patient has stress incontinence with support of the prolapse and her closure pressure is still greater than 20 $cmH_2O$ (Chapter 34).

32. d. Potential genuine stress incontinence. She only has stress incontinence with reduction of the prolapse as may be the case in up to 80% of women with this degree of pelvic relaxation (Chapter 34).

# Subject Index

MIX
Papier aus verantwortungsvollen Quellen
Paper from responsible sources
FSC® C105338

If you have any concerns about our products,
you can contact us on
**ProductSafety@springernature.com**

In case Publisher is established outside the EU,
the EU authorized representative is:
**Springer Nature Customer Service Center GmbH**
**Europaplatz 3, 69115 Heidelberg, Germany**

Printed by Libri Plureos GmbH
in Hamburg, Germany